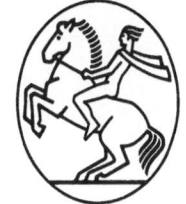

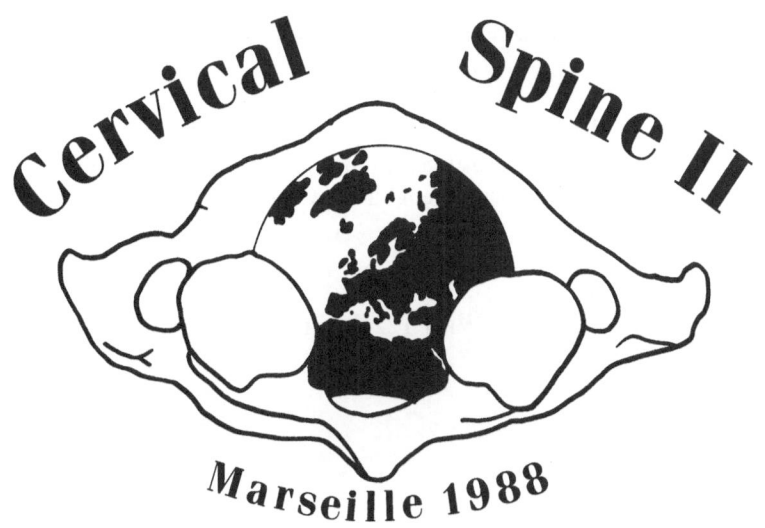

Marseille 1988

Edited by R. Louis and A. Weidner

Springer-Verlag Wien New York

Professor René Louis, M.D.
Service de chirurgie orthopédique et traumatologique, Hôpital de la Conception,
Marseille, France

Priv.-Doz. Dr. med. Andreas Weidner
Department of Neurosurgery, Paracelsus-Klinik, Osnabrück,
Federal Republic of Germany

With 122 Figures

ISBN-13: 978-3-7091-9057-9   e-ISBN-13: 978-3-7091-9055-5
DOI: 10.1007/978-3-7091-9055-5

Preface

The second common meeting of the European Section and the Cervical Spine Research Society took place in Marseille (France) from June 12 to 15, 1988 and was organized by René Louis. More than 130 specialists from every part of Europe, from America and Asia participated, representing, among others, the fields of Orthopedics, Neurosurgery, Traumatology, Neurology, Anatomy, Rheumatology and Radiology.

This meeting again was convincing proof of the growing interest which exists in Europe in research into injuries and diseases of the cervical spine.

The main topics of this meeting were the subluxation of the lower cervical spine (chapter 1) and the infectious diseases of the cervical spine (chapter 2). Chapters 3 and 4 of this volume deal with degenerative lesions and the upper cervical spine. In chapter 5 experimental reports are presented, so that a good synopsis is provided of our present state of knowledge of diseases of the cervical spine.

The European Section of the Cervical Spine Research Society was founded by Mario Boni in 1984, who unfortunately died in 1986 and was proclaimed Honory President of the European Section. There is a European meeting every summer and one every three years with our colleagues from the United States of America, Canada and Japan organized in Europe.

The first combined meeting was organized by Pierre Kehr in Strasbourg (France) in 1985 and the presented papers were published in Cervical Spine I (Springer, Wien-New York, 1987).

The European section of the Cervical Spine Research Society invites all those interested in the clinical and research problems of the cervical spine to join this society. We are interested in a multidisciplinary analysis of the various topics inherent in a specific problem of the cervical spine. This was the idea of the founding members of the Cervical Spine Research Society in the United States. Their purpose is the exchange and development of ideas and philosophies regarding the diagnosis and treatment of cervical spine injury and disease. Membership composition should reflect the varying specialities and disciplines dealing with the cervical spine: biochemistry, bioengineering, neurology, neurosurgery, radiology, orthopedic surgery and others.

We would wish to express our heartfelt thanks to all the organizers of this second meeting which proved to be of excellent scientific value. We extend our thanks to all the authors who prepared papers for publication and to Pierre Kehr (Strasbourg/France) for assistance in editing, and Werner K. Doyle, M.D. (Department of Neurosurgery, New York University).

Without the help and advice of our publisher Springer-Verlag (Wien-New York) it would have been impossible to make available the presented papers to all those who could not attend the meeting. We should like to express our sincere thanks for this cooperation.

Marseille and Osnabrück, August 1989   René Louis, Andreas Weidner

Membership List

ARGENSON, C., M.D., Professor, Orthopedics, founding member, Nice, France.

BONI, M., M.D., Professor, (†) founding member, Honory President.

BRAAKMAN, R., M.D., Professor, Neurosurgery, founding member, Rotterdam, The Netherlands.

CANADELL, J., M.D., Professor, Orthopedics, founding member, Pamplona, Spain.

CHERUBINO, P., M.D., Professor, Orthopedics, General Secretary, Pavia, Italy

DALLE ORE, G., M.D., Professor, Neurosurgery, founding member, Verona, Italy.

DEHOUX, E., M.D., Orthopedics, Reims, France.

DENARO, V., M.D., Professor, Orthopedics, Office member, Catania, Italy.

DIRHEIMER, Y., M.D., Rheumatology, Strasbourg, France.

DOVE, J., M.D., Orthopedics, Stoke-on-Trent, England.

DVORAK, J., M.D., Neurology, Zurich, Switzerland.

EVANS, D., M.D., Professor, Orthopedics, founding member, Ranmoor Shefield, England.

FINESCHI, G., M.D., Professor, Orthopedics, founding member, Roma, Italy.

FUENTES, J., M.D., Neurosurgery, Montpellier, France.

GROB, D., M.D., Orthopedics, Zurich, Switzerland.

GUTMANN, G., M.D., Non-surgical therapy, Bad Saasendorf, Federal Republic of Germany.

HARMS, J., M.D., Professor, Orthopedics, Karlsbad, Federal Republic of Germany.

HOHMANN, D., M.D., Professor, Orthopedics, founding member, Membership Committee, Erlangen, Federal Republic of Germany.

HUSAG, L., M.D., Neurosurgery, Aarau, Switzerland.

JEANNERET, B., M.D., Orthopedics, St. Gallen, Switzerland.

JUNG, A., M.D., Professor, Orthopedics, honorary member, Strasbourg, France.

KEHR, P., M.D., Professor, Orthopedics, founding member, President 1985/86, Education Committee, Strasbourg, France.

KORRES, D., M.D., Professor, Orthopedics, Athens, Greece.

LIEBIG, K., M.D., Professor, Orthopedics, Erlangen, Federal Republic of Germany.

LOGROSCINO, C., M.D., Professor, Orthopedics, founding member, Membership Committee, Roma, Italy.

LOUIS, R., M.D., Professor, Orthopedics, founding member, President 1987/88, Membership Committee, Marseille, France.

MAGERL, F., M.D., Priv.-Doz., Orthopedics, President, St. Gallen, Switzerland.

MARTI, R., M.D., Professor, Orthopedics, Amsterdam, The Netherlands.

O'BRIEN, J., M.D., Professor, Orthopedics, founding member, London, England.

PRIJAMBODO, B., M.D., Orthopedics, corresponding member, Indonesia.

RAUSCHNING, W., M.D., Professor, Orthopedics, Uppsala, Sweden.

ROBLES MARIN, D., M.D., Professor, Anatomy, Valencia, Spain.

RODEGERDTS, U., M.D., Professor, Orthopedics, founding member, Treasurer, Bremerhaven, Federal Republic of Germany.

ROY-CAMILLE, R., M.D., Professor, Orthopedics, Paris, France.

SAVINI, R., M.D., Professor, Orthopedics, Bologna, Italy.

SOLINI, A., M.D., Professor, Orthopedics, Torino, Italy.

VIERA, J., M.D., Professor, Orthopedics, founding member, President 1986/87, Office Member, Lisboa, Portugal.

WACKENHEIM, A., M.D., Professor, Radiology, Research Committee, Strasbourg, France.

WEATHERLEY, C., M.D., Orthopedics, Oswestry, England.

WEIDNER, A., M.D., Priv.-Doz., Neurosurgery, founding member, Editor, Osnabrück, Federal Republic of Germany.

Contents

1. Subluxation and Management of Instability

2. Infection of the Cervical Spine

3. Degenerative Lesions and Management

4. The Upper Cervical Spine

5. Experimental Reports

List of Contributors

ARAND, M., Dr., Klinik für Unfallchirurgie der Universität Ulm, D-7900 Ulm, Federal Republic of Germany.

ARGENSON, C., M.D., Professor, Service d'Orthopédie-Traumatologie, Hôpital Saint-Roch, F-06000 Nice, France.

BENAZZO, F., M.D., Orthopaedic Clinic of The University of Pavia, I-27100 Pavia, Italy.

BENEZECH, J., M.D., Department of Neurosurgery, Clinique Rech, F-34000 Montpellier, France.

BERTALANFFY, H., Dr., Department of Neurosurgery, Klinikum der Albert-Ludwigs-Universität, D-7800 Freiburg, Federal Republic of Germany.

BORROMEO, U., M.D., Orthopaedic Clinic of The University of Pavia, I-27100 Pavia, Italy.

BRAAKMAN, M., M.D., Department of Neurosurgery, University Hospital Rotterdam, NL-3015 GD Rotterdam, The Nertherlands.

BRAAKMAN, R., M.D., Ph.D., Professor, Department of Neurosurgery, University Hospital Rotterdam, NL-3015 GD Rotterdam, The Netherlands.

BUFFATTI, P., M.D., Department of Neurosurgery, University Hospital, I-37100 Verona, Italy.

CASTERA, G., M.D., Service de Chirurgie Orthopédique et Traumatologique, Hôpital De La Conception, University of Marseille, F-13385 Marseille Cedex 5, France.

CECILIANI, L., M.D., Professor, Orthopaedic Clinic of The University of Pavia, I-27100 Pavia, Italy.

CHERUBINO, P., M.D., Professor, Orthopaedic Clinic of The University of Pavia, I-27100 Pavia, Italy.

CHIOE, S., M.D., Department of Neurosurgery, Paracelsus Klinik, D-4500 Osnabrück, Federal Republic of Germany.

CLARK, R., M.D., Department of Orthopaedic Surgery, University of Iowa, Iowa City, IA 52242, U.S.A.

DALLE ORE, G., M.D., Professor, Department of Neurosurgery, University Hospital, I-37100 Verona, Italy.

DE BOECK, H., M.D., Department of Orthopaedic Surgery, Academic Hospital University of Brussels, B-1090 Brussels, Belgium.

DEHOUX, E., M.D., Centre Hospitalier Regional et Universitaire de Reims, F-51092 Reims Cedex, France.

DENARO, V., M.D., Professor, Orthopaedic Clinic, University of Catania, I-95125 Catania – Sicilia, Italy.

DI GIACINTO, G., M.D., Division of Neurosurgery, St. Luke's-Roosevelt Hospital Center, New York, NY, U.S.A.

Dove, J., M.D., F.R.C.S., Spinal Service, Stoke-on-Trent ST4 7EW, England.

Eggert, H., M.D., Professor, Department of Neurosurgery, University Hospital, D-7800 Freiburg, Federal Republic of Germany.

Ehara, S., M.D., Department of Radiology, University of Iowa, Iowa City, IA 52242, U.S.A.

El-Khoury, G., M.D., Department of Radiology, University of Iowa, Iowa City, IA 52242, U.S.A.

Epstein, J., M.D., Professor, Department of Neurosurgery, The Medical School of the State of New York at Stony Brook, Stony Brook, New York, 410 Lake Ville Road No. 100, New Hyde Park, NY 11042, U.S.A.

Epstein, Nancy, M.D., Professor, Department of Neurosurgery, The Medical School of the State of New York at Stony Brook, Stony Brook, New York, 410 Lake Ville Road No. 100, New Hyde Park, NY 11042, U.S.A.

Faccioli, F., M.D., Department of Neurosurgery, University Hospital, I-37100 Verona, Italy.

Fuentes, J., M.D., Department of Neurosurgery, Clinique Rech, F-34100 Montpellier, France.

Griffet, J., M.D., Service d'Orthopédie-Traumatologie, Hôpital Saint-Roch, F-06000 Nice, France.

Hohmann, D., M.D., Professor, Department of Orthopaedic Surgery, University of Erlangen-Nürnberg, D-8520 Erlangen, Federal Republic of Germany.

Hughes, J., M.D., Division of Neurosurgery, St. Luke's-Roosevelt Hospital Center, New York, NY 10021, U.S.A.

Igram, C., M.D., Department of Orthopaedic Surgery, University of Iowa, Iowa City, IA 52242, U.S.A.

Jeanneret, B., M.D., Klinik für Orthopädische Chirurgie, Kantonsspital, CH-9007 St. Gallen, Switzerland.

Kalff, R., M.D., Priv.-Doz., Department of Neurosurgery, University Hospital, D-4300 Essen, Federal Republic of Germany.

Kehr, P., M.D., Professeur d'Orthopédie-Traumatologie à la Faculté de Médecine Chirurgien des Hôpitaux, F-6700 Strasbourg Cedex, France.

Korres, D., M.D., Department of Orthopaedic Surgery, University of Athens, GR-10434 Athens, Greece.

Lestienne, G., M.D., Laboratoire de Physiologie Neurosensorielle, 15, rue de l'Ecole de Médecine, F-75270 Paris Cedex 06, France.

Liebig, K., M.D., Professor, Department of Orthopaedic Surgery, University of Erlangen-Nürnberg, D-8520 Erlangen, Federal Republic of Germany.

Liverneaux, P., M.D., Laboratoire de Physiologie Neurosensorielle, 15, Rue de l'Ecole de Médecine, F-75270 Paris Cedex 06, France.

Logroscino, C., M.D., Professor, Sezione Chirurgia Vertebrale – Policlinico A. Gemelli, I-00136 Roma, Italy.

Louis, R., M.D., Professor, Service de Chirurgie Orthopédique et Traumatologique, Hôpital De La Conception, University of Marseille, F-13385 Marseille Cedex 5, France.

Mähring, M., M.D., Department Unfallchirurgie, Universitätsklinik, A-8036 Graz, Austria.

NAKANO, K., M.D., Department of Orthopaedic Surgery, Chuo Hospital, Hakodate 041, Japan.

NAKANO, N., M.D., Nakano Orthopaedic Hospital, Chuoko, 064 Sapporo, Japan.

NAKANO, T., M.D., Nakano Orthopaedic Hospital, Chuoko, 064 Sapporo, Japan.

NGUYEN, D., M.D., 260-A Main Street, Redwood City, CA 94063, U.S.A.

OPPEL, U., M.D., Orthopädische Universitätsklinik Bochum St. Josef Hospital, D-4630 Bochum, Federal Republic of Germany.

PACHE, T., M.D., Service d'Orthopédie et Traumatologie de l'Appareil Locomoteur, CH-1011 Chuv/Lausanne, Switzerland.

PALIOTTA, V., M.D., Sezione Chirurgia Vertebrale, Policlinico A. Gemelli, I-00136 Roma, Italy.

PRIJAMBODO, B., M.D., Surgical Department of Medical School, Airlangga University, Surabaya, Indonesia.

RAMON, R., M.D., Servicio Coyt, Hopital Clinico y Provincial, 08036 Barcelona, Spain.

RAO, R., M.D., c/o Orthopädische Klinik Seepark, D-2850 Bremerhaven, Federal Republic of Germany.

RAYNOR, R., M.D., Professor, Department of Neurosurgery, St. Vincent's Hospital, New York, NY 10021, U.S.A.

RODEGERDTS, U., M.D., Professor, Clinic of Orthopaedic Surgery, D-2850 Bremerhaven, Federal Republic of Germany.

SAVINI, R., M.D., Professor, Istituto Ortopedico Rizzoli, I-40136 Bologna, Italy.

SCHULITZ, K., M.D., Professor, Department of Orthopaedic Surgery, University Hospital, D-4000 Düsseldorf, Federal Republic of Germany.

SEGAL, P., M.D., Professor, Centre Hospitalier Regional et Universitaire de Reims, F-51092 Reims, Cedex, France.

STAUDTE, H., M.D., Professor, Department of Orthopaedics, D-5102 Würselen, Federal Republic of Germany.

SUNDARESAN, N., M.D., Division of Neurosurgery, St. Luke's-Roosevelt Hospital Center, New York, NY, U.S.A.

SZYSZKOWITZ, R., M.D., Professor, Department of Traumatology, University Hospital, A-8036 Graz, Austria.

THIEL, M., M.D., Department of Orthopacdics, D-5102 Würselen, Federal Republic of Germany.

ULLRICH, C., M.D., Department of Radiology, Charlotte Memorial Hospital and Medical Center, Charlotte, NC 28232, U.S.A.

ULRICH, C., M.D., Priv.-Doz., Unfallchirurgie, Klinik am Eichert, D-7320 Göppingen, Federal Republic of Germany.

VIEIRA, J., M.D., Professor, Department of Orthopaedic Surgery, Lisbon University-Hospital Santa Maria, P-1699 Lisboa Codex, Portugal.

VILLAS, C., M.D., Professor, Department of Orthopaedic Surgery and Traumatology, University Clinic of Navarra, E-31080 Pamplona, Spain.

WEHLING, P., M.D., Orthopädische Universitätsklinik, D-4000 Düsseldorf, Federal Republic of Germany.

WEIDNER, A., M.D., Priv.-Doz., Department of Neurosurgery, Paracelsus Klinik, D-4500 Osnabrück, Federal Republic of Germany.

WHITECLOUD, III, T., M.D., Department of Orthopaedics, Tulane University School of Medicine, New Orleans, LA 70112, U.S.A.

WHITESIDES, T., M.D., Professor, The Emory Clinic, 135 Clifton Road, N.E., Atlanta, GA 30322, U.S.A.

WÖRSDÖRFER, O., M.D., Professor, Department of Traumatology, Städtische Kliniken, D-6400 Fulda, Federal Republic of Germany.

1. Subluxation and Management of Instability

I. Application and Management of Instability

Cervical Spine II
© by Springer-Verlag 1989

1.1. Severe Strains of the Lower Cervical Spine

R. Louis and G. Castera, Marseilles, France

This article deals with ruptures of the structures connecting the vertebrae that may lead to vertebral displacement when exceeding their physiological limits. Severe intervertebral strain, as an entity, is a fairly recent concept and many of the classic European or American texts do not mention it at all or refer to it as the subluxation described by Watson-Jones. The cervical spine, with its 20 articulations, is much more likely to suffer strain with ligamentous rupture during severe injury than the rest of the locomotor system. Moreover, the problems are different, for very often simply transporting the patient in a position of rest restores articular alignment and disguises the ligamentous rupture. In the evaluation of cervical trauma ligamentous injury must be routinely investigated. Furthermore, when there is vertebral displacement the cervical spine threatens the 3 structures its bony canals are intended to protect: the spinal cord in the vertebral canal, the spinal nerves in the foramina and the vertebral artery in the transverse foramina.

The case-histories that form the basis of this study are derived from the symposium on acute injuries of the cervical spine conducted by M. Bombart and R. Roy Camille (Paris, 1983), which has facilitated our work on severe strains. This symposium on severe lesions of the lower cervical spine without neurological complications makes reference to 310 cases, and among these there were 67 severe strains. These severe strains comprised 21% of the severe injuries of the lower cervical spine, all with identifiable radiological lesions.

Two pathological types can be initially distinguished: severe strain due to a mechanism of extension-distraction in 6% of these cases and strain due to flexion-distraction in 94%. Severe extension-distraction strain is associated with, in all cases, rupture of the anterior longitudinal ligament and of that part of the annulus fibrosus anterior to the nucleus pulposus. Sometimes the ligamentous rupture may extend to the posterior ligamentous structures. The severe flexion-distraction type of strain is characterized by rupture of all the structures connecting the vertebrae posterior to the nucleus pulposus, i.e., the posterior longitudinal ligament, the posterior articular capsules, the ligamenta flava, the interspinous ligaments and the nuchal ligament. Sometimes the rupture may extend to the anterior part of the intervertebral disc, which may then be completely fissured horizontally or detached from a vertebral body. The description of these lesions were characterized mainly by operative findings. The lesions of severe strains are distributed unequally from C2 to T1:

C2–3: 9%; C3–4: 19%; C4–5: 22%; C5–6: 36%; C6–7: 12%; C7–T1: 2%. It is evident that severe strains of the cervical spine may involve any one of the 6 intervertebral discs, thus distinguishing them from the luxations of the inferior cervical spine which are localized exclusively to the three lower cervical discs. The explanation of this difference is that the presence of the mandible at the level of the mobile segments of C2 to C5 in forced flexion of the head prevents these segments from suffering flexion of sufficient degree to dislocate the vertebrae. On the other hand, the three lower segments are subject to a greater range of flexion and dislocation which may result in articular disengagement following ligamentous rupture. The vertebral displacement produced by severe strain at the moment of injury, even if reduction has occurred spontaneously or after the patient has been stretched out horizontally, may bring about lesions of the neurovascular structures protected by the vertebral canals, causing injury to the spinal cord, the spinal nerves and the vertebral artery. We shall not deal with the cord lesions here, since this is discussed in another chapter. Nor will we discuss lesions of the vertebral artery which were not specifically studied in the case-records of the symposium. However, certain syndromes of headache and vertigo may be posttraumatic manifestations of vertebral artery lesions.

We are left with radicular lesions of the spinal nerves, which are relatively common in severe strains since they were present in 46% of cases. We found that 22% of cases exhibited only subjective pain in the distribution of one cervical root, 9% showed signs of sensory or motor deficit in the distribution of a root, and 15% demonstrated combined subjective symptoms of pain with signs of motor or sensory deficit. The changes in caliber of the intervertebral foramina, as well as rupture of the adjacent ligaments in front at the level of the disc and of those behind at the level of the ligamentum flavum and the articular capsules, account for the possibility of root lesions due to edema, compression or direct injury. But very often, pain referred along a radicular dermatome may be evidence of an injury of the dorsal branch of the radicular nerve at the site of the ligamentous lesions. This is not a direct lesion of the spinal nerve but represents referred pain.

Diagnosis

While standard radiographs sometimes reveal obvious signs of a vertebral subluxation, these films may unfortunately only show minor signs at the limit of normality. Only flexion-extension films in moderate flexion and extension

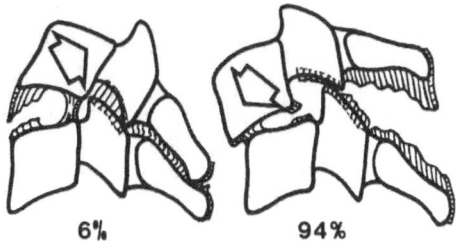

6% 94%

Fig. 1. Diagram of pathological lesions in severe strains of the inferior cervical spine: 6% of lesions are due to extension-distraction mechanism and 94% are secondary to flexion-distraction injuries

under medical supervision are capable of displaying unsuspected ligamentous lesions.

Severe extension-distraction strains are demonstrated by the presence in extension of an anterior gaping of the intervertebral space, with or without avulsion of a fragment of the vertebral margin. A monodiscal retrolisthesis and loss of articular parallelism in the same position are also pathognomonic signs of this type of strain. We can list 5 pathognomonic signs of severe flexion-distraction strain (Fig. 2). The presence of at least three of these signs if sufficient for a diagnosis of ligamentous rupture:

1. anterolisthesis of 3.5 mm or more
2. an interspinous gap wider than the adjacent interspinous spaces above and below
3. loss of parallelism of the articular facets
4. loss of contact of the articular facets of 50% or more,
5. angular disruption of vertebral body alignment, as seen from the line of projection of the posterior wall of the vertebral bodies, is also an excellent pathologic sign if equal to 15° or more.

These last criteria cited are derived from our experimental studies on cadavers and from studies of severe strains. However, there are several diagnostic traps which must be recognized if a false diagnosis of severe strain is to be avoided. First, physiological anterolisthesis must not be confused with displacement due to ligamentous rupture. Forced flexion of the normal cervical spine may produce a physiological anterolisthesis of 3 mm or less above C4 and of 2 mm or less below C4. This physiological phenomenon is due to displacement of the centre of rotation in cervical flexion-extension well below the nucleus pulposus in the subjacent vertebral body. Angular displacement also produces an antero-posterior displacement of the vertebral bodies. Nor should an inversion of the cervical curvature due to compensation for reversal of the normal dorsal curvature be confused with ligamentous rupture resulting in loss of vertebral body alignment. Flexion-extension films in hyperflexion clearly distinguish the two conditions. The third trap is confus-

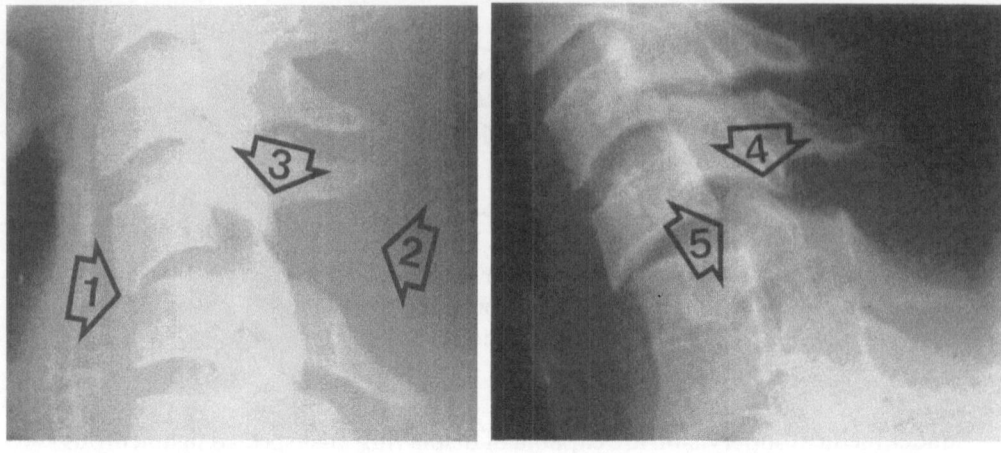

Fig. 2 a, b. The five pathognomonic signs of flexion-distraction evaluation in severe strain injury: (a) anterolisthesis of 3.5 mm or more (*1*), interspinous gap (*2*), loss of articular parallelism (*3*); (b) loss of contact of articular surfaces by 50% or more (*4*), angular disruption of vertebral body alignment of 15° or more (*5*)

ing joint instability, due to some articular laxity, with a severe strain. The hinge action of certain discs affected by a discarthrosis above a physiological or congenital vertebral fusion may allow a range of joint movement in hyperflexion and hyperextension greater than normal. Overriding of joints leads to progressive stretching of the connecting structures. However, the loss of contact of the joint surfaces is always less than 50% in cases with chronic ligamentous lesions.

In addition to these false-positive diagnoses, it is important to stress false-negatives, particularly when the films show a fracture of the spinous process or an avulsion of a corner of the vertebral body. These fractures are often simple incidental findings and the addition of flexion-extension films is necessary to demonstrate a possible severe strain injury. However, it often happens that the initial pain at the time of injury, together with some degree of muscle spasm, hinders the performance of the flexion-extension films. In suspicious cases, and if the painful syndrome persists, flexion-extension films should be repeated in several days or weeks following the injury.

Natural Course

In order to clarify the therapeutic indications, it is important to know the natural history of severe strains of the spine. Severe sprain injuries can be placed into two different categories. Certain cases of rupture of the intervertebral connecting structures may end in spontaneous healing after immobilization with the formation of calcification resulting in a spontaneous fusion, which is solid enough to prevent any secondary vertebral displacement. In approximately half of the cases, however, this does not occur.

As an example we present the case of a 37 year old woman, who sustained in September 1976 a severe injury to the cervical spine with nondisplaced fractures of the spinous processes of C5 and C6 and without any changes in the vertebral bodies or articular facets (Fig. 3). This patient was treated for 6 weeks in a Thomas collar and developed a progressive syndrome of chronic cervico-brachial pain in the C7 distribution with hyperreflexia in the lower limbs. The radiographs 2 years later showed malalignment with an 80% anterolisthesis, bilateral luxation and nonunion of the spinous processes. To manage this patient, we performed a vertebral osteotomy in a single-stage combined anterior and posterior approach.

Of the 18 cervical vertebral osteotomies performed to date, 4 were for this type of injury. We conclude from these observations that spontaneous healing of severe strains of the spine is problematic, and that the development of malunion with stenosis of the vertebral canal and of the intervertebral foramina is the major risk of conservative management.

Treatment

During our symposium we came to an unanimous agreement in asserting that the treatment of choice for severe strain of the cervical spine is surgical stabilization. Of course, if there are contraindications to operation, or if the patient refuses, treatment will have to be bracing. In this case the stability of the lesion must be checked 3 months later with flexion-extension films and a late operation may then be indicated, if instability is found. Before operation, it is important to reduce displacements by orthopaedic means, i.e., by light traction and hyperlordosis. We use controlled orthopaedic reduction in a frame used for correction of scolioses, and we hold the spine in a minerva plaster jacket until the time of operation, which can then be done electively within several days. In the cases studied in the symposium, preoperative orthopaedic reduction was performed in 18%. It was successful in only ⅔ of cases. In the successful cases the interval between injury and reduction was 4 days, while in the failures it was 23 days. All the patients underwent operation, 67% by the anterior route and 33% by the posterior route. All patients operated by the anterior route had an intervertebral or intravertebral fusion with iliac graft, 92% and 8% respectively. Eighty three percent of these fusions were combined with an osteosynthesis with plate and screws of the Sénégas type or our own type.

All severe strains operated upon by the posterior route (Fig. 4) underwent osteosynthesis, either by two plates screwed into the articular columns (89%)

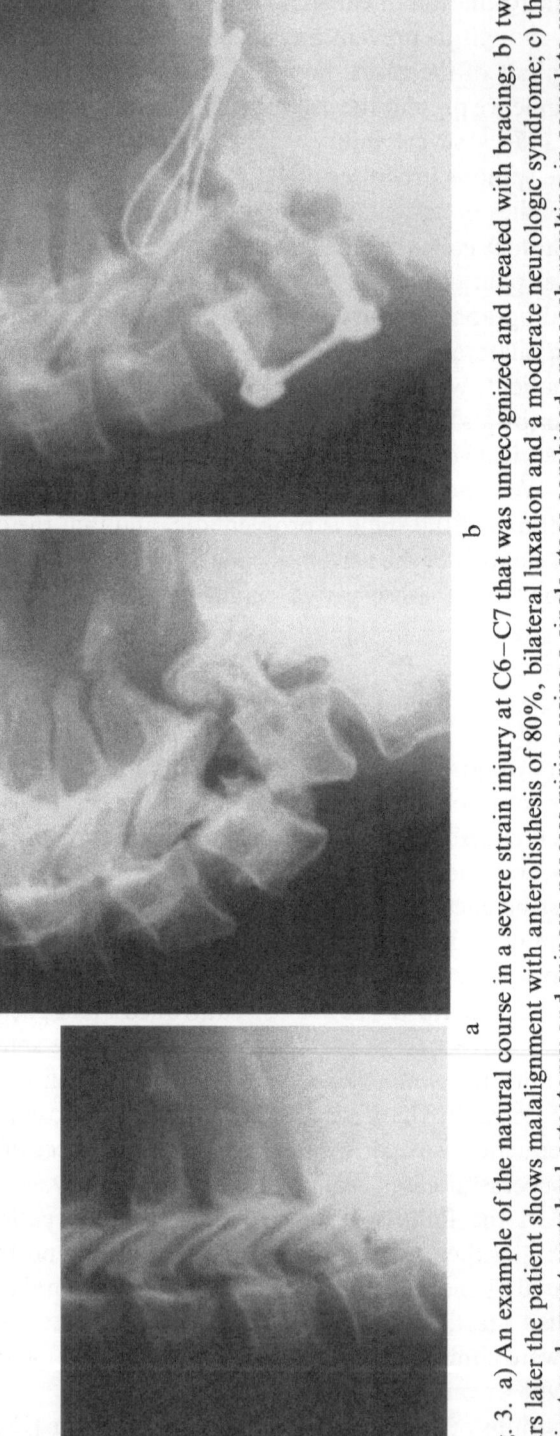

Fig. 3. a) An example of the natural course in a severe strain injury at C6–C7 that was unrecognized and treated with bracing; b) two years later the patient shows malalignment with anterolisthesis of 80%, bilateral luxation and a moderate neurologic syndrome; c) the patient underwent vertebral osteotomy and spinous process wiring using a single-stage combined approach resulting in complete cure

or by interlaminar-spinous wiring (11%). Only 44% of these patients underwent supplementary fusion with iliac bone grafting. The extent of the stabilization was limited to one level in 89% of cases and to two levels in 11%. Our own preference is for the addition of a graft in every cervical stabilization for severe strain to ensure fusion and definitive stabilization. If osteosynthesis alone does not result in callus formation or solid healing, the risks are obvious. If healing is unsound, micro-movements lead to disruption of the fixation. Or, if the metal is subsequently removed, a pseudarthrosis may develop.

Results

All results were assessed 6 months after operation. From the functional aspect, they were considered good in 61% of cases operated by the anterior route and in 67% of cases operated by the posterior route. The results were considered fair in 25% of the anterior and 28% of the posterior cases, and were judged poor in 14% of the anterior and 6% of the posterior cases. Thus, there seems to be no significant difference between the two techniques. The overall result was satisfactory in some 85% of cases. From the structural aspect, i.e., the restoration of the appearance of the vertebral bodies, articulations and calibre of the spinal canal, the results were judged good or fair in, 91% of cases operated from in front and in 100% of cases operated posteriorly. Loss of stability was found in 3% of the anterior cases and was absent in the posterior operations. These differences in structural results may be explained in that posterior surgery allows better articular adjustment, which automatically re-establishes more normal alignment and lordosis of the vertebral bodies. As far as the nerve roots are concerned, anterior surgery produced deterioration in 3% versus 0% in posterior surgery.

The aggravation of root symptoms by anterior surgery is probably due to the interbody grafts. If the graft is poorly positioned, it may threaten the spinal nerves in their foramina. On the other hand, improved cases amounted to 58% in those operated by the anterior route, and only 17% for the posterior route. So, the posterior route seems much less effective than the anterior route for radicular syndromes. This difference may be due to the anterior approach which allows better restoration of the height of the intervertebral foramina, since the embedding of an interbody iliac graft restores the normal height of the intervertebral space.

In conclusion, we stress the importance of routine assessment of severe strains of the lower cervical spine with flexion-extension films. Their natural course does not result in a satisfactory prognosis in a high percentage of cases. Therefore, the treatment of choice is surgical stabilization by either the anterior or posterior route. It seems important to safeguard the spinal nerves

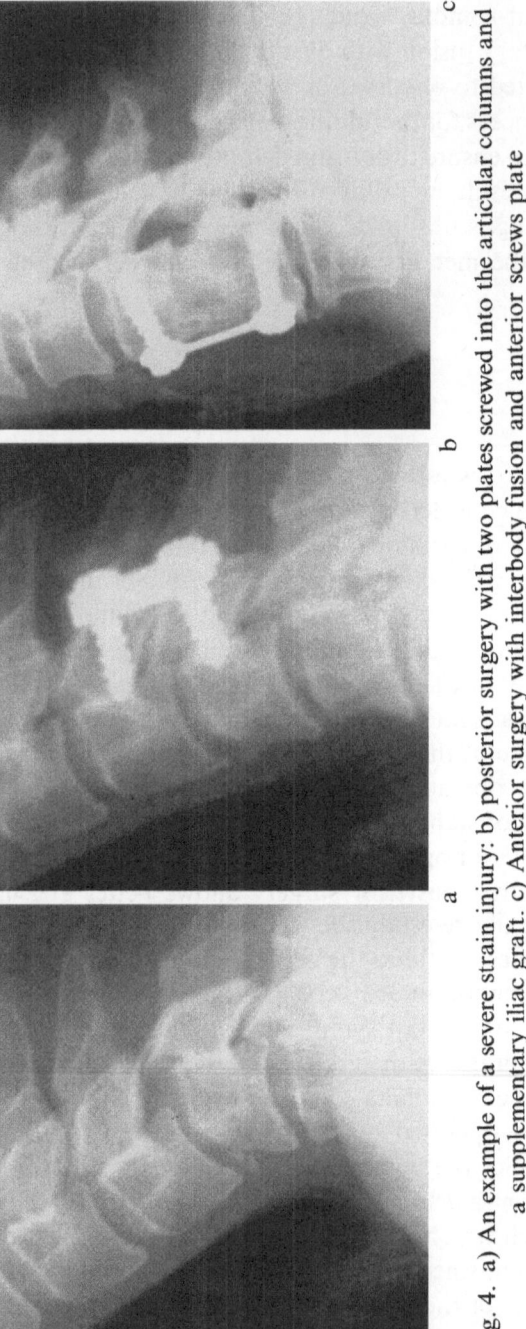

Fig. 4. a) An example of a severe strain injury: b) posterior surgery with two plates screwed into the articular columns and a supplementary iliac graft. c) Anterior surgery with interbody fusion and anterior screws plate

by restoring the height of the intervertebral foramina, and to ensure definitive stabilization by combining fusion with grafting and osteosynthesis. The anterior route seems preferable for severe strains with root lesions.

References

1. Ectors L, Achslogh T, Saintes MJ (1960) Les compressions de la moelle cervicale. Masson et Cie, Paris, pp 101–115
2. Hardy AG (1977) Cervical spinal cord injury without bony injury. Paraplegia, 14:296–305
3. Jung A, Kehr P (1972) Pathologie de l'artère vertébrale et des racines nerveuses dans les arthroses et les traumatismes du rachis cervical. Masson et Cie, Paris
4. Louis R (1978) Les entorses graves du rachis cervical (Table ronde). Actualités chirurgicales. 79ᵉ Congrès français de Chirurgie, Masson et Cie, Paris pp 142–156
5. Louis R (1979) Traumatismes du rachis cervical. I. Entorses et hernies discales. La Nouv. Presse Med 8.22:1843–1849
6. Louis R, Castera G (1984) Les entorses graves du rachis cervical inferieur. In: M Bombart, R Roy-Camille (eds) Traumatismes recents du rachis cervical inferieur. Symposium. Rev chir orthop T.70-7:527–532
7. Mitsou A (1976) An usual case of subluxation of C3–C4. Acta Orthop Scand 47:629–631
8. Perna E (1975) Tetraplegia from trauma of the cervical spine in the absence of fractures and luxations. J Neurosurg Sci 19:171–175
9. Raynor RB (1977) Compression de la moelle cervicale par protrusion discale aiguë traumatique. Spine 2:39–43
10. Rothman R, Simeone F (1975) The spine. WB Saunders, Philadelphia
11. Roy-Camille R, Saillant G (1972) Chirurgie du rachis cervical. Luxation pure des articulaires. Nouv Presse Méd 1:2330–2332
12. Roy-Camille R, De la Caffinière JY, Saillant G (1973) Traumatismes du rachis cervical supérieur C1–C2. Masson et Cie, Paris
13. Ruge D, Wiltse L (1977) Spinal disorders. Lea et Febiger, Philadelphia
14. Senegas J, Gauzere JM (1976) Plaidoyer pour la chirurgie antérieure dans le traitement des traumatismes graves des cinq dernières vertèbres cervicales. Rev Chir Orthop 62 [suppl] 11:123–129
15. Wilson DH (1977) Anterior cervical discectomy without bone graft. Report of 71 cases. J Neurosurg 47:551–555

Cervical Spine II
© by Springer-Verlag 1989

1.2. Hyperflexion Sprain of the Cervical Spine

R. BRAAKMAN and M. BRAAKMAN, Rotterdam, The Netherlands

Definition

The hyperflexion sprain of the cervical spine has already been described by Malgaigne (1885), Archer (1945) and Watson-Jones (1955) as incomplete, self-reducing and momentary dislocation of the spine respectively. Watson-Jones introduced the designation of anterior subluxation for those cases of dislocation in which the articular processes are not interlocked. Hyperflexion sprain is characterized by partial dislocation of the intervertebral joints with rupture of the posterior ligaments and joint capsules in one or two motion segments.

The hyperflexion sprain is usually due to disruptive hyperflexion, but it may also be part of a hyperflexion injury with compressive forces acting along the axis of the cervical spine [10, 11]. The skeletal system, however, should remain largely preserved.

Diagnosis and Missed Diagnosis

The diagnosis is a radiological one. The smooth cervical curvature is interrupted in one or two segments by a marked kyphotic angulation (Fig. 1). The diagnosis should not be made in cases of small angulations, which may be due to spondylosis and which can also be seen in apparently normal spines of completely healthy persons [7].

Flexion-extension studies are commonly not necessary and may be dangerous. We saw, for example, two cases in which during the flexion manoeuvre facet interlocking occurred. The best "functional" investigation is a lateral X-ray in the sitting position, in which the gravitational centre of the skull is situated anteriorly to the vertebral axis of the spine. In this position a lesion of the dorsal ligaments will become manifest in the form of a kyphotic angulation between two vertebrae. The angulation should disappear if the neck is completely extended in the recumbent patient with a hanging head position [4].

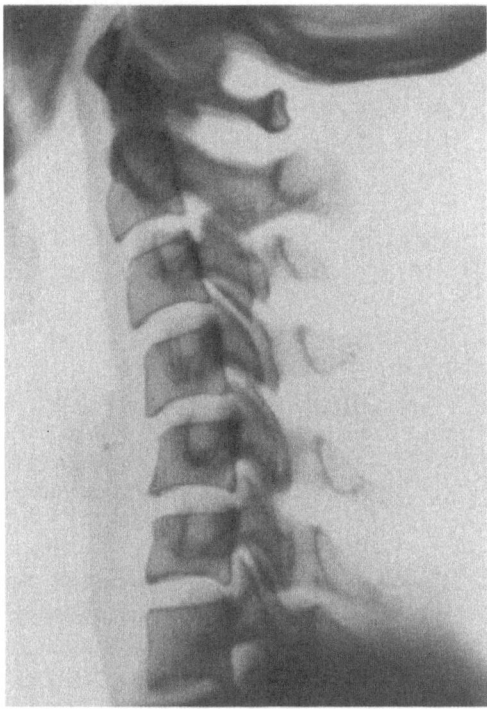

Fig. 1. Hyperflexion sprain in a 40 year old female with characteristic kyphotic angulation C4 – C5

The diagnosis may initially be missed in cases of posttraumatic muscle spasm resulting in arcual kyphosis, particularly in children. This usually develops some hours after the injury. The kyphotic angulation is then not detected, but is revealed as soon as the normal lordosis of the cervical spine has recurred (Fig. 2). The diagnosis may also be missed in unconscious patients in supine position, in whom the cervical spine sags, again assuming a kyphotic curve [4, 11].

On the other hand, in children, more or less marked step formation between vertebral bodies, especially in the C2 – C3 and C3 – C4 regions may be wrongly diagnosed as subluxation, although it is a normal phenomenon in flexion and in arcual kyphosis in children (pseudo-subluxation) [5, 10].

Personal Series

The hyperflexion sprain is a relatively rare injury. We observed 50 cases in 25 years. In the same period 150 cases of facet interlocking of the cervical spine were seen. In children under the age of 18 years the lesion is commonly

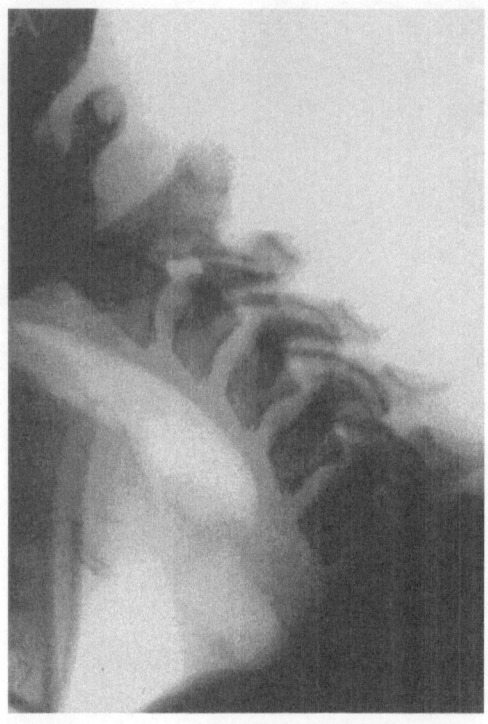

a

Fig. 2. 13 year-old female injured in a traffic accident. a) Note the severe arcual kyphosis the day after injury: muscle spasm disguises the hyperflexion sprain at C2–C3, revealed later when lordosis recurred. b) Two months later: development of calcifications in the interspinous ligaments of C2–C3, resulting in the c) elongation of the spinous process of C2 2 years later. Mobility in the segment C2–C3 was preserved

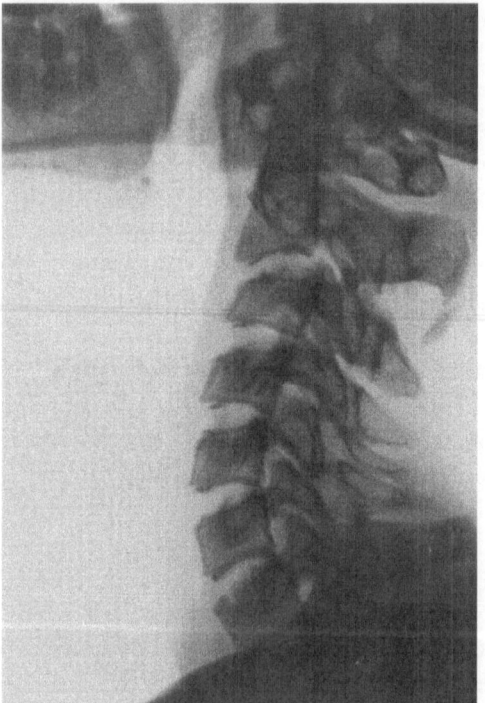

b

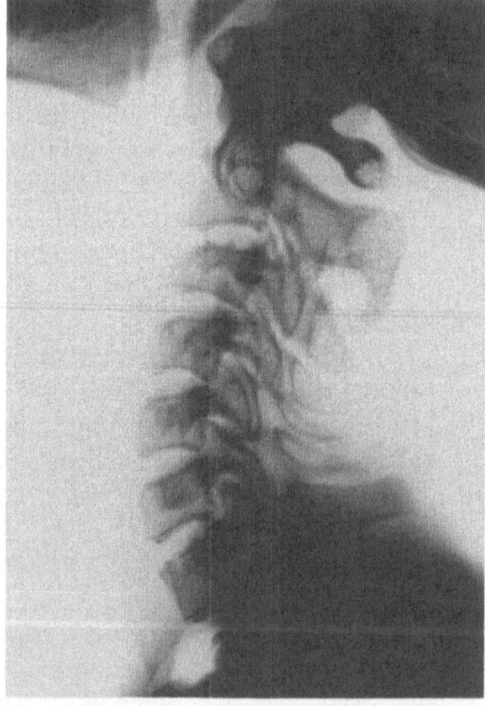

c

Table 1. *Results of Non-operative and Operative Treatment for Hyperflexion Sprain of the Cervical Spine. Number of cases subjected to secondary operative treatment in parenthesis*

Segment	Non-operative						Operative			
	Excellent		Good	Poor		Unknown	Primary		Secondary*	
	normal mobility		immobile				Good	Moderate	Good	Moderate
	no angulation	mild kyphosis		progr. kyphosis	inter-locking		1 segm. immobile	2–4 segm. immobile	1 segm. immobile	2–4 segm. immobile
C2–C4 13	3	1	5	4 (4)					1	3
C4–C7 37	3	3	5	9 (7)	2 (1)	2	1	12	1	7
Total 50	6	4	10	13	2	2	1	12	2	10

* In the case of failure of non-operative treatment.

Excellent = normal lordosis or mild kyphosis ($<8°$) with normal mobility at the injured level.

Good = normal alignment or mild kyphosis but with an immobile segment.

Moderate = in the case of fusion of two or more segments but without complaints.

Poor = in the case of progessive kyphosis or unilateral interlocking.

localised at the C2–C3 or C3–C4 level, and in adults the majority occur between C4 and C6 [3].

This relationship between age and level has also been reported by others in smaller series [1, 6, 9]. Neurological deficit is mild and reversible and usually consists of a root lesion. Only one patient had a persistent mild cervical cord lesion.

Treatment

The experience with treatment in our series is presented in Table 1. We learned that application of a Minerva jacket, a Halo-cast or a brace and subsequent mobilization invariably leads to recurrence of the angulation. Prolonged bedrest or the application of external mobilizers is of no use in hyperflexion sprain.

However, in children under 16 years of age, the long-term results without treatment are good. Gradually the angulation disappears and with simultaneous calcification of parts of the posterior ligaments, the cervical lordosis is restored. The spinous process of the vertebra above the lesion is transformed and elongated (Fig. 2b–c) [3]. The mobility of the affected segment may nevertheless remain normal. Fusion in patients under 16 years of age is indicated only in cases with more than 20° of angulation [3].

In adults a policy of wait and see may be adopted in minor angulation. Many of these patients have no persistent complaints, despite their persistent kyphotic angulation. In moderate or severe angulation the failure rate with conservative management in adults is, however, more than 50% (failure being permanent angulation and/or complaints). Primary fusion by bone grafting seems preferable. Fusion may be effected either by a posterior or anterior approach. Wiring without bone grafting results in recurrence of the angulation [3, 9, 12]. The aim of this operation is mainly to prevent the onset of a late myelopathy, due to stretching of the cord over the angulation.

Summary

The hyperflexion sprain or anterior subluxation of the cervical spine, characterized by a localized disruption of the posterior ligaments and joint-capsules in one or two motion segments is a relatively rare injury. On radiographs the smooth cervical curvature is interrupted in one or two segments by a marked kyphotic angulation. Neurological involvement is rare and usually reversible. In patients under 16 years of age usually the C2–C4 level is involved. Spontaneous realignment of the cervical spine is common and primary surgical treatment should be restricted to children with a kyphotic angulation of more than 20°.

Although in adults with persistent relative mild angulation initial complaints may disappear, primary surgical treatment is commonly necessary, because kyphosis may progress during conservative management and may even result in unilateral facet interlocking. Wiring alone is insufficient and leads to a recurrence of angulation. Bone fusion either by anterior or posterior approach gives good results.

References

1. Allen BL Jr, Ferguson RL, Lehmann TR, O'Brien RP (1982) A mechanistic classification of closed, indirect fractures and dislocations of the lower cervical spine. Spine 7(1):1–27
2. Archer VW (1945) The osseous system: a Handbook of Roentgendiagnosis. Yearbook Publ, Chicago
3. Braakman M, Braakman R (1987) Hyperflexion sprain of the cervical spine. Follow-up of 45 cases. Acta Orthop Scand 58:388–393
4. Braakman R, Penning L (1968) The hyperflexion sprain of the cervical spine. Radiol Clin Biol 37:309–320
5. Cattell HS, Filtzer DL (1965) Pseudosubluxation and other normal variations in the cervical spine in children. A study of one hundred and sixty children. J Bone Joint Surg (Am) 47:1295–1309
6. Chagnon S, Blery M (1982) Entorses et luxations du rachis cervical chez l'enfant. A propos de 17 cas. J Radiol 63:465–470
7. Juhl JH, Miller SM, Roberts GW (1962) Roentgenographic variations in the normal cervical spine. Radiology 78:591–596
8. Malgaigne JF (1855) Traité des fractures et des luxations. Tome II. Baillière, Paris
9. Pennecot GF, Leonard P, Peyrot des Gachons S, Hardy JR, Pouliquen JC (1984) Traumatic ligamentous instability of the cervical spine in children. J Pediatr Orthop 4:339–345
10. Penning L (1964) Non-pathological and pathologic relationships between the lower cervical vertebrae. Amer J Roentgenol 78:591–598
11. Penning L (1983) Obtaining and interpreting plain films in cervical spine injury. In: Bailey et al. (eds) The cervical spine. JB Lippincott Co, Philadelphia, pp 262–295
12. Scher AT (1979) Anterior cervical subluxation: an unstable position. AJR 133:275–280
13. Watson-Jones R (1955) Fractures and joint injuries. Vol II, 4th ed. Livingstone, Edinburgh London

Cervical Spine II
© by Springer-Verlag 1989

1.3. Serious Cervical Distortions (so Called Subluxations)

V. Denaro, Catania, Italy

The 'cervical distortions' are injuries in which the related pathologies, anatomic-pathology, and clinical picture have been clarified only in recent years, since they have become very frequent both in sports traumatology and accidents.

They are classified according to the seriousness of the injury and given the anatomic pathological description of 'simple' or 'serious distortion' (or progressive and neuraggressive distortions).

The *simple cervical distortions* are the most frequent and they occur when the traumatic event only causes an extreme motion in 'distraction' and there aren't significant tears of ligament structures of the 'motion segment' of the cervical spine. The most common is the traumatic distortion known as 'whiplash'.

In these cases the clinical picture varies and at times is rather complex and characterized by pain (referred to the arms, shoulders and lateral regions of the neck) often with vertigo, dysphagia, and vision disturbances. Emotional changes often appear, which are evidenced by a neurosis that dominates the clinical picture. Clinically there is a stiffness and the disappearance of the physiological lordosis of the cervical spine.

The *serious cervical distortions* occur less frequently. They are determined by an injury causing a 'loss of continuity' of the complex ligament system of the 'cervical motion segment'. However, the injury to the ligament structures is not complete and immediate, as in a dislocation, but it is partial such that it causes the loss of strength and therefore loss of the normal relation of the segments in a gradual, slow and progressive way. This results in modification of the diameter of the cervical spinal canal and involves the spinal cord (such injuries can therefore be called 'neuroaggressive').

Leaving out the simple cervical injuries that we have already reviewed [2], we will only deal with the 'serious cervical distortions'. Due to the differences that exist in the embryological, biomechanical, and therapeutic aspects it is possible to distinguish the upper distortions, affecting the first two cervical vertebrae, and the lower distortions, affecting the remaining five cervical vertebrae.

Serious Upper Cervical Distortions (C1–C2)

The ligament structures which guarantee the stability of the upper cervical spine are well known (tectorial membrane, lateral ligaments in 'Y', cruciform ligament, occipito-atlantal or alar ligaments, atlanto-odontoid joint and lateral C1/2 joint).

As far as biomechanics are concerned, according to experimental studies [4, 5, 7, 8, 10] one can say that the alar ligaments and those in 'Y' control the rotation; the cruciform ligament controls the rotation and the stability of the dens with the anterior arch of the atlas.

In clinical practice, the mechanism of the trauma results in specific injuries of the ligament system (as it has been experimentally demonstrated). The common injuries are rotary dislocation, antero-posterior dislocations and rarely lateral dislocations.

The clinical picture is characterised, in addition to pain, principally by muscular concentration with torticollis. Early in the course of the injury the contractions can hide an acute ligament lesion. It will suffice to immobilize the patient and give him analgesics and muscle relaxant drugs and then reevaluate the patient within a few days.

The X-ray signs associated with a 'cervical serious distortion' with routine radiology are: a) in the antero-posterior transoral projection, assymetry between the epistropheal axis and the lateral parts of the atlas, which suggests a rotary dislocation (or a lateral dislocation); b) in the lateral projections in static conditions a 'serious distortion' with injury of the atlanto-epistopheal ligaments can be invisible, but if dynamic X-rays are taken, where the patient moves actively in maximum flexion and extension the signs of instability will appear (it is advisable that the patient performs the movements in flexion and extension by himself in the presence of the surgeon).

In lateral view X-rays one must consider the distance between the epistropheal axis and the anterior arch of the atlas, which generally must not be more than 1–2 mm in adults, and 3–4 mm in children (where the presence of the growth cartilage is to be considered). Higher values are expressions of a pathologic instability of C1–C2 (Fig. 1).

Besides the traditional X-rays, nowadays a CT scan of the segment in question will easily prove the suspected instability. In fact a rotatory instability will be immediately evident by a CT scan even during the first few days following the trauma. It is important to keep in mind the differential diagnosis that it is possible to find patients suffering from collagenous disease (such as rheumatoid arthritis) which presents with instability that could simulate a posttraumatic state.

Once the diagnosis of 'serious distortion' with initial dislocation has been made, the treatment will depend on the seriousness of the instability.

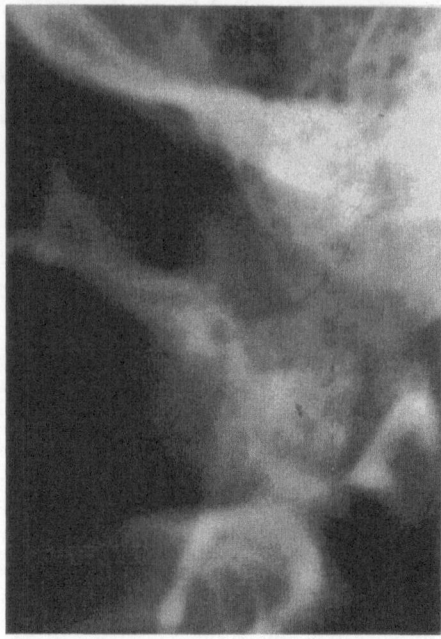

Fig. 1. X-ray showing a severe distortion affecting C1–C2. The atlanto-dental interval is more than 3 mm

1. In rotary dislocations reducible by traction the treatment will be conservative with a halo for three months. We underline that it is possible to
verify the reduction by a CT-scan with the patient in traction, or by traditional X-rays, having put the patient in Halo-cast or vest traction.

If the rotary dislocation is not reducible a surgical reduction should be
attempted, followed by wiring and fusion with modelled autogenous bone
graft of C1–C2–C3 (Fig. 2). Surgical reduction of recent injuries is simple,
whereas it is difficult and involves a certain amount of hazard in old injuries.
In such cases it is always necessary to be cautious and to terminate attemps
of reduction if during the reduction alterations in Somato-Sensory Evoked
Potentials (SSEP) appear (it is necessary to use intraoperative SSEP monitoring). In one case we were satisfied by a partial reduction since the above
mentioned SSEP alteration occurred.

2. In C1–C2 dislocations in the antero-posterior direction, if the diastasis
between the epistropheal axis and the anterior arch of the atlas is about
2–3 mm and it is reducible, the treatment will not necessarely be surgical.
After the reduction has been performed, treatment in a halo or in a minerva
cast for at least three months will suffice. If the diastasis of the axis-arch is
more than 3 mm or if neurological signs are present, the treatment must be
surgical, consisting of posterior fusion of C1–C2–C3 (Fig. 2).

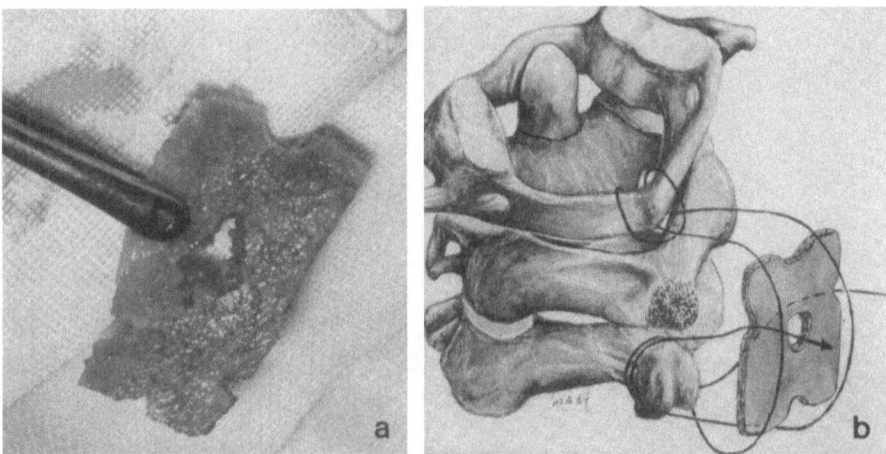

Fig. 2. Fusion technique C1 to C3: a) moulded autologous bone graft and b) technique of suturing with synthetic non absorbable material

Serious Distortion of the Lower Cervical Spine (C3–C7)

It is well known that the lower cervical spine has a fundamental role in maintaining cervical stability. The biomechanical functional unit called 'motion segment' is composed of:
– the anterior longitudinal ligament
– the intervertebral disc
– the posterior longitudinal ligament
– the posterior articular joints
– the ligamentum flavum
– the interspinosus ligaments
– the nucal ligaments
– the intertransversal ligaments (scarcely developed, are often mistaken for the intertransversal muscles).

It has long been discussed and quite an amount of research and experimental work has been done on the role of the single ligament in maintaining vertebral stability [4, 5, 7, 8, 10].

In other words we can say that in order to maintain the cervical vertebral stability, even admitting the fundamental importance of all the ligament structures, the main stabilizing role is attributable to by the posterior longitudinal ligament and to its connection with the posterior wall of the intervertebral disc (Fig. 3a). So, when the ligament system is injured by trauma involving the posterior longitudinal ligament or its connection with the disc, even if we will not have an immediate vertebral dislocation, within a short period of time we will observe a slow, gradual and progressive dislocation of

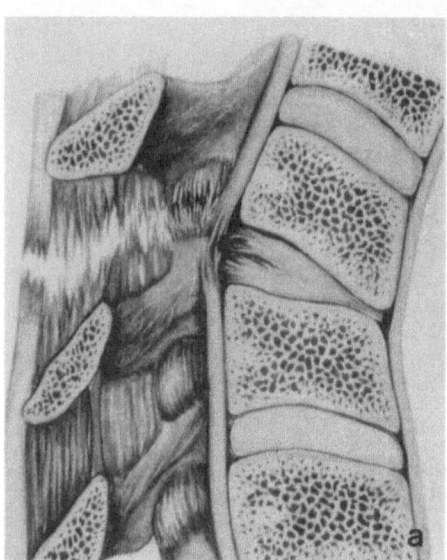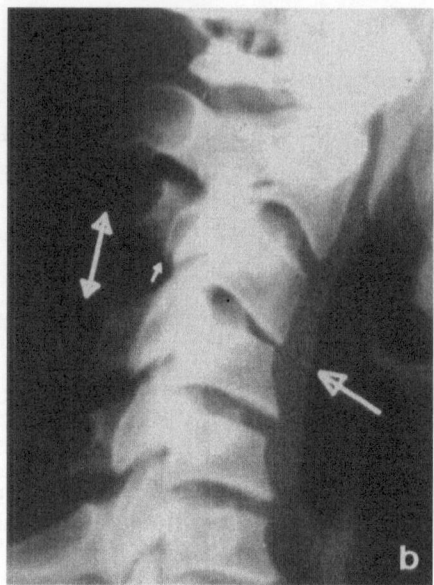

Fig. 3. a) Ligamentous lesions in distorsion. b) X-ray showing a severe distortion

the mentioned vertebrae with consequent loss of relation between the contiguous vertebrae and possible serious spinal cord damage.

It is understandable that it is always necessary to suspect a 'serious distortion' of the cervical spine, especially if the patient presents with cervical pain, or torticollis, or serious contractions of the neck masses, or feeling of instability of his spine. Therefore an accurate X-ray study is fundamental. We recommend, in absence of bone injuries, to look for a C1–C2 injury in studying the first X-rays in static and dynamic conditions in order to uncover the hidden signs of a 'serious distortion'. The important X-ray elements in order to prove a serious latent distortion, are the following (Fig. 3):

1) an anomalous diastasis of the apophysis-spinous
2) an inclination, even a minimal one of the vertebrae with partial exposure of the articular surfaces
3) an anterior inclination (kyphosis) of the disc in question
4) a horizontal sliding of a vertebrae on the other more than to 3 or 4 mm.

All these X-ray findings can be present together or separately.

But if these findings are not clear, due to serious muscle contraction that limits the active movements of the neck, it will be necessary to immobilize the patient using a brace. After one or two weeks the dynamic X-rays are repeated (in the presence of the surgeon and with the patient completely conscious and awake).

Once the muscular contractions have diminished in the setting of a 'serious distortion', the eventual instability will be identified by the dynamic studies (in maximum flexion and extension).

The treatment strategy in these injuries can be the following:

A – For recent injuries:

– if the injury is reducible, it is possible to try conservative treatment (Halo traction followed by immobilization in Halo-cast or -vest). The reduction often does not last long. That is why we prefer to carry out a posterior fixation after reduction, with plate and screws in the articular process according to Roy-Camille's procedure.

B – For old injuries:

– if the dislocation is reducible with dynamic tests, then a posterior fixation utilizing Roy-Camille plates with bone-graft can be performed

– if the dislocation is irreducible, then gradual cranial traction is applied (up to 12 kg). If the dislocation is reduced by the traction a posterior fixation using Roy-Camille plates and screws associated with bone-graft will be done. At times, if there is a morphological alteration of the vertebral bodies and spinal cord disturbances, a decompression and anterior fusion will be done during the same surgical session.

– but if the dislocation has created a serious morphological alteration of the bodies with neurological damage, it will be necessary to use a combined approach with the patient lying on his side. In this case it is possible to perform an anterior and posterior approach during one procedure. Anteriorly a large somatectomy is performed and posteriorly the posterior articulations are released. In this way it is possible to first reduce and then fix the segment posteriorly with plates. This is then followed by an anterior fusion with modelled bone-graft.

As usual all these operations are followed by an immobilization with brace for 2–3 months.

Case Reports

Our personal experience consist of 21 operated cases from 1979 to June 1988 (8 of which were performed at the Clinica Ortopedica e Traumatologica dell' Universitá di Pavia). The patient ages ranged from 14 to 52 years. There were 7 C1–C2 serious distortions and 14 in C3–C7.

The procedure was:

A. Among the seven C1–C2 injuries, 4 were rotary dislocations and were treated without surgery, three of them by traction and fixation in Halo-jacket. All of them recovered without movement impairment except for a slight limitation in extreme rotation of the neck.

The other case was an old rotary dislocation with serious torticollis (which occurred 8 months after the trauma). After halo-traction the patient

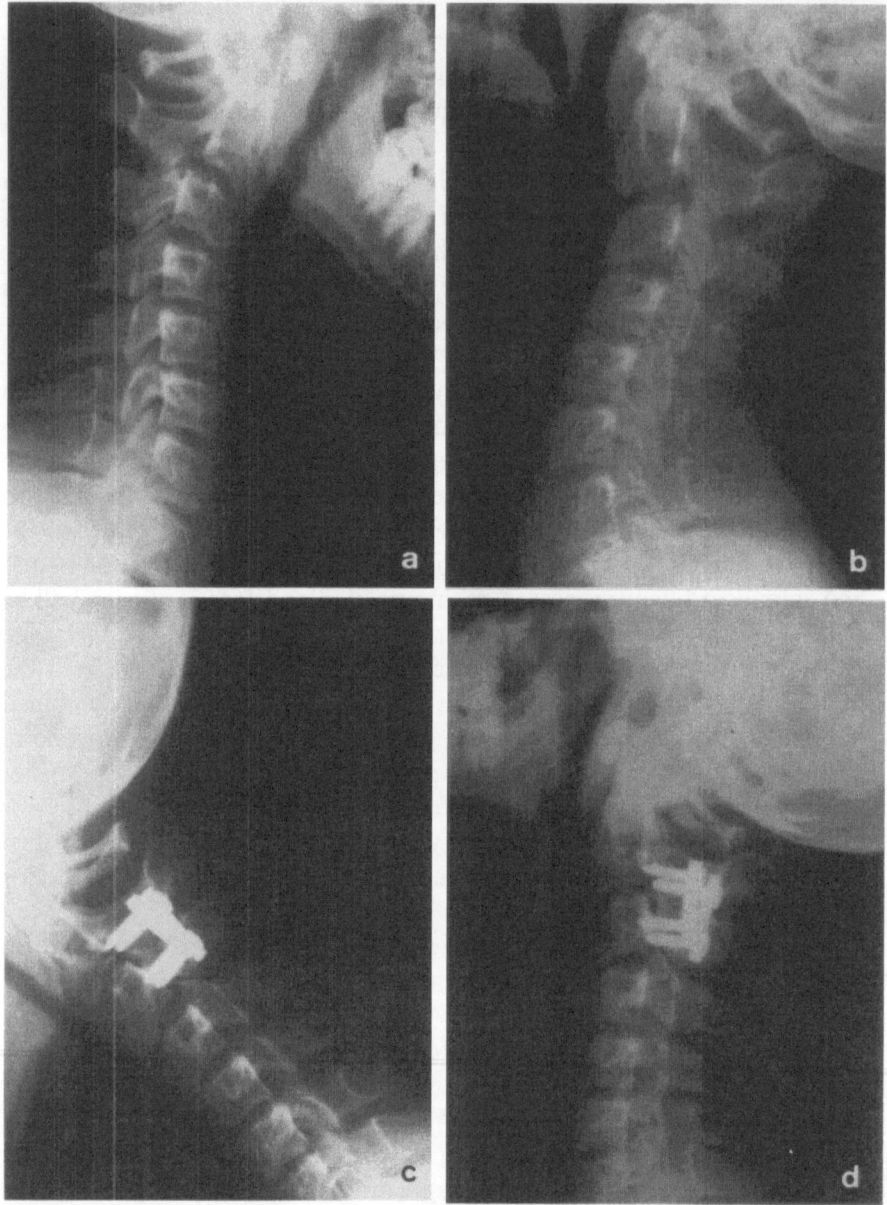

Fig. 4. Severe distortion of C2–C3 in a 16 year old young man a) in flexion b) in extension. After reduction and dorsal osteosynthesis: c) flexion and d) extension. Note there is no evidence of instability. A second serious distortion occurred 8 months later, causing C4–C5 subluxation and spastic tetraparesis. e) and f) Dynamic X-rays. g) Reduction in halo-traction. h) Stabilization with additional dorsal osteosynthesis

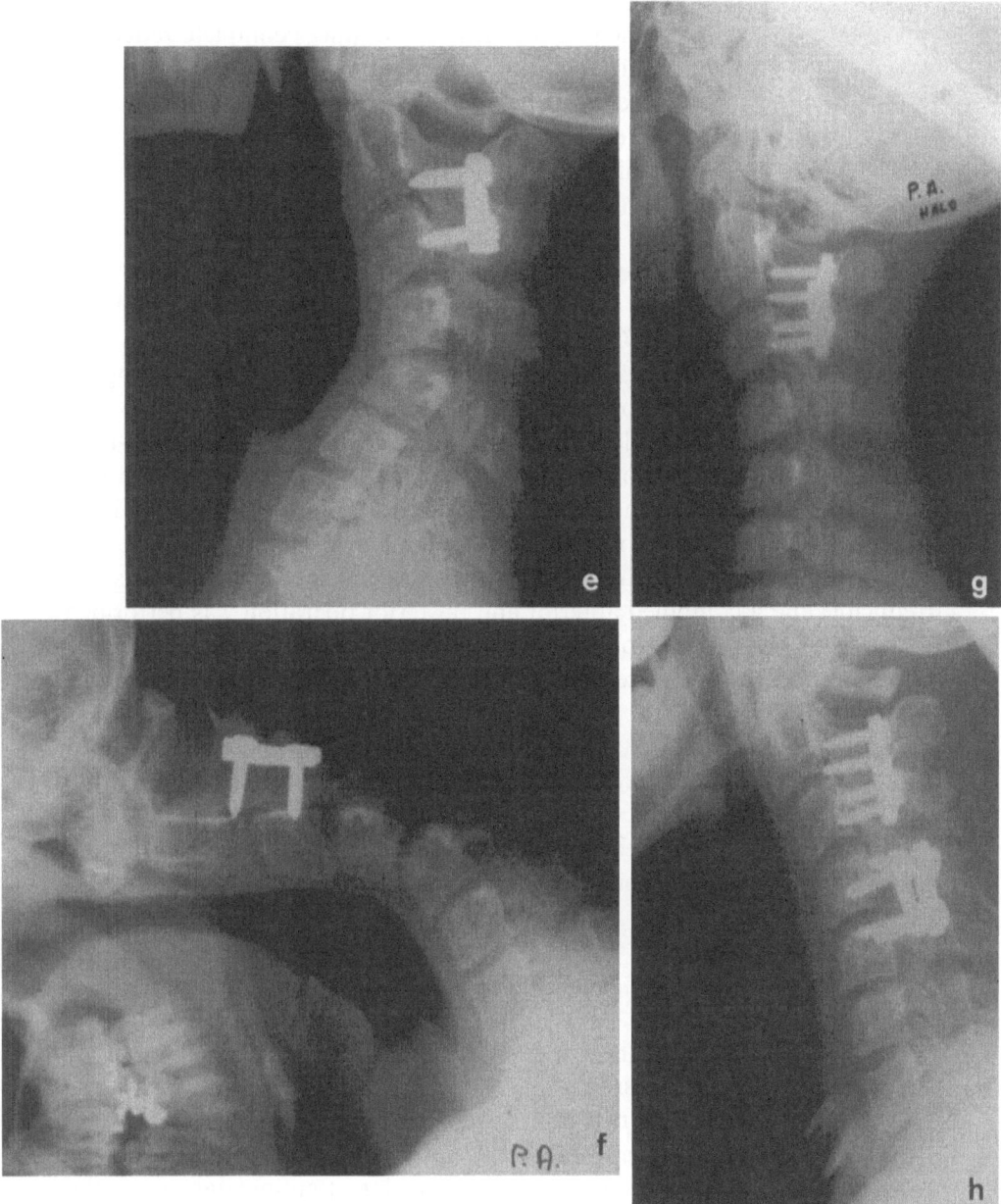

was operated, with posterior fusion with only partial reduction (due to the appearance during the maneuvre of SSEP disturbances complete reduction was abandoned). The result was satisfactory with respect to stability and aesthetics, also relieving the serious torticollis.

In the other three cases of serious antero-posterior dislocation with diastasis between the epistropheal-axis and atlas arch of more than 3 mm, a reduction and fixation was carried out with wire and modelled bone graft of C1–C2–C3.

B. C3–C7 'serious distortions' included 14 cases (7 C5–C6, 3 C4–C5, 2 C6–C7, 1 C3–C4, 1 C2–C3), 9 of which were operated by reduction and fixation according to Roy-Camille's procedure with bone-graft.

Two old distortion cases with significant dislocation and morphological alteration of the vertebral bodies and with increasing pyramidal spinal cord disturbances were operated through an anterior approach after Halo-traction treatment (during halo traction improvement of the spinal cord injury was witnessed). The procedure involved a wide anterior decompression, large corpectomy and fusion and somatic reconstruction with bone-graft. One case with serious anterior dislocation and with increasing spastic tetraparesis was irreducible and a combined anterior and posterior operation was performed in the same surgical session, carrying out an anterior corpectomy, large decompression, posterior release and therefore a reduction and posterior-anterior fixation.

One case with a C2–C3 'serious distortion' was operated with posterior fixation with plates and screws. 8 months later he had further trauma that caused a new distortion of C4–C5 (Fig. 4).

In all these cases a perfect surgical fixation was the result with neurological recovery. There were neither local nor general complications worth mentioning.

Conclusive Considerations

As a consequence of the experience gained from the small series of patients observed, it is possible to state:
1. 'Serious distortions' are rare injuries and they risk being overlooked during initial evaluation. Since they are serious, progressive and neuraggressive they are to be investigated with particular attention right from the initial presentation.
2. The pathogenesis is due to lesions of the important ligament structures that guarantee stability to the upper (C1–C2) and lower spine (C3–C7). It is important to underline that the loss of stability is not immediate but gradual, slow and progressive.
3. The diagnosis is essentially made through X-rays both traditional X-ray with dynamic tests and CT scan.

4. The goal of the treatment is to reduce the dislocation and to get a firm fixation of the injured segment.

The reduction and fixation produce excellent clinical results (disappearance of the symptoms and neurological improvement). Biomechanically the results were also excellent (the segments that underwent surgery were all firmly stabilized).

References

1. Babin S, Katzner M, Schvingt E (1975) Entorses graves du rachis cervical inferieur et leurs consequences, un cas de luxation ancienne et meconnue. Nouv Presse Med 4:2033
2. Denaro V (1974) Distorsione del rachide cervicale a colpo di frusta. Atti e memorie della SOTIMI, vol XXVIII
3. Fielding JW (1964) Normal and selected abnormal motion of the cervical spine from the second cervical vertebra to the seventh cervical vertebra based cineroentgenography. J Bone Joint Surg 46A:1779–1781
4. Louis R (1982) Chirurgie du rachis. Springer, Berlin Heidelberg New York Tokyo
5. Louis R, Goutallier D (1977) Symposium sur les fractures instables du rachis. Rev Chir Orthop 63:417
6. Fielding JW, Hawkins RJ (1977) Atlanto-axial rotary fixation. J Bone Joint Surg 59A:37–44
7. Roy-Camille R, Saillant G, Berteaux D, Lartat-Jacob A, Bisserié M (1977) Entorse grave par lesion traumatique du segment mobile rachidien (SMR) de la colonne cervicale. J Chir (Paris) 113:121
8. Roy-Camille R, Saillant G, Berteaux D, Bisserié M (1978) Entorses graves du rachis cervical. Rev Chir Orthop 64:677
9. Roy-Camille R, Saillant G, Denaro V, Mamoudy P, Bisserié M (1981) Distorsioni gravi del rachide cervicale negli sportivi. It Journ Sports Traumatology 3:203
10. White AA, Panjabi MM (1978) The clinical biomechanics of the spine. J.B. Lippincott Company, Philadelphia

Cervical Spine II
© by Springer-Verlag 1989

1.4. A Momentary Documentation of a Cervical Vertebrae Fracture

M. THIEL and H. W. STAUDTE, Aachen, Federal Republic of Germany

Introduction

Countless articles with experimental, clinical-roentgenographic and autopsy findings have been published dealing with the mechanism of injuries caused by whisplash and snapping of the cervical spine [1, 5, 9, 11, 17, 19]. They range from mild distortions with no morphological signs of injury to fatal lesions with complete rupture of the spinal cord [16, 20].

In spite of the abundancy of literature on this theme, we feel that this short article is of special interest because it is accompanied by a photo documentation of the chronological injury process and because of the slow tempo of the event it allows an exact reconstruction of the pathogenesis.

Case History

While rough-housing in the party-den at a friend's house, a strong, healthy 18 year old male (M.H.) suffered a depressed fracture on the anterior edge of the 7th cervical vertebra with rupture of the posterior articular process and subluxation of the right vertebral joint (Fig. 1).

M.H. had a muscle spasm causing deviation of the cervical vertebrae and complained of ulnar dysaesthesia in both forearms and hands more severe on the right side. In addition, his ability to make a fist with his right hand was weakened. Later it was found that the exact moment of injury had been photographed.

In Fig. 2 one can see the process taking place. The person standing behind M.H. executed a maximal flexion of the cervical spine. M.H. said he first attempted a muscular opposition to this force but then his strength gave out. He then heard a cracking sound in his neck, followed by a ripping feeling in the anterior part of his throat accompanied by an electric "shock" in both arms.

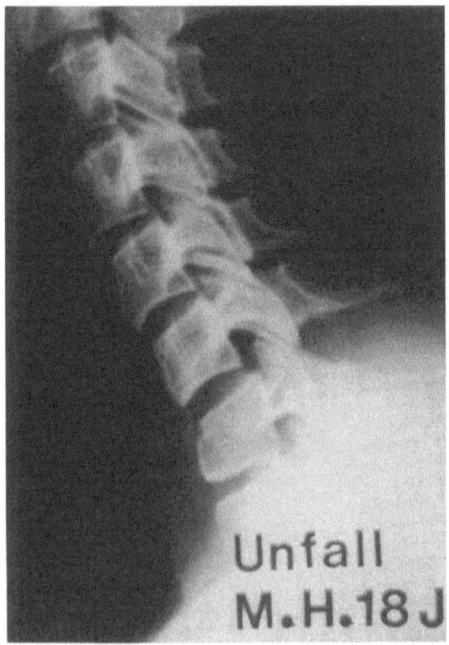

Fig. 1. X-ray showing fracture of the anterior edge of C7. Subluxation C6/7

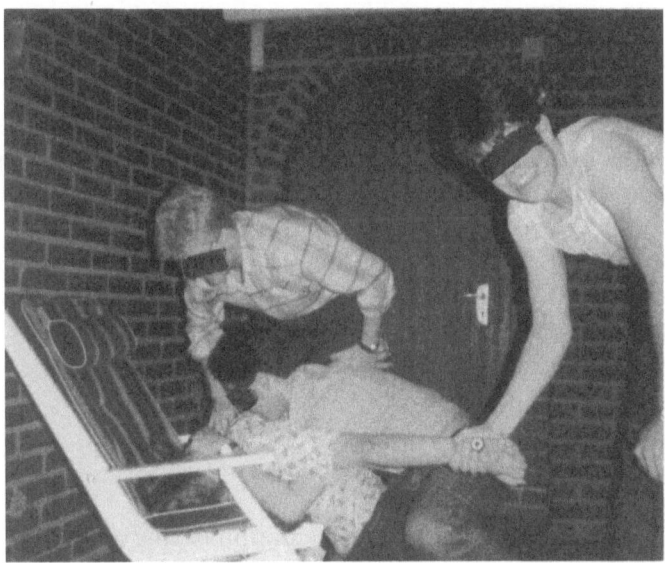

Fig. 2. Documentation of the injury

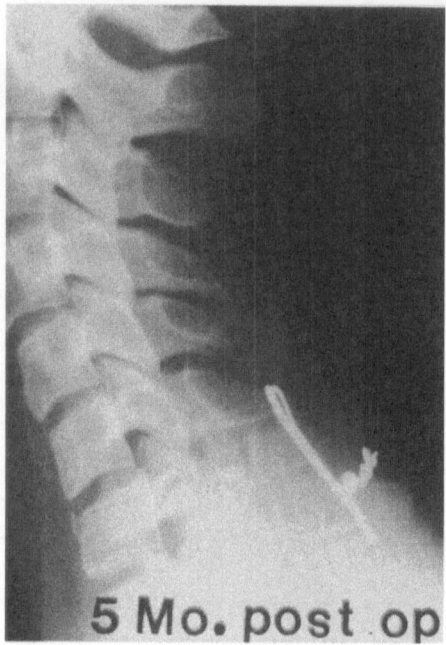

Fig. 3. Postoperative X-ray of the dorsal fusion of C6/7

Therapy

M.H. presented to us about 20 hours after the trauma with a history of progressing injury of the right 8th cervical nerve root.

On the next day we performed an open reduction followed by a posterior fusion with hip-bone chip and wire loop (Fig. 3).

The external fixation was carried out for 8 weeks with a Camp-apparatus. In the 5th postoperative month the bone graph was calcified and the cervical body fracture had healed with a slightly wedged deformity.

The neurological symptoms were diminishing. In the 8th month following the operation, M.H. still complained of uncomfortable sensations and dull pains in the palm of the right hand. These were of no pathological importance. The EMG and nerve conducting velocity were normal.

Discussion

Aside from the photographic documentation of this event, this case is of special interest also for the fact that one sees that the process of injury took an unusually long time. Each phase was consciously registered by the victim and precisely reconstructed in the pathogenesis. A fracture of a cervical body

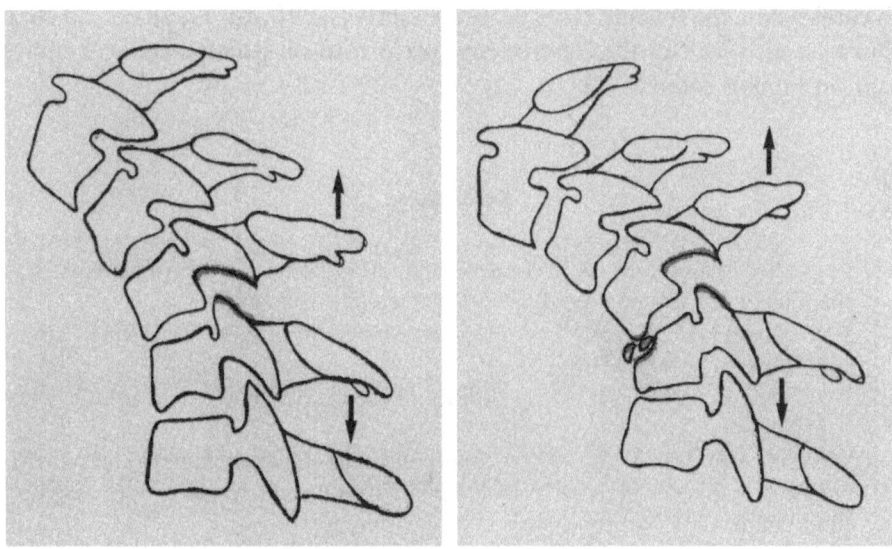

a   b

Fig. 4. a) Rupture of the joint capsule and ligamentum flavum, b) tear-drop fracture

is often the result of a whiplash which causes a flexion/retroflexion of the cervical spine. In our case, the fracture was due mainly to the slackening of tension resulting from the rupture of the posterior structures and to the axial compression. The latter arose as the perpetrator employed his body weight in addition to the strength of his arms. Because of the position of the head on the seat of the chair, the body weight was transferred to the cervical spine like an axial weight. Thus, it indirectly intensified the bending force causing the posterior ligaments to strain and the capsule apparatus and the ligamentum flavum to rupture (Fig. 4).

This corresponds to the testimony of the victim who reported that he immediately experienced a posterior pain. Thereafter, a ventral break in the anterior edge of the cervical body (tear-drop fracture) resulted (Fig. 4b).

Along with so-called hyperanteflexion fractures (named by Braakman) one often sees tuft fractures of the cervical body. The most common location is the lower cervical spine below the 5th cervical body [2, 10, 17].

In a large-group study, Bohlmann [2] found that in approximately 20% of the cases in which nerve-root lesions following cervical spine trauma were accompanied by subluxation or luxation deviations in the articular processes, a fracture in the cervical body was also present.

Taking the documentation of our victim into account and observing the unusually long time development of the events of this accident, one can conclude that here the process of injury was biphasic [6−8].

We were not able to find any comparable chain of events in the literature. It is interesting to note that this pattern of injury is very similar to that found in cases where the trauma takes place instantly [see 10, 14, 17, 18, 21, 22 etc.]. Our case also verifies the experiments performed on isolated cervical spines and on human cadavers [4, 13, 22].

References

1. Bauze RJ, Ardran GM (1978) Experimental production of forward dislocation in the human cervical spine. J Bone Joint Surg 60B:239–245
2. Bohlman HH (1979) Acute fractures and dislocations of the cervical spine. J Bone Joint Surg 61A:1119–1142
3. Braakman R, Penning L (1971) Injuries of the cervical spine. Excerpta Medica, Amsterdam
4. Clemens HJ, Burow K (1972) Experimentelle Untersuchungen zur Verletzungsmechanik der Halswirbelsäule beim Frontal- und Heckaufprall. Arch orthop Unfall Chir 74:116–145
5. Erdmann H (1973) Schleuderverletzungen der Halswirbelsäule. In: Junghanns H (Hrsg) Die Wirbelsäule in Forschung und Praxis, Bd 56. Hippokrates, Stuttgart
6. Fabricius B (1969) Stoßartige Beschleunigung von Fahrzeuginsassen bei Auffahrunfällen. Inaug. Diss. Berlin
7. Fiala E (1969) Zur Verletzungsmechanik bei Verkehrsunfällen. H Unfallheilk 98:31–52
8. Gögler E (1969) Biomechanik des Verkehrsunfalls. H Unfallheilk 99:235–240
9. Hinz P (1970) Die Verletzung der Halswirbelsäule durch Schleuderung und durch Abknickung. In: Junghanns H (Hrsg) Die Wirbelsäule in Forschung und Praxis, Bd 47. Hippokrates, Stuttgart
10. Hinz P (1972) Verletzungsmuster der Halsorgane in Abhängigkeit zur Impulsrichtung. H Unfallheilk 110:15–20
11. Jefferson G (1940) Discussion on fractures and dislocations of the cervical spine. Proceedings of the Royal Society of Medicine 33:657–660
12. Jeffreys E, McSweeney T, Roaf R (1980) Disorders of the cervical spine. Butterworth, London
13. Lange W (1972) Die Reaktion des Systems Kopf–Halswirbelsäule bei stoßartiger Beschleunigung des Torsos. H Unfallheilk 110:8–15
14. McCall IW, Park WM, McSweeney T (1973) The radiological demonstration of acute lower cervical injury. Clin Radiol 24:235–240
15. Penning L (1976) Dynamische Aspekte der Halswirbelsäulenverletzung. Unfallheilk 79:5–10
16. Rompe G (1987) Kritische Stellungnahme zum aktuellen Stand der Beschleunigungsverletzung der HWS und ihre Begutachtung. Im Druck
17. Saternus KS (1979) Die Verletzungen von Halswirbelsäulen und von Halsweichteilen. In: Junghanns H (Hrsg) Die Wirbelsäule in Forschung und Praxis, Bd 84. Hippokrates, Stuttgart
18. Schaafsma SJ (1970) Plexus injuries. In: Vinken PJ, Bruyn GW (Hrsg) Handbook of clinical neurology, Bd 7. North Holland Publishing Co, Amsterdam, pp 402–429

19. Schmaus H (1890) Beiträge zur pathologischen Anatomie der Rückenmarkser-
schütterung. Virch Arch Pathol Anat 122:470–495
20. Thiel M (1982) Kausalfaktoren für Extremverletzungen der Halswirbelsäule. Z
Rechtsmed 88:249–256
21. Whitley JF, Forsyth HF (1960) Classification of cervical spine injuries. Am J
Roentg 83:633
22. Ziffer D (1967) Das Verhalten der Halswirbelsäule in Verbindung mit der
Schädelbasis und der oberen Brustwirbelsäule bei schlagartiger Druck-
beanspruchung (Stürze auf unnachgiebige Hindernisse – Stahlplatten –) und bei
schlagartiger Zugbeanspruchung (Zerreißung). Zbl Verkehrs-Medizin, Verkehrs-
Psychologie, Luft- und Raumfahrt-Medizin 4:194–217

1.5. Acute Disc Protrusion in Severe Trauma of the Lower Cervical Spine

R. B. RAYNOR, New York, N.Y., U.S.A.

The initial management of the more severe injuries of the lower cervical spine depends on their type. A Halo apparatus may be used for fracture or soft tissue disruption. If the injury has caused an unstable condition, fusion may be the treatment chosen. In most cases this will be of the posterior type. The usual diagnostic studies done for evaluation consist of plain X-rays and a CT scan, though tomography may be done at some institutions. A myelogram with CT scan is usually not considered necessary even though soft tissue detail is difficult to evaluate by CT scan without the presence of contrast.

When anterior fusion is done, it is usually for stabilization, especially if the primary pathology is disruption of the anterior bony elements. Since these can be well visualized by CT scan, a contrast study may not be part of the pre-operative evaluation.

Though the possibility of acute disc protrusion in injuries of the cervical spine is mentioned [1, 4, 7-9, 11] there is little data on their occurrence and importance. Most authors mention their occurrence only in passing [2, 6].

The group studied consisted of twenty patients, all seen shortly after injury occurred. All had moderately severe to severe neurological deficit. Moderate deficit was defined as at least a 25% loss of motor power in both arms or hands and leg weakness. Five patients had physiologic transection of the cord with no demonstrable motor or sensory activity below the level of injury. The majority of patients had deficits somewhere between these extremes.

Sensory deficit was also graded and evaluated.

In this group there were twelve patients with significant fractures of a vertebra. A significant fracture was defined as either a compression, pedicle, or body fracture or dislocation. Cracks in a laminal arch or spinous process were not considered of major importance for this study.

All patients were carefully evaluated neurologically and skeletal traction instituted. The patients were observed for changes in neurological signs. As soon as their condition was stable and it was technically feasible, diagnostic studies including contrast were done. On average this was seven to ten days following injury, but sometimes this was as early as 3 days post injury. Recently some patients have been evaluated on admission when the conditions and circumstances were appropriate.

Results

Eleven patients had no evidence of disc protrusion demonstrated by radiographic examination. Of the remaining nine patients, seven had disc protrusions large enough to impinge on the spinal cord and exert significant pressure. In one instance the disc was clearly not exerting pressure on the spinal cord, and in one patient the findings were unclear. All patients exhibited a central cord syndrome with more involvement of the upper extremities as compared to the lower.

Anterior disc excision and fusion were performed in eight patients. Of the seven patients with definite cord pressure, four had major improvement in their neurological status immediately following surgery (Table 1). Improve-

Table 1. *Disc Excision. Immediate Improvement*

Age	Neuro-logic level	Lesion	Motor status			Sen-sory	Follow up	
			Arms	Hands	Legs			
17	C6	Compound C6 Fracture	3	1 −	1 proximal 0 distal	poor	Day 2	toes 1+ legs 3 arms 3 (ambulated)
49	C5	Spondylosis	3	1	3	good	Day 2	arms 3+ hands 3
26	C6	C6−7 Dislocation	3	1 −	1 −	poor	Day 5	hands 3 legs 2
56	C5	Spondylosis	3	1 −	2+	good	Day 2	arms 3+ hands 2 legs 3+

Grading Scale:
0 – no movement seen or felt.
1 – slight movement observed.
2 – movement present, but not against gravity.
3 – movement against gravity but unable to maintain position against additional force.
4 – normal power.

Table 2. *Disc Excision. No Immediate Improvement*

			Motor status				
Age	Neurologic level	Lesion	Arms	Hands	Legs	Sensory	Follow up
61	C5	C5–6 Dislocation	2	1	3	good	no change
42	C6	C6 Compression fracture	2+	1	0	fair	no change Died of pneumonia 3rd day
62	C6	Spondylosis	3	1	2	good	no change
44	C7	C6–7 Dislocation	3	0	0	good	ambulatory with crutches at 1 year
35	C5	Cord contusion	2	0	3	good	no surgery minimal protrusion

ment was measured by changes in motor function and had to be at least 25% improved to be considered significant. The improvement had to manifest itself within the first five days to be attributed to the surgical decompression.

If rapid neurological improvement was not evident by the fifth post-operative day, no major changes occurred other than the slow improvement frequently seen in patients with central cord injury [10] (Table 2). Usually, the increase in neurological function was evident by the second or third day. Surgical decompression was not considered to have altered the normal course of the disease if this improvement did not occur. Three patients with definite cord pressure did not improve, nor did one with questionable cord compression.

There did not appear to be any significant difference in the initial presentation of patients to distinguish any of the three groups. Before a definitive diagnostic study was done, there was no way of separating those patients who had cord compression due to a disc protrusion from those that did not. We were also unable to predict which patients with disc protrusion would benefit from decompression and which would not.

Discussion

Of the twenty patients studied, twelve had significant fractures. In three cases these were compression fractures, one of whom had an extruded disc. Two had normal discs (Table 3). There were eight patients with no fracture but severe neurological involvement. Two had significant disc protrusions.

Table 3. *Fractures* vs. *Disc Status*

	Dislocation	Compression	No fracture	Total
Disc protrusion	4	1	4	9
No protrusion	5	2	4	11

The remaining nine fracture patients had vertebral body dislocations. Of these, four had disc protrusions, five did not. A recent study noted an 8.8% incidence of disc protrusion in patients with facet subluxations [1], but their neurological status was not noted.

Mirvis *et al.* observed herniated disc material in eleven of twenty-one patients after cervical trauma [6]. In seven patients the herniated disc was associated with a fracture or dislocation. No correlation was made between the severity of the neurological deficit and the disc herniation, though the authors do note that the disc herniation could be related to the neurological findings.

This study indicates that, though small, there are a significant number of disc protrusions that occur with cervical spine injury, especially when fractures and neurological deficit are present. These can produce major neurological deficit. Removal of these disc fragments results in immediate neurological improvement. In this series half the patients with disc protrusion showed such improvement following surgery. The series is too small to evaluate the true incidence of cord pressure due to disc protrusion. However, we feel that all patients with neurological deficit should have a myelogram followed by CT scan at the earliest convenient time. It is possible that magnetic resonance imaging will replace the CT myelogram, but at this time we do not feel confident enough with this test to use it as the basis for deciding whether or not a disc protrusion causing pressure on the spinal cord is present.

References

1. Arena MJ, Eismont FJ, Green AB (1987) Intervertebral disc extrusion associated with cervical facet subluxation and dislocation. Presented at the Cervical Spine Research Society, Dec. 3, 1987, Washington, D.C.
2. Bohlman HH, Ducker TB, Lucas JT (1982) Spine and spinal cord injuries. In: The spine, 2nd ed. W.B. Saunders Company, Philadelphia, USA
3. Braakman R (1970) Neurological and neurosurgical aspects of injuries of lower cervical spine. Acta Neurochir (Wien) 22:245–260
4. Cloward RB (1973) Skull traction for cervical spine injury: Should it be abandoned? JAMA 226:1008
5. Cloward RB (1961) Treatment of acute fractures and fracture dislocations of the cervical spine by interbody fusion. J Neurosurg 18:201–209
6. Macnab I (1982) Acceleration extension injuries of the cervical spine. In: The spine, 2nd ed. W.B. Saunders Company, Philadelphia, USA
7. Mirvis SE, Geisler FH, Jelinek JJ, Joslyn JN, Gellad F (1988) Acute cervical spine trauma: evaluation with 1.5 T imaging. Neuroradiology 166:807–816
8. Raynor RB (1968) Severe injuries of the cervical spine treated by early anterior interbody fusion and ambulation. J Neurosurg 28:311–316
9. Schneider RC (1962) Surgical indications and contra-indications in spine and spinal cord trauma. Clin Neurol 8:157–184
10. Schneider RC, Thompson JM, Bebin J (1958) The syndrome of the acute central spinal cord injury. J Neurol Neurosurg Psychiatry 21:216–227
11. Wilson CB (1965) The role of the anterior interbody fusion in acute injuries of the cervical spine. Kentucky Med Assoc J 63:260–264

Cervical Spine II
© by Springer-Verlag 1989

1.6. Unilateral Dislocation of the Lower Cervical Spine

D.S. Korres, K. Stamos, El. Velikas, An. Andreakos,
and Chr. Hardouvelis, Athens, Greece

Acute trauma to the cervical spine is the main cause leading to serious permanent disability or to death in a considerable number of patients.

The lower cervical spine due to its position and its characteristic bio-mechanical behavior, is exposed to a great deal of trauma. Among the different patterns of injuries which involve the lower cervical spine, unilateral dislocation appears to provoke great concern; this may be due to its instability. There is controversy about the natural history of this injury and its managment as well (Roraback 1987). What is the best method of obtaining and maintaining a reduced unilateral dislocation? What is the indication for surgical stabilization? Is the anterior or the posterior approach recommended? Is the development of spontaneous fusion always the proper solution to this problem?

Many authors suggest that reduction can be obtained by skeletal traction (Romadier and Bombard 1964); others prefer an open reduction (Bailey 1961; Bohlman 1979); reduction by manipulation under general anesthesia is also advocated (Evans 1961; Cheshire 1969).

In spite an agreement defining the instability of this injury (Beatson 1963; White *et al.* 1976) the problem of management remains cloudy. Cloward (1961) is in favor of an anterior stabilisation, while others (Stauffer 1977) advocate a posterior approach. However the presence of late complications is also a very important problem which is related to the initial management.

Material

From Jan. 1970 to Dec. 1985, 368 fractures, dislocations or fracture-dislocations were admitted to the Orthopaedic Department, Athens University, K.A.T. Hospital.

Fifty-nine of the previously mentioned patients (16.03%) were classified as having sustained a unilateral dislocation at the lower cervical spine. There were 39 men and 20 women with an average age of 42 years. Road traffic

D. S. Korres et al.

Table 1. *Levels of Unilateral Dislocation*

C_2-C_3 :   2 (03.3%)
C_3-C_4 :   8 (13.5%)
C_4-C_5 : 20 (33.8%)
C_5-C_6 : 16 (27.1%)
C_6-C_7 : 12 (20.3%)
C_7-T_1 :   1 (01.6%)

Table 2. *Neurological Status in 36 Patients*

Initial status (36 pts)	Surgical group (6 pts)	Conservative group (30 pts)
Fr A: 4	(2): 1 Fr A, 1 Fr C	(2): 2 Fr A
Fr B: –	–	–
Fr C: 2	(1): 1 Fr E	(1): 1 Fr E
Fr D: 7	(3): 3 Fr E	(4): 3 Fr E, 1 Fr D
Fr E: 23	–	(23): 2 Fr D, 21 Fr E

accidents were responsible for this injury in just over half of the patients (50.8%), while falls from heights, diving, sport injuries or other causes were responsible for the remaining cases.

Table 1 shows the levels involved with a clear predominance at C4–C5 level.

Neurological signs were found in 13 cases (22%) but in only 4 patients was serious neurological symptomatology present (Table 2). Associated injuries of the skeleton were present in 4 patients (6.7%) and in the spine, in particular, in 3 cases (5%). Facial and or head injuries were detected in 18% of the patients.

Fifty-two patients (88.1%) were treated conservatively and 7 patients (11.8%) with operation. In all cases an attempt was made to reduce the dislocation by a closed method. No general anesthesia was given for this purpose. Reduction with traction and with or without manipulation was successful in 48 patients (81.3%). Conservative treatment consisted of application of skeletal or Glisson traction in bed for six weeks; this was followed by the application of a Minerva or a four post brace for a period of 8 to 10 weeks. Operative treatment consisted of an anterior interbody fusion in all cases. In two cases this was done in situ.

Three out of 59 patients (5%) died while in the hospital, from reasons related to their cervical trauma.

Patients stayed in the hospital for an average period of 8 weeks.

Method

Twenty-three patients (33.3%) were lost to follow-up or the data available was inadequate. The medical records of 30 patients treated conservatively and 6 patients treated by operation were analysed. The average follow-up time for those 36 patients was 9.4 years (2 to 18).

In all 36 patients a meticulous clinical and radiological examination was performed in order to exclude any instability. X-ray examination included AP, lateral, left and right oblique views as well as dynamic x-ray.

Accordingly, the patients were classified into three groups: (a) in group A are those patients having an excellent result which means being asymptomatic with an anatomical reduction and good alignment of the cervical spine, with some osteo-arthritic changes, (b) group B contains those patients having a satisfactory result, which means being asymptomatic but with an unsatisfactory radiological picture, showing malalignment of the spine and or extensive osteo-arthritic alterations. And (c) in group C are those patients having a poor result both clinically and radiologically.

Results

It appears that in the present series the final results were related to the stability obtained. Table 3 summarise the results.

From the conservative group (30 pts), twelve patients (40%) were classified in group A, six more patients (20%) were classified in group B and the remaining twelve patients (40%) having a poor result were classified in group C. In Table 2 we can see the neurological evaluation of those patients presented. From the surgically treated group of six patients, three had been classified in group A, two in group B and one with a poor result was classified in group

Table 3. *Clinical and Radiological Evaluation of 36 Patients with Unilateral Dislocation*

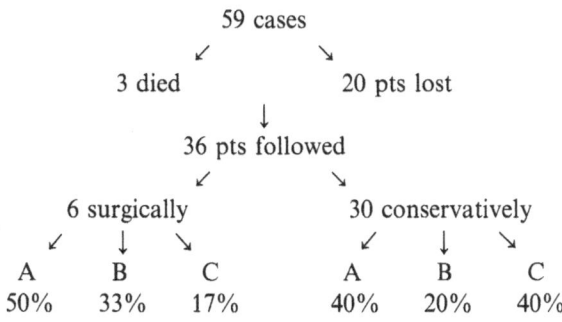

A: excellent result, B: satisfactory result, C: poor result.

C. The neurological evaluation of these patients is also shown in Table 2. Spontaneous fusion was seen in 11 cases (36.6%); in 8 cases it occurred in patients classified in group C, while two cases were detected in patients of group B and one in a patient of group A.

Discussion

Unilateral dislocation is a common injury, with a tendency to be missed at the initial examination (Evans 1976). In this series the frequency of this lesion was found to be 16% of all cervical spine injuries. Its mechanism is attributed to bending forces associated with a rotatory element (Roaf 1960; Brakman 1967); this was confirmed in the present series by a high rate of associated head injuries (18.6%). Road traffic accidents were found to be responsible for nearly half of the cases showing the complexity and the violence of forces required for this kind of injury. The most involved levels are C4–C5 and C5–C6 because these are the most mobile segments (Table 1). Neurological injury was also detected with frequency similar to that reported in the literature (Beatson 1963), being about 22%. Lesions of the cord are not so common; the commonest type of lesion being root involvement. In all cases an attempt to reduce the dislocation was made as soon as possible after their admission. Reduction of the dislocated joint is of great importance. We do not use general anesthesia, following Bailey's (1961) and Durbin's (1957) statements for existing dangers. We prefer to do it using traction, alone or with gently manipulation.

In case of failure, we suggest reduction by an open method. Reduction was not always successful by either closed or open methods because of delay or of the inadequacy of the approach used; the latter obliged us to fuse the cervical spine, in two cases, in a displaced position. Roraback (1987) suggests that reduction is difficult. In our series it was shown that the reduction was easier if it was performed early. In this series the interval from injury to reduction was 3 days (1 to 18) and the rate of success was almost 81%.

In unilateral dislocation, both the anterior and posterior elements are affected making it an unstable injury. Instability is defined as "acute" and "subacute" or "late", and each have their clinical and radiological manifestations (White et al. 1975, Herkowitz and Rothman 1984). Late instability may be manifested years after the injury in spite of a spontaneous fusion. It was shown from this series that nearly all the patients who had an unsuccessful reduction or who presented with redisplacement, developed a spontaneous fusion which was proved to lead to unsatisfactory results.

If the reduction was successful spontaneous fusion was less frequent. The incidence of radiologically evident spontaneous fusion after cervical spine trauma is reported to be between 36–66% (Roraback 1987). In our series it was found to be 36.6%. We think that the development of spontaneous fusion indicates a more extensive injury than had been appreciated at the initial examination. Spontaneous fusion was shown to be related to more late complications. This is explained by the fact that the slowly developing spontaneous fusion permits a gradual narrowing of the foraminae with all the consequences this may provoke.

This is not so in surgically treated patients where the height of the intervertebral space is restored and preserved. The presence of either form of instability (clinical or radiological) at follow up may indicate a failure in the management of the injury. This was found in almost 60% of the conservatively treated patients in our series. This result is compared to the high rate of success (83%) in the patients treated surgically. As far as the clinical results are concerned this difference is also impressive as only 17% of the surgically treated patients had clinical complaints as opposed to 40% of the patients treated conservatively.

The method of treatment does not appear to influence the outcome of a complete neurological lesion as it does for the incomplete one; the latter may be better managed by operative means. Conservative treatment in the long term may result in neurological deterioration as in two of our patients.

Because of increased instability, redisplacement or neurological impairment, we decided to treat 7 patients by an anterior interbody fusion. The need for surgical management may be in question, considering that almost 36% of these injured spines are going to stabilize spontaneously; but we should not rely on spontaneous fusion alone, especially when displacement persists and deformity of the cervical spine is noted to progress.

We suggest that it is of great importance not to allow a spontaneous fusion to develop in a displaced position and to try to prevent this by early open reduction and stabilization. An anterior approach will be helpful but is not strongly recommended as the main lesion on this specific injury is in the posterior elements.

References

1. Bailey RW (1961) Fractures and dislocations of the cervical spine. Surg Clin North Am 41:1357–1366
2. Beatson T-R (1963) Fractures and dislocations of the cervical spine. J Bone Joint Surg 45-B:21–35
3. Bohlman HH (1979) Acute fractures and dislocations of the cervical spine. J Bone Joint Surg 61-A:1119–1142
4. Braakman R, Vinken PJ (1967) Unilateral facet interlocking in the lower cervical spine. J Bone Joint Surg 49-B:249–257
5. Cheshire DJE (1969) The stability of the cervical spine following the conservative treatment of fractures and fracture-dislocations. Paraplegia 7:193–203

6. Cloward RB (1961) Treatment of acute fractures and fracture dislocation of cervical spine by vertebral body fusion. J Bone Joint Surg 18:201–209
7. Dourbin FC (1957) Fracture dislocations of the cervical spine. J Bone Joint Surg 39-B:23–38
8. Evans DK (1961) Reduction of cervical dislocation. J Bone Joint Surg 43-B:552–555
9. Evans DK (1976) Anterior cervical subluxation. J Bone Joint Surg 58-B:318–324
10. Herkowitz HN, Rothman RH (1984) Subacute instability of the cervical spine. Spine 9,4:348–357
11. Ramadier JO, Bombarom (1964) Fractures et luxations du rachis cervical sans lésions médullaires. 2me. partie. Rev Chir Orthop 50:3
12. Roaf R (1960) A study of the mechanics of spinal injuries. J Bone Joint Surg 42-B:29–33
13. Roraback CH, Rock MG, Hawkins RS, Bourne RB (1987) Unilateral facet dislocation of the cervical spine. Spine 12,1:23–27
14. Stauffer ES, Kelly EG (1977) Fracture-dislocation of the cervical spine instability and recurrent deformity following treatment by anterior inter-body fusion. J Bone 59,7:45–48
15. White AA, Panjabi MM, Southwick WD (1976) Clinical instability in the lower cervical spine. A review of past and current concepts. Spine 1:15–27

Cervical Spine II
© by Springer-Verlag 1989

1.7. Subluxation of the Lower Cervical Spine: a Challenge for Diagnosis and Treatment

J.M. FUENTES and J. BENEZECH, Montpellier, France

Subluxation of the lower cervical spine (C3–C7) is a challenge for diagnosis and treatment.

In clinical practice the diagnosis of a subluxation is not always obvious and quite often the typical displacements occur with some delay after the trauma (subacute cervical spine instability). We reviewed our clinical material with respect to the various situations and kinds of treatments, and we report 4 main forms of diagnosis and 2 principles of treatment. Circumstances of diagnosis were: *missed diagnosis* (at the early stage), *neglected subluxation* (untreated sprain), *suspected subluxation* (insufficiency of plain lateral X-rays and necessity of further radiologic investigations), and *inadequate treatment* (worsening subluxation by inadequate treatment). In all cases we advocate *surgical treatment* with anterior fusion and osteosynthesis using plates after reduction by external traction in acute subluxation, and double approach in cases of mishapen callus or if reduction doesn't occur after traction.

Clinical Material

Fifteen cases of subluxations are been treated in our institution (Clinique RECH, Montpellier) from January 1985 to June 1988.

The level of the subluxation was: C4–C5: 3 cases, C5–C6: 7 cases, and C6–C7: 5 cases. Anterior approach with interbody fusion (Robinson) and additional anterior osteosynthesis by plate was performed in 9 cases, a combined approach with posterior osteosynthesis and anterior graft in 5 cases, and posterior approach alone in 1 case. The 5 following cases are particularly illustrative.

Summary of 5 Cases

Case 1: Missed diagnosis or hidden sprain.

The first patient was a young radiologist (30 years-old) who after a diving accident complained of cervical pain with numbness in his right thumb. The

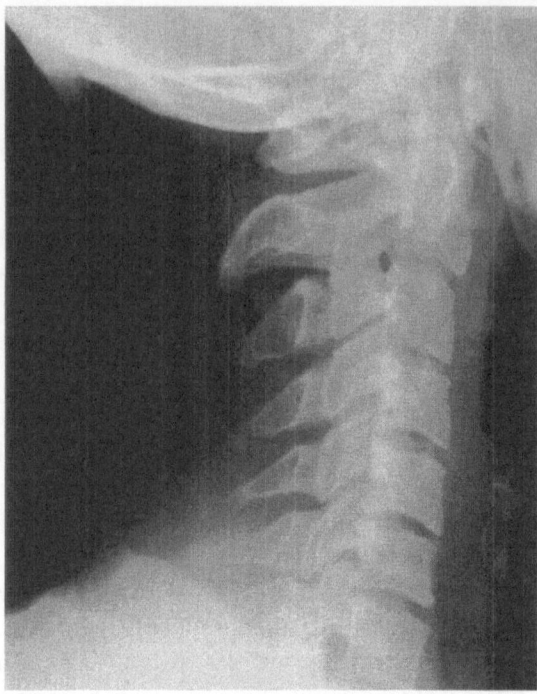

Fig. 1. Case 1. Initial lateral X-ray. The C5–C6 disk was found narrowed. No loss
of the alignment

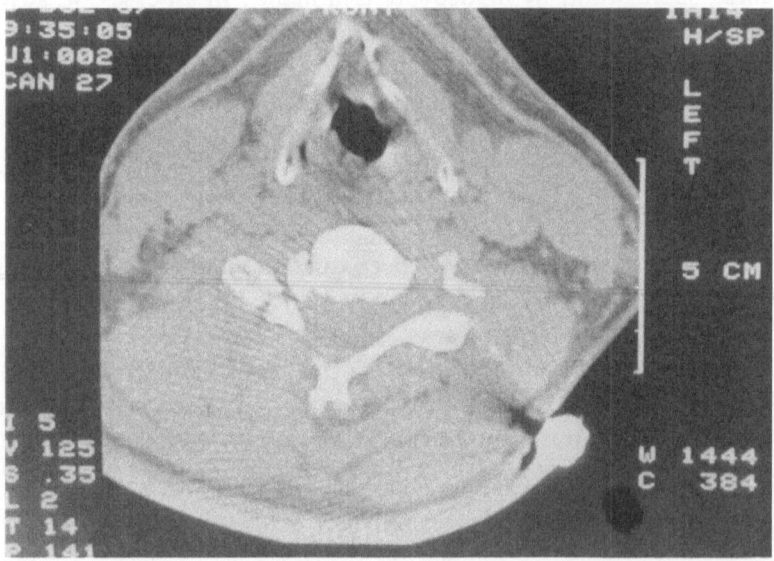

Fig. 2. One day later, a subluxation at the same level was present with forward
displacement of C5 and the CT Scan permitted a correct diagnosis of a severe sprain
by hyperextension mechanism in association with a right articular process fracture
of C6

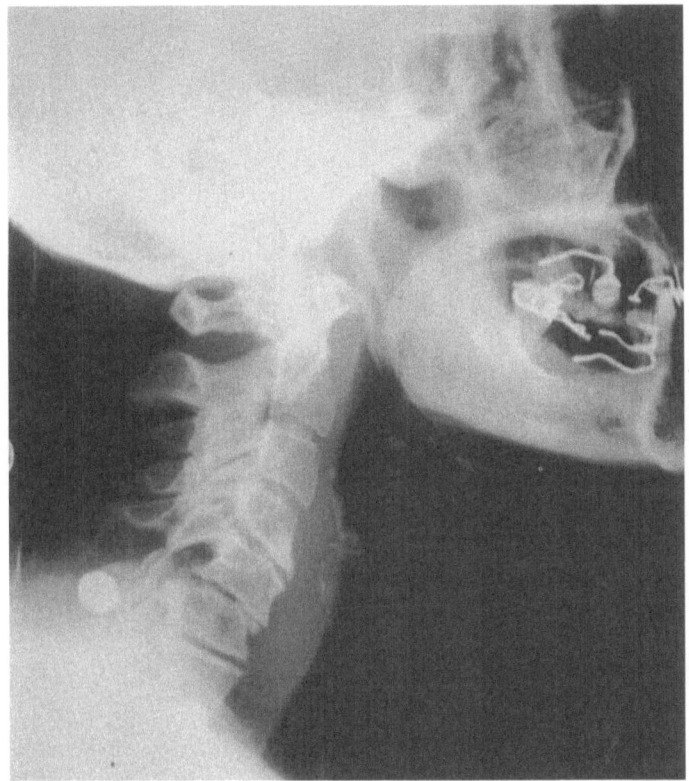

Fig. 3. Case 4. Initial X-ray findings: Subluxation at the C5–C6 level. 1987, July 19th

initial lateral view X-ray indicated a loss of the height at the C5–C6 level (Fig. 1).

On the following day, a CT Scan was done and showed a subluxation at the same level (scout-view) with an articular process fracture of the right C5 posterior pillar by a mechanism of hyperextension (Fig. 2). In this case the first X-ray examination was so-called normal but a second cervical roentgenogram taken a few days later showed an obvious subluxation. It was a delayed subluxation due to subacute cervical spine instability.

Case 2: Worsened and neglected subluxation.

A 25 year old woman received a radiological examination of her cervical spine after a car crash because she had cervical pain and paresthesias in both arms. The initial lateral view demonstrated a slight and forward displacement of C5/C6 less than 2.5 mm. Ten days later the displacement had reached 3 mm and required a surgical stabilization (Fig. 6).

Case 3: Suspected subluxation or subluxation proved by other methods.

Very often the early change after sprain is only a disc-pinch because muscle spasm prevents acute subluxation. In this case, radiological investigation including *dynamic examination,* will demonstrate an obvious instability.

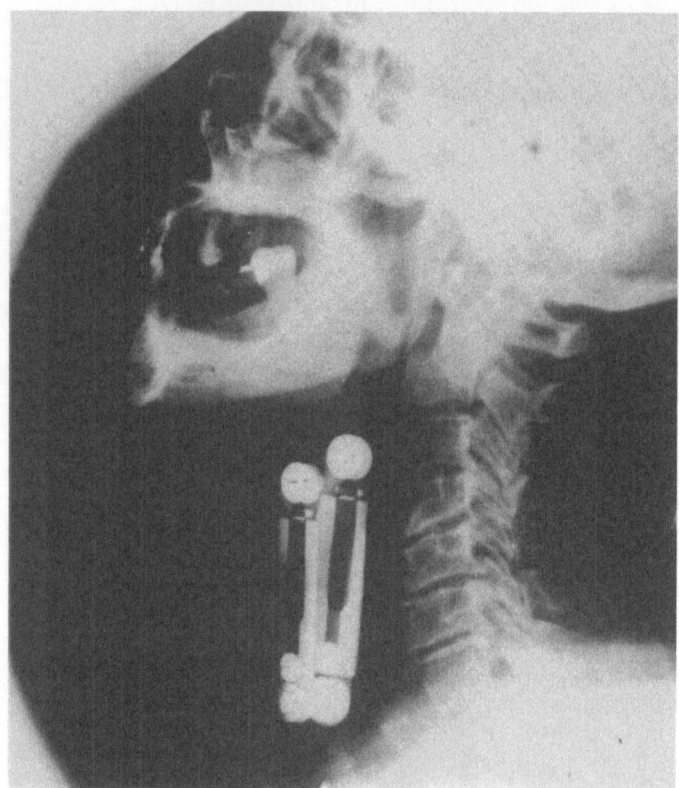

Fig. 4. Good reduction by external immobilization. August 5th

A 65 year old woman complained of cervical pain after falling down-stairs. She received a lateral X-ray which was considered normal. Because of a brachial neuralgia which occurred a few days later a flexion-extension examination was carried out and a sprain injury was discovered.

In some cases the instability of a severe sprain is proved by the X-ray follow up during conservative treatment. The following cases emphasize the necessity of careful attention when conservative treatment is choosen because treatment failure can always occur.

Case 4: Inadequate treatment by external immobilization.

A 60 year old woman presented with subluxation of the lower cervical spine (Fig. 3). With a good result of the closed reduction she was immobilized with a hard-collar for 3 months (Fig. 4). After the removal of the external immobilization, recurrence of the displacement was obvious (Fig. 5).

Case 5: A 22 year old male sustained cervical trauma 6 months prior to presenting to us. No treatment except a hard collar was given in another institution. He was referred to us because he had neck pain and weakness in

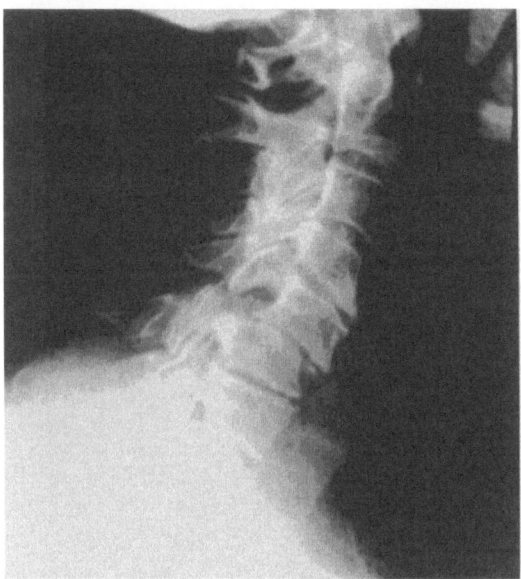

Fig. 5. After removal of the cervical hard collar, recurrence of the displacement. November 8th

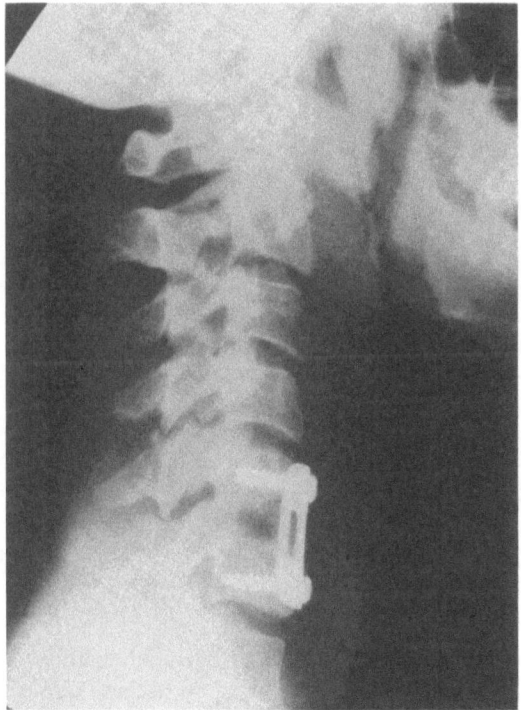

Fig. 6. Case 2. Routine procedure: interbody fusion according to Robinson and anterior osteosynthesis with a plate

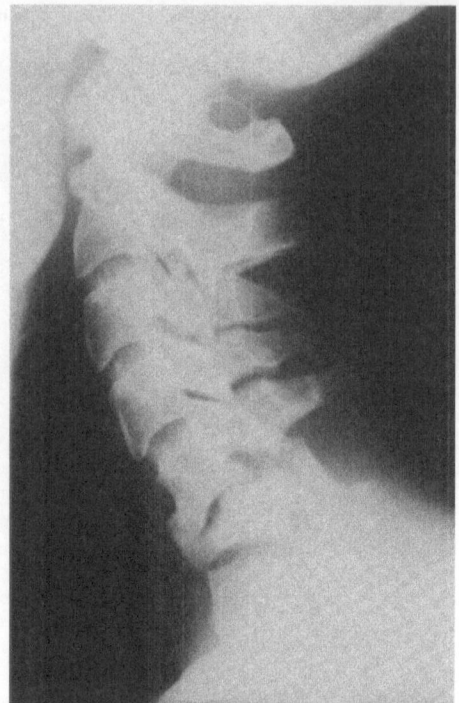

Fig. 7. Case 5. Double approach in old and fixed subluxation. a) Mishapen callus after neglected cervical trauma 6 months prior. b) Because facetectomy for posterior reduction was necessary, articular plate fixation was not feasbile and posterior wiring was done. Anterior iliac crest graft with additional anterior plating was performed in the same operation with an anterior procedure

both arms. A mishapen callus between C5–C6 was present (Fig. 7a) and a combined approach was used for surgical management (Fig. 7b).

Discussion

The term "sprain" is used to describe the tearing of the ligamentous and discal intervertebral joints, by an acute flexion-stress.

A subluxation can also occur by an extension mechanism, like in case 1, when an articular process fracture may be associated. The main anatomical findings are a complete loss of the posterior ligament stabilization complex by tearing of the interspinous ligament, ligamentum flavum and inter-articular joints at the level of the subluxation. Anteriorly, the posterior ligament is commonly ruptured, as well as the posterior part of the disc. The anterior ligament usually remains intact and this fact is the main reason explaining the "missed" sprain: This is because the displacement can reduce by itself like a book closed along its binding [2].

In this situation either correct alignment of the spine is preserved by muscles spasm, or a subluxation exists immediately or subluxation may be delayed up to 3 weeks after the initial trauma (subacute instability). According to White and Panjabi [4], the diagnosis of sprain is accurate, when all these following signs are present:

1) the forward displacement of a vertebra at least 3.5 mm in front of the lower cervical vertebra.
2) an angle of local kyphosis of 11° at the level of the subluxation.
3) a posterior articular process overlapping less than 50% (according to Roy-Camille [3] and Louis [1].

But often these signs are missing in the first X-ray examination because:

1) muscle spasm hides the sprain, 2) X-ray examination is performed in the supine position and in this situation the intact anterior ligament permits a good reduction in extension of the displacement producing a good realignment of the vertebral body. *Flexion-extension dynamic X-ray* under the control of the physician is necessary but more often a correct diagnosis is made by repeat X-ray investigation within 1 month following the injury [2]. *CT-Scan (high resolution scanner)* with, if necessary, small doses of metrizamide introduced by C1–C2 puncture to define intraspinal structures may be an alternative to search for disc herniation or associate bony fractures. CT also avoids excessive cervical manipulation. From a surgical point of view a posterior approach with osteosynthesis can reduce the subluxation (osteosynthesis by plates or wiring osteosynthesis with interspinous bony graft or acrylic) when no fracture of the vertebral body exists or if there is no fragment within the anterior portion of the canal [3]. But in our experience, the posterior osteosynthesis can fail. In our practice we preferred an anterior

approach in the 9 last cases after reduction had been obtained by external traction. A total discectomy using the operative microscope and Gardner-Wells traction is performed. An interbody fusion according to Robinson, with iliac bone graft is done with an additional anterior osteosynthesis (Fig. 6).

Postoperatively, immobilization by a collar is kept for 3 months. When a patient presents with an old displacement with a mishapen callus, or when reduction is not feasible by cervical traction, a combined antero-posterior approach is performed because reduction cannot occur with a single anterior procedure done (Fig. 7a and b).

References

1. Louis R (1987) Stability and instability of the cervical spine. In: Kehr P, Weidner A (eds) Cervical spine I. Springer, Wien New York, pp 21–27
2. Rifkinson-Mann St, Mormino J, Sachdeo VP (1986) Subacute cervical spine instability. Surg Neurol 26:413–416
3. Roy-Camille R, Saillant G, Berteaux D, Lortat-Jacob A, Bisserie M (1977) Entorse grave par lésion traumatique du segment mobile rachidien (S.M.R.) de la colonne cervicale. J Chir 113:121–130
4. White A, Panjabi M (1978) Clinical biomechanics of the spine. JB Lippincott Company, Philadelphia, USA

1.8. Unusual Evolution of Bone Graft in Misdiagnosed C7 Fracture: Case Report

F. BENAZZO, P. CHERUBINO, and C. CASTELLI, Pavia, Italy

Case Report

D.A., a 46 year old male, was involved in a motor vehicle accident in October, 1986, during which he reported a hyperflexion injury of the cervical spine. The patient immediately began complaining of persistent neck pain, and after several weeks left arm pain and paraesthesia of the 4th and 5th fingers of the left hand appeared, and he consulted a doctor. The first x-rays taken in January 1987 were considered negative, although in retrospect, an initial alteration of the body of C7 was quite evident (Fig. 1). Because of persistent pain, a second set was taken in February 87, which showed a crushed and deformed vertebral body at C7 (Fig. 2). A minerva cast was applied for 4 months, but despite this a definite lower limb spastic paralysis appeared. CT scan, performed on May 87 showed no extrinsic medullary compression, but the body of C7 looked like an empty bony shell interrupted anteriorly and posteriorly. 4 months had elapsed since the crushed vertebra was diagnosed. The patient was admitted to our Clinic in June 1987. Initial physical examination revealed obvious signs of medullary and radicular compression. Myelography was performed and showed complete interruption of the dye column at the inferior border of C7. That night the neurologic picture suddenly worsened and the patient became quadriplegic. An emergency operation was performed with decompressive somatectomy of C7 by an anterior approach, and arthrodesis of C6–T1 using a tricortical cancellous graft taken from the iliac crest [1]. The body of C7 had almost disappeared, reduced to a shell of cortical bone which contained a soft encephaloid substance. The curved posterior wall had caused the compression of the spinal cord.

The histological diagnosis of the encephaloid tissue was: "cartilagineous and discal tissue with nonspecific degenerative phenomena. No neoplastic lesion".

The patient was placed in a halo-vest and his neurological conditions improved rapidly. Within a week he recovered full sphincteric control and

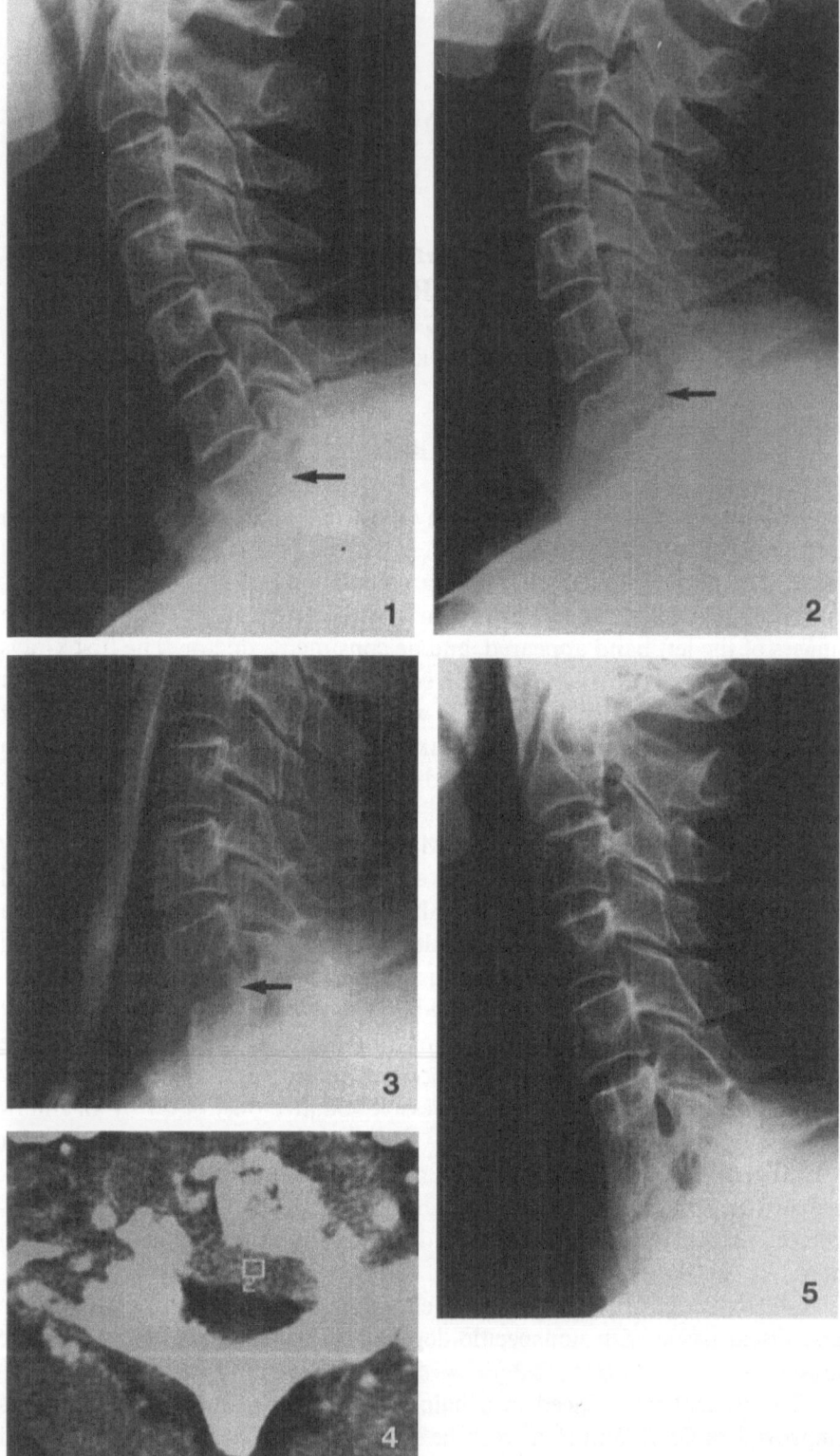

upper and lower limb strength, with a complete neurological recovery. The patient was then released with the halo-vest, and followed monthly in our out-patient clinic.

Two months after surgery x-rays showed fusion between the lower part of the graft and the body of T1, while in the upper part an almost complete reabsorption was evident. The osteolysis was accompanied by proliferation of osseous tissue which formed an anterior wall separated from the vertebral bodies (Fig. 3). CT scan at this time showed extensive lysis of the graft with invasion of the anterior paravertebral muscles by newly formed tissue. The latter had a homogeneous aspect and the injection of intravenous dye showed a clear uptake (Fig. 4). A series of tests were performed to reveal a possible neoplastic nature of the tissue: bone scan (which showed an intense uptake at the lower cervical level); C.T. scan of abdomen and chest; sonograms of abdomen and thyroid gland. All proved negative.

The patient's clinical condition remained excellent during this time, without any sign of further medullary compression.

In October 1987 a new operation was performed, in order to biopsy the tissue, and eventually to stabilize the spine. The lower portion of the graft was well consolidated but the upper part had been completely reabsorbed. Behind a very thin shell of cortical bone there was a soft, greyish, encephaloid tissue similar to that found during the first operation but more abundant. There was no pathological material in or among the prevertebral or scalene muscles as had been shown by CT. The soft tissue was completely removed, and a new tricortical cancellous graft was taken from the iliac wing and solidly inserted in the gap. An intraoperative histological examination found that the material was composed of "fibro connective tissue with rich lymphocyte infiltration". It was not possible however to determine whether this was due to a chronic inflammatory process or to a lymphoproliferative disease. Subsequent histological examination however excluded a lymphoid tumor. After

Fig. 1. The alteration of the body of C7 was difficult to assess, at the time of the first X-ray examination

Fig. 2. One month later, C7 appeared crushed and deformed

Fig. 3. The upper part of the graft was almost completely reabsorbed two months after surgery

Fig. 4. CT scan showed the lysis of the graft and the invasion of the muscles by the well vascularized, newly formed tissue

Fig. 5. Fusion of the new graft, after the second operation

4 months the graft was completely fused, and the lower cervical spine was stable (Fig. 5). The patient's neurological and clinical condition were excellent.

Discussion

There are several aspects of this clinical case which can be discussed: 1) the time which elapsed between the trauma and the appearance of the lesion of C7; 2) the type of lesion, that is a progressive collapse of the vertebral body with secondary medullary compression; 3) the osteolysis of the upper portion of the graft with fusion of the lower third and the appearance of newly formed bony wall.

We can hypothesize that the cervical spine sprain had no pathogenetic relationship with the subsequent clinical story. In other words, that the collapse of the body was ongoing, due to another cause, and that its evolution was accelerated by the trauma. The large number of lymphocytes found in the newly formed tissue at the time of the second operation could have been the expression of a lymphoma of low malignancy. However, no other signs of lymphoma (or of other tumors), were present in other organs or in the peripheral blood.

Secondly, and more probably, there could have been an initial misdiagnosed crush fracture of the vertebral body of C7 since the first X-ray were taken two months later.

As a matter of fact, the tissue removed from the body of C7 during the first operation showed necrotic bony trabeculae and degenerated discal tissue without any sign of infection or tumor. We can hypothesize that the disk material may have penetrated into the body of C7, creating a local disturbance in the repair phenomena inducing a focus of chronic aseptic inflammation with associated lymphocyte infiltration and newly formed inflammatory tissue which could have caused bone reabsorption. This phenomenon can be observed in an aseptic inflammatory process of bone. The fact that no tumor-like infiltration was found despite the CT image favors the possibility of an aspecific inflammatory process, whose surgical removal was sufficient to stop bone reabsorption and induce formation of new bone and transplant fusion.

Reference

1. Boni M, Cherubino P, Denaro V, Benazzo F (1984) Multiple subtotal somatectomy: technique and evaluation of a series of 39 cases. Spine 9,4:358–362

Cervical Spine II
© by Springer-Verlag 1989

1.9. Cervical Spine Injuries: Radiographic Evaluation

CH. R. CLARK, C. M. IGRAM, G. Y. EL-KHOURY, and SH. EHARA, Iowa City, Iowa, U.S.A.

Radiographic evaluation of a cervical spine injury can be problematic. It often may be difficult to visualize an injury on the initial emergency room radiograph. This is particularly true at the occipito-cervical and cervical-thoracic junctions where there is a great deal of overlap of structures. In addition, certain fractures, particularly those involving the posterior elements, may be difficult to visualize on plain films. Severe osteopenia may be problematic. The *extent* of the injury may be difficult to determine on the initial radiograph. The plain film may give a *clue* to the diagnosis but additional studies are necessary to *delineate* the injury in its entirety.

Certainly the most serious problem is the failure to make the diagnosis. A high index of suspicion is the key to proper diagnosis.

The purpose of this study was to evaluate the patterns of cervical injury in a large series of patients in order to determine a rational approach to further diagnostic workup. Our goals therefore, are to provide accurate diagnosis, eliminate redundant radiographic studies and be cost effective in the process.

There has been a moderate amount of work published in the radiographic and trauma literature. Doris [4] determined that the Five View series, that is the AP, open mouth odontoid, lateral and both obliques, was the gold standard for evaluation of the cervical spine. Bachulis [2] felt that if the patient was alert, neurologically intact, and complained of no neck pain, cervical x-rays were not indicated. We certainly do question this recommendation. Bachulis [2] preferred the CT scan for further evaluation.

Harris [5] reviewed a large series and favored the CT scan as the advanced radiographic procedure of choice. He felt that the tomogram was not useful in facet dislocations and dens fractures. Interestingly, our study determined that polytomography was very helpful in both of these injuries.

This manuscript is a condensation of a paper which was recently published [3].

Materials and Methods

Our study involved a follow-up of 227 patients with cervical spine injuries between 1978 and March 1986 at the University of Iowa Hospitals and Clinics. We encountered multiple common fractures and dislocations including: dens fractures, Jefferson fractures, hangman fractures, burst and compression fractures, unilateral/bilateral facet fractures and/or dislocations, laminar fractures, pedicle fractures, occipito-atlantal dislocations, and atlantoaxial rotatory dislocations.

In order to evaluate this group of patients, we further divided our study population into three groups. Patients in group I were those who had plain radiographs which were *sufficient* to make the diagnosis. Patients were placed in group II if additional studies changed either the *extent* of the injury or the *type* of the injury. Patients in group III were those who had initial radiographs interpreted as normal. The diagnosis was only made on subsequent radiographic workup.

An example of a group I injury is one in which the plain films were sufficient to make the entire diagnosis. A common example of a group I injury is a compression fracture of a vertebral body which is well seen on the AP lateral and oblique views. A group II injury is one in which the plain radiographs suggest the injury but additional studies were necessary to fully evaluate the injury. An example of this would be evidence of anterior-posterior subluxation on a lateral radiograph which required tomography to clearly point out whether indeed a dislocation of a facet existed as well as the possibility of an associated fracture. A group III injury is one in which the plain radiographs are initially normal. A good example of this is a dens fracture in which the plain x-rays were interpreted as normal. AP and lateral tomograms are required to make the diagnosis.

Results

This monograph summarizes our findings which are discussed in more detail in our recently published paper [3]. There were 50 patients who sustained 51 dens fractures. Out of this group 27 were Anderson and D'Alonzo [1] type II and 21 were type III. A large percentage of patients with dens fractures fell into group II. That is, additional studies changed the extent or type of the injury. We found tomography to be the most helpful advanced radiographic study. Not only does it determine the fracture type which is very important when planning the therapeutic approach to the patient, but it rules out additional associated fractures. In this group, we found that the CT scan provided less information.

Facet fractures comprised the largest single fracture type in our study. There were 63 patients who sustained 70 injuries. A significant finding in this group of patients was that 10 patients had a delay in diagnosis averaging 11 days. Neurological deficits included four patients with cord injuries and nine patients with root deficits. In addition, there were 24 associated cervical fractures. Once again the majority of patients were in group II. Of this group, additional information was provided by tomography in 28 patients and by CT scan in nine. Overall, we found tomography to be most useful.

We encountered 20 patients with hangman's fractures. Seven of these patients had associated teardrop fractures. We found that, in general, plain films were sufficient to make the diagnosis.

There were many different types of vertebral body fractures encountered in our study. Twenty-six had burst fractures, 25 compression fractures, and 31 had teardrop fractures. Additional studies were helpful. We found the CT scan and tomography both useful to differentiate the type of injury, that is distinguishing between a burst fracture and a compression fracture, and also to determine the presence and/or extent of bony fragments in the vertebral canal.

Fifty-one patients sustained posterior element fractures including fractures of the transverse processes, laminar fractures, posterior spinous process fractures and pedicle fractures. In this group, additional studies were required to determine the extent of the injury and most importantly the associated injuries. We found that CT scan and tomogram were each helpful. We also found a high incidence of associated fractures in this group of patients.

Jefferson fractures can be diagnosed on plain films but the CT scan is most helpful to determine the extent of the injury.

We found 34 patients with facet dislocations. Approximately ⅔ were unilateral and ⅓ bilateral. In our series none were missed initially. Associated fractures were common and we found additional radiographic studies to be helpful with unilateral dislocations but we found the plain films to be sufficient with bilateral dislocations. The tomogram provided the most additional information in this series of patients.

Neurological deficits were most common in bilateral facet dislocations with 3 out of 11 patients having a cord injury and 6 out of 11 having root involvement.

Occipito-atlantal dislocations comprised a small group. Two patients had this injury and the plain films were sufficient. Both of these patients died early on after their injuries.

We found the CT scan useful in quantitating the degree of atlantoaxial rotatory dislocation. It was very important however, to orient the cuts of the scan in the plane of the ring of C1.

Summary and Conclusions

Plain radiographs are the primary studies when approaching a patient with a cervical spine injury. They must be carefully scrutinized by the treating physician. All seven vertebral bodies must be seen. The key to diagnosis is the suspicion of a cervical spine fracture/dislocation. Secondly, we found polytomography to be particularly advantageous in patients with facet injuries and dens fractures.

The CT scan is particularly advantageous in patients with Jefferson fractures, atlantoaxial rotatory dislocations, posterior element injuries, and body fractures.

In summary, efficient radiographic diagnosis is the key to safe and timely patient care.

References

1. Anderson LD, D'Alonzo RT (1974) Fractures of the odontoid process of the axis. J Bone Joint Surg 56A:1663–1674
2. Bachulis BL *et al.* (1987) Clinical indications for cervical spine radiographs in the traumatized patient. Am J Surg 153:473–478
3. Clark CR, Igram CM, El-Khoury GY, Ehara E (1988): Radiographic evaluation of cervical spine injuries. Spine 13:742–747
4. Doris PE, Wilson RA (1985) The next logical step in the emergency radiographic evaluation of cervical trauma: The five view trauma series. Radiology 3:371–385
5. Harris JH (1986) Radiographic evaluation of spinal trauma. Ortho Clin North Am 17:75–86

Cervical Spine II
© by Springer-Verlag 1989

1.10. Motion-segment Changes Following Fusions of Traumatic Instabilities in the Lower Cervical Spine

M. Mähring and R. Szyszkowitz, Graz, Austria

Although there are more and more papers on operative fusion for traumatic instabilities in the lower cervical spine, there is no real answer about the effects on the non-fused motion-segments.

We know from radiologists and neurosurgeons about rapid degeneration and sometimes hypermobility in adjacent motion-segments after fusions for spondylosis. We therefore investigated to determine, if these changes also occur after posttraumatic cervical spine fusions.

Since March 1977 we have performed 140 fusions in the lower cervical spine without or with neurologic deficit of all grades. In 1986 we reviewed 60 patients [1], the follow-up period ranged between 8 and 1 year with an average of 3.9 years postoperative; the mean age was 33 years. Most of the fusions reported here were performed from the front, using cortico-cancellous bone grafts from the iliac crest and H-plates for fixation.

45 patients had one-level fusions and 11 had two-level fusions. 4 patients were excluded from this study: one had a deep infection, and the X-rays from 3 patients were not adequate for our purpose.

Most fusions were carried out in C5/6 and C6/7 which are the most mobile segments.

All patients underwent a clinical and radiological examination, total range of spinal motion was recorded, radiologic disc appearance and spondylophyte formation were also classified. Assessment of motion-segment function was made according to the method of Penning [3].

Because of the differences in physiologic segment motion we introduced the term of "relative function" by considering the mean value of each motion-segment function to be 100% of function. So it became possible to compare all motion-segment functions despite their different motion.

Since operative damage or increased stresses had to be expected in the segments next to fusions, they were separated from the non-adjacent ones.

We analyzed 235 non fused motion-segments, 101 of them were adjacent to fusions and 134 were non-adjacent.

169 out of 235, which is 72%, were found to be normal (Fig. 1). But looking to the segments above and below fusions, only 48% had normal radiological appearance. Relative function was reduced to 74%.

The most striking findings were nose-like and bridging spondylophytes in the anterior aspect of adjacent segments, in previous normal motion-segments. We consider these spondylophyte formations to be the reaction to an intraoperative stripping of the anterior longitudinal ligament in adjacent segments, and the use of excessively long plates (Fig. 2). The disces remain normal and function even after years of impaired motion. In two cases a bridge broke after 2 and 3 years resulting in improved function; even here the disces remained quite normal, an important difference to deforming spondylosis [4].

Noses and bridges were exclusively found next to fusions (Table 1). That there was still some function even in bridges may be due to the fact that they are anchored only to one side of the fusion, possibly a positive effect of early functional treatment.

Spondylosis was only found in 20 adjacent motion-segments of which 10 were unchanged compared to the initial X-rays. Relative function was significantly decreased (mean age in this group was 51 years). There were only 5 increased and 8 unchanged degenerations in the non-adjacent segments, which is the normal finding in this age group [2] and in this usually multisegmental disease.

Table 1. *Radiological Findings in Motion-segments of 56 Patients Above, Below and Non Adjacent to Fusions*

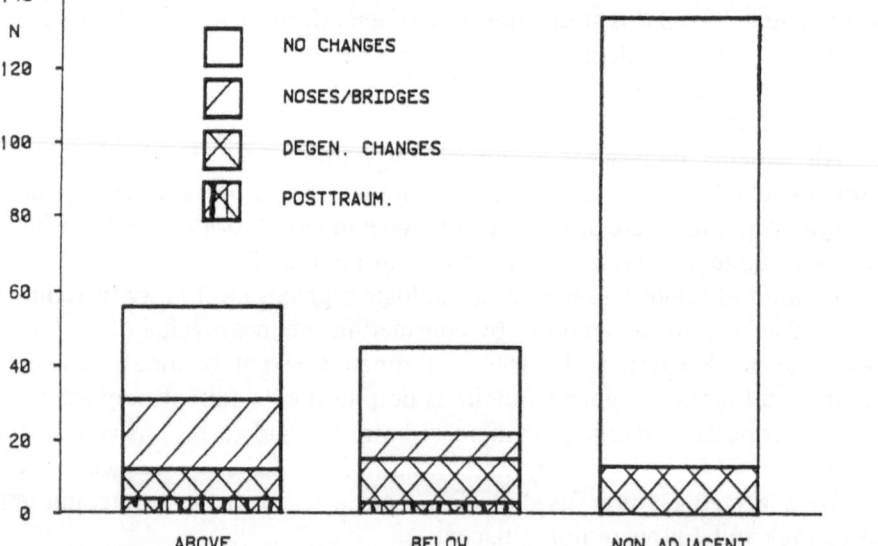

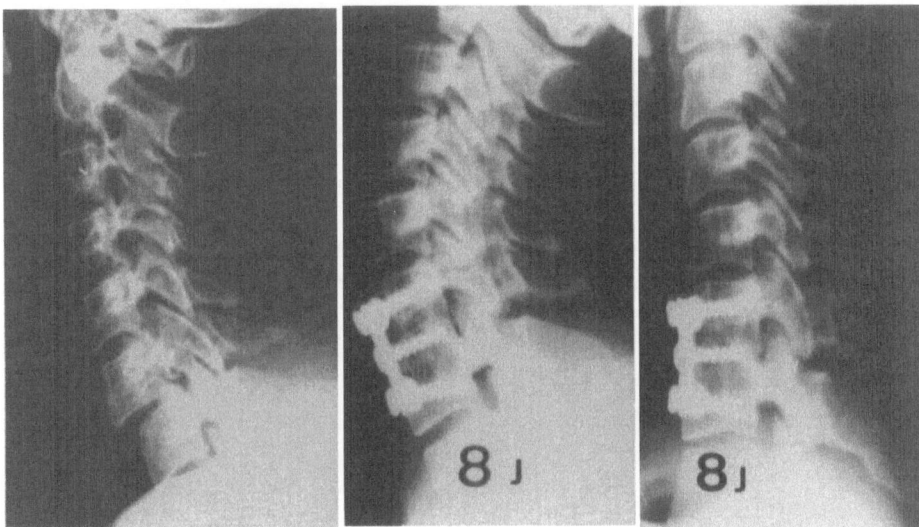

Fig. 1. 35 year old female: 8 years after fusion the adjacent motion-segments are free
from degenerative changes with good function

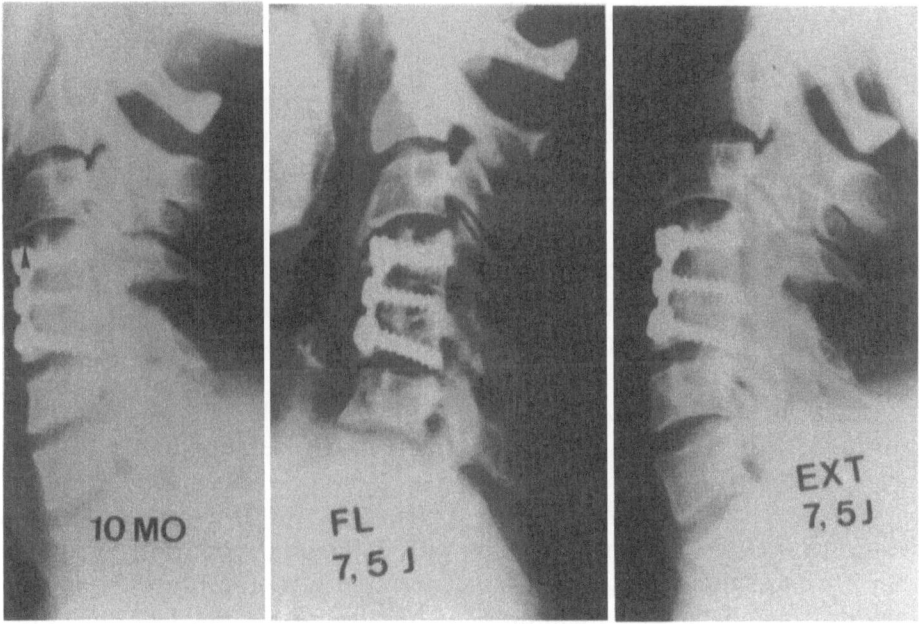

Fig. 2. 28 year old female: nose-like spondylophyte above fusion due to an excessively
long plate; normal disc, good motion

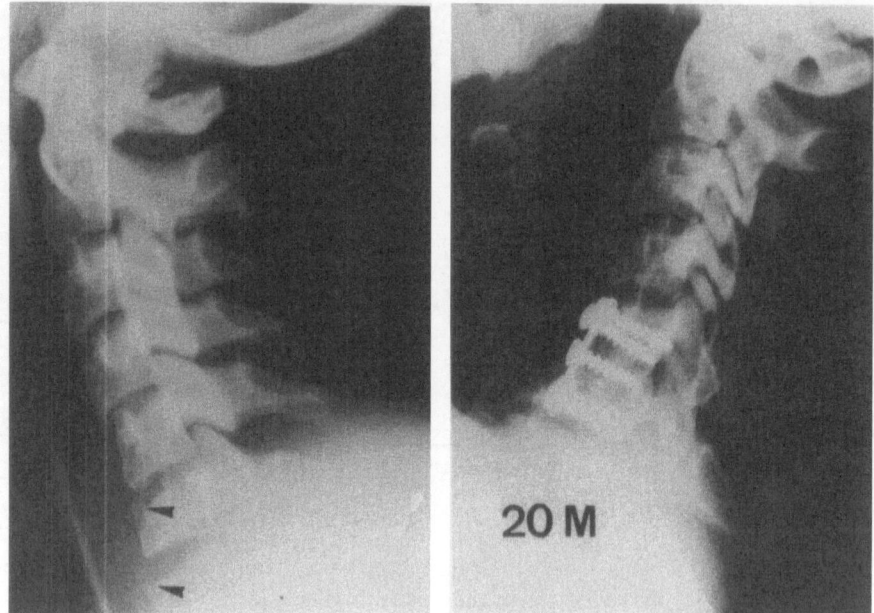

Fig. 3. 40 year old male: 20 months after fusion of C5/6 with rapid degeneration in C6/7 including the disc due to an unrecognized injury also in C6/7

In 7 cases rapid development of degenerative change was attributed to previously undetected additional trauma to a normal motion-segment. This was followed by rapid degeneration including the disces (Fig. 3), resulting in significant loss of function.

Hypermobility could not be found in any case. The maximum motion found in three cases at C6/7 was 142%, which is still normal.

Healthy motion-segments, as usually found in trauma patients, compensate in the neighborhood of the fusions in contrast to fusions for degenerative spondylosis.

An analysis of radiological findings and function clearly showed the bad functional effect of spondylophyte formation, degeneration and posttraumatic reactions.

Cervical fusions for trauma carry a higher risk for the adjacent motion-segments, but lower than in patients with deforming spondylosis. Careful operative technique can offer a distinct decrease in postoperative spondylophyte formation; special attention must be payed to restrict detachment of the anterior longitudinal ligament to the injured disc, which is best achieved by fenestration and by avoiding the use of excessively long plates.

It took mother nature quite long time to develop our highly specialized spine, and we are obliged to preserve as much function as possible by careful operative technique.

References

1. Mähring M (1988) Segmentveränderungen der Halswirbelsäule nach cervikalen Spondylodesen instabiler Verletzungen. Unfallchir (In press)
2. Nathan H (1962) Osteophytes of the vertebral column. J Bone Joint Surg 44A:243–286
3. Penning L (1978) Normal movements of the cervical spine. Am J Roentgen 130:317–326
4. Schmorl G, Junghanns H (1957) Die gesunde und die kranke Wirbelsäule in Röntgenbild und Klinik. Thieme, Stuttgart

1.11. Management of the Cervical Spine Injury in Surabaya (Report of 75 Cases)

B. Prijambodo, C. Abdurrahman, and T. Sunartomo,
Surabaya, Indonesia

Introduction

Cervical spine fracture, dislocation or fracture dislocation is found more and more often with the increase of accidents or occupational accidents. Although trauma of the vertebra is associated in 80% without neurologic deficit, in cervical trauma it is not uncommon to find spinal cord injuries. In my series, 45 cases (60%) among 75 cervical injuries were associated with spinal cord injury.

There are two goals of cervical injury management [7]. The first goal is achieving a painless stable vertebra and the second is the prevention of the complication of spinal cord injury. So, knowledge about pathological anatomy of vertebral fracture, ligamentous disruption or dislocation is required to determine rational management. All treatment measures are directed toward obtaining maximal benefit for the patient with a minimal associated risk.

Spine Instability [1, 2, 4, 5]

Spinal instability has been characterized by some authors based on the 2 column concepts of Holdsworth and the 3 column concepts of Louis (one anterior and two posterior) and of Denis (anterior, medial and posterior).

According to Louis, vertebral stability is based on 3 vertical columns; specifically, one anterior column and two posterior columns. Each column contributes 1 point to stability. Instability is defined by injury to two or more columns, producing a coefficient of instability of ≥ 2.

In the author's clinic, this theory is very helpful to determine the surgical approach. Anterior, posterior or a combined approach is used depending on which column is injured.

There Are Two Instabilities:

1. Temporary Instability

In general a lesion of the vertebrae classified in this category, is treated by orthopaedic or conservative methods, for example by a minerva jacket.

However, there are several exceptions like burst type fractures with narrowing of the medullary canal because displacement of the vertebral body fragment may require anterior decompression even if the coefficient of instability is 1. Another example is a vertical fracture.

2. Permanent Instability

When a lesion occurs through the disc or if there is any ligamentous disruption, recovery is always poor because of inadequate healing of the fibrous tissue. So there will be a risk of "late secondary displacement". For example, this is true for bilateral facet dislocation and tear drop fracture. In these cases the author believes that stabilization is absolutely necessary to prevent secondary displacement.

Diagnosis

Important in the treatment of cervical injury is taking care of the patient when he arrives. In the author's clinic all patients who are diagnosed with possible cervical injury are treated as if cervical injury is present until it can be ruled out.

In the suspicious cervical injury, in which AP and lateral X-rays are normal, due to autoreposition or spontaneous reduction post trauma, we carry out dynamic X-ray with flexion and extension in lateral projection. The image intensifier is very useful here to avoid overdistraction or overcorrection.

Several authors use a stress test which is gradual application of about 30–40 pounds of cervical traction and direct visualization on lateral radiography. Then we can test the stability of the segment that was suspicious. This test is especially useful for late instability [7].

In the dynamic X-rays instability exists when vertebral body displacement is more than 3.5 mm, facet joint displacement is more than 50%, or angulation between vertebrae is more than 11° [2, 4, 5].

These criteria are for the lower cervical spine. In the case of a burst fracture the role of tomography (CT scan) is to find out if there is any compression from anterior or posterior causing narrowing of the medullary canal.

General Management

Operative Indication

In the author's clinic, operative indications of cervical injury are:
1. Instability
2. Narrowing of the medullary canal
3. Neurologic deficit (progressive)

In the patient with a neurologic deficit which is complete or incomplete and with a stability problem or narrowing canal, the author carried out operative decompression and stabilization.

Anatomical reposition of the cervical dislocation means we had performed a decompression because by doing this we recreated the diameter of the medullary canal. So in each dislocation or fracture-dislocation we perform a closed manipulation without general anesthesia and with control by image intensifier. If the dislocation is reduced we perform stabilization as the second phase. When it can not be reduced due to facet locking we carry out an emergency operation.

The surgical techniques of the anterior, posterior or a combined approach (anterior and posterior) will depend on which column has been damaged. For example, in the case of a burst fracture, we perform anterior decompression, bone graft and anterior plating. Whereas, in fracture-dislocation cases we carried out anterior and posterior fusion.

We never carry out laminectomy because we are sure that laminectomy decompression will result in instability of the spine.

The patient with temporary instability is treated conservatively by minerva jacket or cervicothoracic brace.

Serious attention is required for cervical injury cases with neurologic deficits (tetraplegia). These cases need a multidisciplinary approach because in addition to the spine injury there are related problems of the cardiovascular system, respiratory system, g.i. system, skin, and associated psychological problems.

The main purpose of stabilization in complete tetraplegia is early mobilization and facilitation of treatment. In summary, the goal of medical treatment is a stable and painless spine. The second goal is the prevention of or continued injury to the spinal cord.

Surgical Techniques of Reduction, Stabilization and Fusion

Anterior Fusion [3, 7]

Anterior fusion is indicated for comminuted anterior vertebral fractures without posterior ligamentous instability. The anterior aspect of the mid and lower cervical spine is approached through a transverse or longitudinal incision of the left anterolateral aspect of the neck.

The left-sided approach offers better exposure and visualization of the lower vertebra (C4–5–6–7) and is less likely to damage the recurrent larynged nerve in the lower cervical spine. The incision is made in the skin and platysma muscle, exposing the mid cervical fascia layer. Mid cervical fascia is incised along the border of the anterior aspect of M. Sternocleidomastoideus and then the muscle is retracted laterally by blunt dissection.

The space between the retracted carotid sheath laterally and the strap muscle, trachea and oesophagus medially is developed down to the prevertebra tissue fascia plane. The prominent portion of the anterior spine are intervertebral discs and the depressed areas identify the vertebral body.

Identification of the vertebral level is confirmed by placing a needle in the disc and obtaining a lateral radiograph or using the image intensifier. The disc above and below the vertebral fracture should be removed. When most of the disc has been removed, the comminuted vertebral body is removed with the rongeur. The posterior part of the body is removed with curets. Bone should not be removed to far laterally otherwise the vertebral artery may be injured. When all comminuted fragments and disc material have been removed, the central portion of the inferior cervical endplate of the vertebra above and the superior endplate of the vertebra below the fracture level should be decorticated. Angle curets should be used for decortication. An iliac crest graft is used; the graft should be shaped to fit into the defect. The graft plug is gently introduced into the defect while traction is increased on the skull tongs temporarily. After the graft is seated in the proper position cervical traction is released. The head is then brought from its slight extension into a slight flexion position and the graft becomes locked. Routinely we use a plate and screws to fix it.

Postoperatively we used a suction drain for 24–48 hours and the neck is immobilized with a cervical collar brace.

A radiographic control check of the position of the graft, plate and screws is made before closing the wound. The day after surgery the drain is removed. The collar brace is used for a 8–12 week period.

Posterior Fusion

Posterior fusion operation is most commonly performed for facet fracture, dislocation, looked facets, posterior ligamentous disruption or subluxation instability. When performing the posterior approach, I prefer to operate with the patient's head stabilized by tong traction. This provides more control of the cervical spine and is very helpful during reposition. A midline incision is made in the muscle insertion into the bifid spinosus processus of

C3, 4, 5, 6 and then the elevator, which has a sharp edge, is used to elevate
the spine's extensor muscles from the lamina, out to the lateral aspect of the
facet joint.

I prefer many different techniques for posterior fusion:
– Sublaminar wiring with H graft
– Modified segmental spinal instrumentation with K-nail
– Plate and screw fixation

Material (see Tables 1–6)

The author took care of 75 cervical injury cases from 1982 to 1987 in
which 56% (42 cases) were operated. 17.3% were female and 82.7% were
male. The youngest was 15 years old and oldest was 55 years old; 49% were
between 25–35 years old. The majority of the patients had a neurologic
deficit, 61.3% (46 cases) with both complete tetraplegia (34.6%) and incomplete neurologic deficit (26.6%); (Table 2).

Table 1. *Incidence and Sex Distribution. Cervical Injury in Surabaya 1982–1987*
(75 cases)

Year	Male	Female	Total
1982	10	2	12
1983	2	–	2
1984	8	–	8
1985	10	2	12
1986	18	6	24
1987	14	3	17
Total	62	13	75

Table 2. *Cervical Injuries in Surabaya (1982–1987)*

Root compression	1
Paraparesis superior paraplegia inferior	5
Tetraparesis	14
Tetraplegia	26
No neurologic deficit	29
Total	75

Table 3. *Surgical Procedure for Cervical Injuries (42 Cases) 1982–1987*

Year	Anterior fusion	Posterior fusion	Ant + post fusion
1982	7	–	–
1983	2	–	–
1984	2	1	1
1985	2	3	1
1986	5	5	3
1987	3	3	4
	21 (50%)	12 (28,5%)	9 (21,5%)

Table 4. *Orthopaedic Treatment 1982–1987*

Year	Glisson traction	Cruthfield traction	Collar brace	Minerva jacket
1982	2	–	3	–
1983	–	1	–	–
1984	1	2	–	–
1985	1	2	3	–
1986	2	1	5	4
1987	1	1	5	1
	7	7	16	5

From 75 cervical injury cases, 42 cases (56%) required reduction and several techniques. Anterior fusion or anterior osteosynthesis were performed in 21 cases (50%), posterior fusion in 12 cases (28.5%), anterior and posterior fusion/osteosynthesis in 9 cases (21.5%) as shown in Table 3.

The rest of the injuries were managed conservatively with cervical traction, immobilization with collar brace, or minerva jacket.

Results

The comparison of the operative and conservative treatment is shown on Tables 5 and 6. The average follow up was 12 months with the longest at 4 years.

Of the 42 cases that were operated 31 cases (74%) had neurologic deficit and of these 52% demonstrated recovery. The mortality rate was 29% (9

Table 5. *Surgical Procedure of Cervical Injury (with Neurologic Deficit) (31 Cases)*

	Permanent	Recovery	Death	Unknown
Paraparesis sup. Paraplegia inf.	–	3	–	1
Tetraparesis	–	11	–	–
Tetraplegia	1	2	9	4
	1 (3%)	16 (52%)	9 (29%)	5 (16%)

Table 6. *Orthopaedic Treatment of Cervical Injury (with Neurologic Deficit) (15 cases)*

	Permanent	Recovery	Death	Unknown
Root compression	1	–	–	–
Paraparesis sup. Paraplegia inf.	–	–	–	1
Tetraparesis	–	1	1	1
Tetraplegia	–	–	7	3
	1 (6.6%)	1 (6.6%)	8 (53%)	5 (33%)

cases). In the conservatively managed group the mortality rate was high at 53% and the recovery rate was low at 6.6%.

The cause of the death was usually due to complications of respiratory tract infection, urogenital tract infection and one patient expired because of bleeding from prolonged respirator tracheostomy.

The longest ventilator requirement was 16 weeks.

Conclusion

In my series operative treatment gave better results compared to conservative treatment, especially in cases with neurologic deficit. In many cases, I modified the osteosynthesis of the posterior cervical spine with sublaminar wiring with H-graft or segmental spinal instrumentation with Küntscher nail. These methods were much cheaper and therefore advantagous in my country because of economic reasons. However, the biomechanical results are also very acceptable in our series with Küntscher nail (375 cases of spinal trauma) [5].

References

1. Denis F (1984) Spinal instability as defined by three column concept in acute spinal trauma. Clin Orthop 189:65–76
2. Louis R (1977) Symposium sur les fractures instables du rachis. Rev Chir Orthop 63:423–425
3. Louis R (1983) Surgery of the spine. Springer, Berlin Heidelberg New York, pp 142, 168–172
4. Louis R (1987) Stability and instability of the cervical spine. In: Kehr P, Weidner A (eds) Cervical spine I. Springer, Wien New York, pp 21–27
5. Prijambodo B, Kadaroelah S, Ichwan P, Radjamin P (1986) Stabilisation for the thoracolumbar fractures. Original paper, Department of Surgery, School of Medicine Airlangga University, Surabaya, Indonesia
6. Roy-Camille R, Mazel RCH, Saillant G (1987) Treatment of cervical spine injuries by posterior osteosynthesis with plates and screws. In: Kehr P, Weidner A (eds) Cervical spine I. Springer, Wien New York, pp 163–174
7. Shannon Stauffer E (1986) Management of cervical injury C3–C7. Orthop Clin North Am 7:45

1.12. The Posterior Approach in the Treatment of Lower Cervical Spine Subluxations

P. BUFFATTI, F. FACCIOLI, G. PINNA, and G. DALLE ORE, Verona, Italy

Introduction

Traumatic disruption of the posterior ligaments of the cervical spine, generally caused by hyperflexion of the neck, whether associated or not with hyperextension – the whiplash injury –, may result in vertebral instability. This condition is not always recognized when injured patients are seen in the emergency room. X-ray examination of the cervical spine usually discloses minor abnormalities that are easily overlooked. However, the appearance of the spine may be normal even to the experienced eye. Some radiological findings have been suggested to represent clues to impending vertebral instability due to posterior ligament lesions [3]: a) widening of the articular surfaces; b) increase of the interspinous distance; c) initial kyphotic appearance with a hinge at the lesion level; and d) reduction of the intervertebral disc space. Dynamic studies may confirm the diagnosis, showing an abnormal mobility of the vertebral bodies with loss of the normal articular relationships. If this condition is not recognized, the continuous movements of the neck lead to anterior subluxation, sometimes weeks or months after the injury [2, 3].

We present our experience with surgical treatment of these vertebral instabilities.

Materials and Methods

In the four-year period 1984–1987, 62 patients, suffering from whiplash cervical injuries, were operated on in the Department of Neurosurgery in Verona. Ten of these patients presented with subluxation of the lower cervical spine. Eight were male, 2 female. Their mean age was 52 years (range 18–73). The causes of cervical injury were motor vehicle accidents in five cases, mountain-climbing falls in two and an accidental fall in the other three. Two patients were first seen in our institution; the remaining were referred from other centers. On admission, x-ray films of the cervical spine were not taken in four cases. In the other four, normal appearance or minor abnormalities in the X-rays were observed. In only two cases was subluxation evident on admission radiographs. In the other eight patients subluxation was demonstrated later, sometimes after a considerable time from the injury. This period ranged from 3 days to 4 months in our series.

Examination showed neurological disturbances in 7 patients (either spinal cord or nerve root compression signs). Six patients suffered from neck pain, in two this was the sole complaint. In one patient, who also suffered from a severe head injury and was comatose on hospital admission, the subluxation was discovered incidentally with x-ray follow-up of the cervical spine after his complete neurological recovery.

Dynamic studies revealed an instability of the cervical spine with reduction of the subluxation in 7 patients while in 3 patients with late referral, only a partial reduction could be obtained after trans-cranial traction.

Surgical Treatment

All patients were operated through the posterior route. In the first two patients of this series fixation of the spine was achieved by insertion of Roy-Camille plates. In the others, stabilization was obtained by insertion of Knodt hooks adapted to the cervical spine (Fig. 1). A second type of smaller hook was developed in our institution (Fig. 2), which is easier to insert and proved to be as reliable as the others. Satisfactory intraoperative reduction of subluxation and fixation were achieved by unilateral Knodt instrumentation in 4 cases. Bilateral Knodt instrumentation was necessary in 3 cases. In one patient, after an initial wiring of the spinous processes, Knodt hooks were inserted after breakage of the steel wires.

Results

Post-operative radiographic follow-up showed a complete realignment of the vertebral bodies in seven patients. In the 3 others, who had a pre-operative non-reducible chronic subluxation, a partial but satisfactory correction of the anterolisthesis of the upper vertebral body was obtained. At follow-up (range: 1 to 4.5 years) all patients with neurological disturbances showed an improvement, with complete recovery in five cases. Painful neck sensations disappeared in all patients.

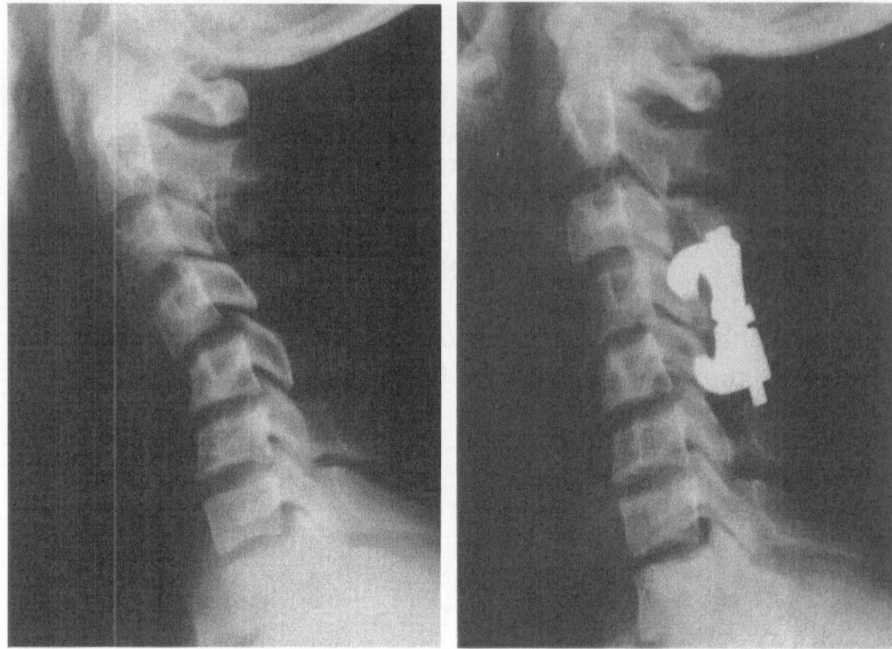

a   b

Fig. 1. a) C4/C5 subluxation, b) complete realignment after Knodt hook insertion

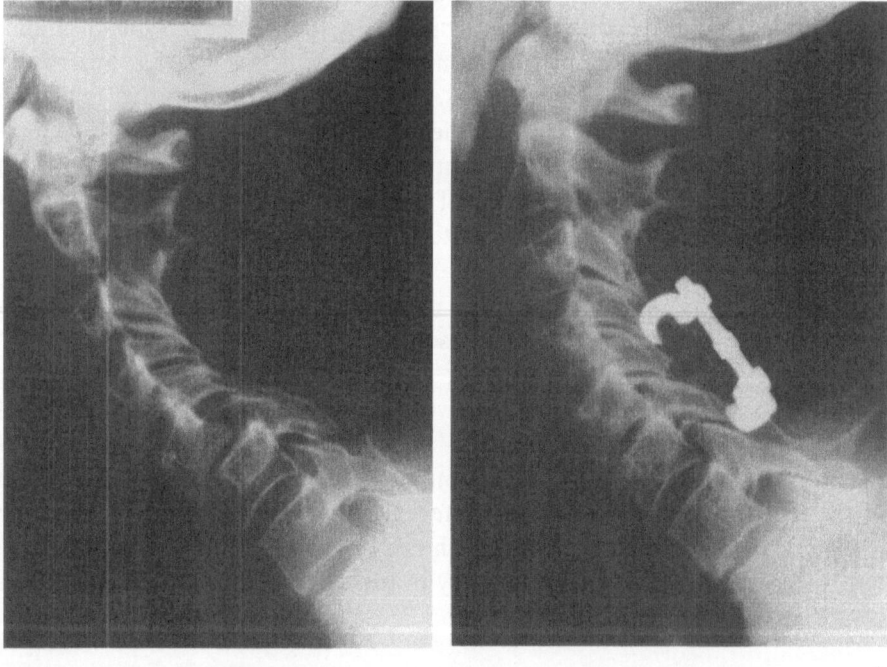

a   b

Fig. 2. a) C5/C6 subluxation, b) after insertion of modified Knodt hook

Discussion

The early diagnosis of cervical subluxation is difficult. The patients often complain only of neck pain or have reduced neck mobility and paresthesiae without neurological signs. X-ray abnormalities are often minimal and are easily missed if not searched for. A considerable experience in spinal injury is therefore needed to suspect a posterior ligament tear from subtle radiological signs such as a widening of articular surfaces or an increase of the interspinous distance. Moreover, it has also been demonstrated that an instability may develop in the absence of radiological abnormalities immediately after the injury [1, 4]. The degree of instability is initially low due to incomplete tear of the soft spinal tissue but increases with movements of the neck. Dynamic studies (flexion-extension radiographs) are recommended if a posterior ligamentous lesion is suspected.

Once established, the subluxation may usually be reduced with trans-cranial traction and immobilization with plaster cast. Conservative treatment, however, usually fails to stabilize the spine.

Lower cervical spine subluxations are best treated with surgical stabilization. Because the site of the lesion is posterior (interspinous ligaments, ligamentum flavum, posterior longitudinal ligaments, articular ligaments) the posterior route is the preferred approach.

Wiring of the spinous processes and/or laminae may be dangerous and does not guarantee firm stability because of frequent rupture of the steel wires. Although the Roy-Camille plates are excellent fixating devices, there is a small risk of vertebral artery or cord injury when inserting the screws into the articular masses.

Our preference for a fixation device is the Knodt hook. The hook-shaped extremities are easily slipped under the laminae and when the threaded bolt that joins the hooks is screwed, they fasten the laminae tightly by slow progressive compression. This allows a realignment of the vertebrae if a preoperative reduction was not obtained. We have recently adopted a smaller type of Knodt hook (Fig. 2) which is more easily inserted with less protrusion into the canal and which offers the same degree of stability and fixation. This fixating technique that we use in all the posterior cervical stabilization procedures is, in our experience, easy, safe and reliable. The stabilization achieved is excellent and no instrument failure has been observed to date with follow-up radiographs.

References

1. Dorr LD, Harvey JP, Nickel VL (1982) Clinical review of the early stability of spine injuries. Spine 7:545–550

2. Penning L (1962) Aspects radiologiques dans les traumatismes de la colonne cervicale. Neurochirurgie 8:279–289
3. Roy-Camille R, Saillant G, Berteaux D, Lortat-Jacob A, Bisserie M (1977) Entorse grave par lésion du segment mobile rachidien (S.M.R.) de la colonne cervicale. J Chir 113:121–130
4. Roy-Camille R, Saillant G, Judet T, Mammoudy P (1982) Traumatismes récénts des cinq dernières vertebres cervicales chez l'adulte (avec et sans complication neurologique). Ann Chir 36:735–744

1.13. Internal Fixation of the Cervical Spine: the Hartshill System

J. Dove, Stoke-on-Trent, U.K.

The Hartshill system is a modification of the Luque system for posterior segmental wiring of the spine and has for five years been our routine means of posterior spinal fixation throughout the spine from skull to sacrum and for all varieties of spinal disorders. This paper presents our experience of the use of the Hartshill system in the cervical spine. There has been 34 cases with minimum two year follow up (trauma 11, rheumatoid 8, facet osteoarthritis 7, tumour 5, congenital 2 and myelopathy 1). There has been only one serious complication. The system is essentially simple and inexpensive but nonetheless attention to detail in technique is important. With proper attention to detail the Hartshill system provides a secure, adaptable, posterior fixation system that can be used throughout the cervical spine.

For many years the Harrington rod was virtually the only fixation system for the spine. It does however suffer from a number of disadvantages and in particular it is not appropriate for use in the cervical spine.

Lange [5] first reported the use of segmental wires in the cervical spine but the first serious attempts at segmental internal fixation of the spine came from the Iberian peninsula. Hernandez-Ros [4] was segmentally wiring tibial grafts to the spinous processes for deformity in Spain in the 1950's and the Portuguese developed a segmental wiring system for deformity using a malleable rod [1]. However the current explosion of interest in segmental wiring for the spine was the result of the work of Luque [6, 7] who popularised the use of segmental sublaminar wires.

In the Stoke-on-Trent Spinal Service we began to use the Luque double 'L' rod system routinely for posterior fixation of the spine but we did encounter a number of practical problems [2]. To overcome these problems we developed the Hartshill rectangle (Figs. 1 a and b). The rectangle is made from a stainless rod which is welded. There is a 100° roof in each end of the rectangle to ensure that the terminal wires slide down the shoulder of the rectangle to lie in the corners thereby giving much increased rotational stability [3]. There are two calibres of rectangle being made either from 5 or 6 mm diameter stainless steel. The 5 mm calibre rectangle is appropriate for use in

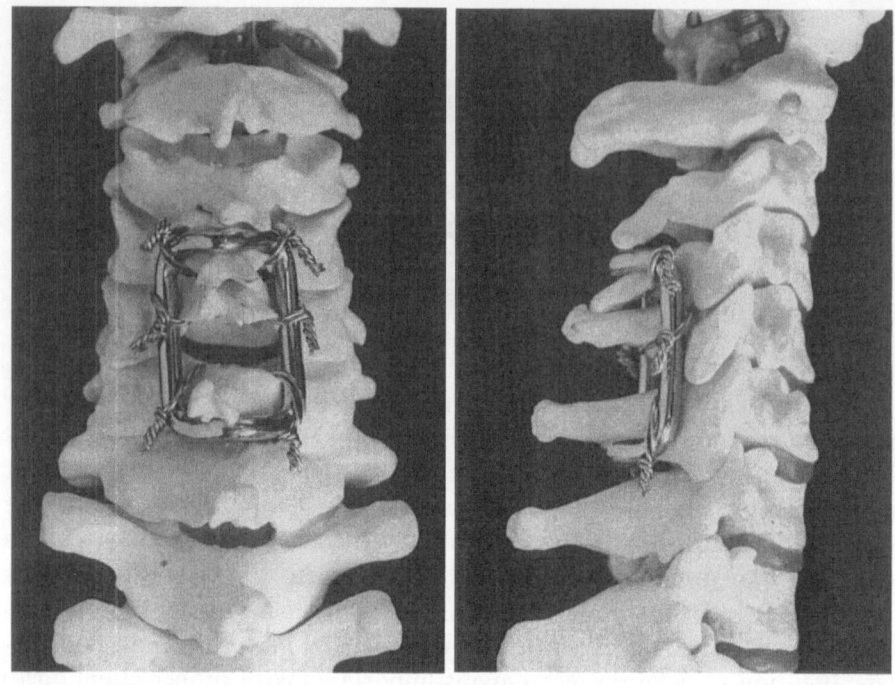

a   b
Fig. 1. a) Posterior view of Hartshill rectangle wired into a model cervical spine.
b) Lateral view of Hartshill rectangle wired to a model spine

the cervical spine. The rectangles are supplied in a range of lengths and the
Hartshill system is supplied by A. W. Showell (Surgicraft UK Limited).

Indications

If the cervical spine is unstable and if the surgeon decides that posterior
stabilisation is appropriate then the Hartshill system can usually be used to
provide that stabilisation.

Surgical Technique

A mid-line posterior approach to the cervical spine is used. The levels
appropriate to the case are identified and whatever surgery is necessary to
deal with the primary pathology is first carried out. Then at each level which

is to be fixed the interspinous ligaments are removed and a small window is made in the ligamentum flavum. The window need be only just large enough to allow the passage of wires.

A rectangle of appropriate length is then chosen. In general with the Hartshill system a rectangle is selected the upper limb of which lies at or immediately below the leading edge of the upper most lamina and the lower limb of which lies at or just behind the trailing edge of the lower most lamina (Figs. 1a and b). In the cervical spine the choise of lengths of rectangle is particularly important. If in any doubt the surgeon should choose the slightly longer rather than a slightly shorter rectangle. The reason for this is that as the wires are tightened, if a shorter rectangle has been chosen there will be a compressive effect with narrowing of the intervertebral foramen and the risk of iatrogenic nerve root compression.

Once a rectangle of appropriate length has been selected it is contoured as appropriate using Hartshill benders.

Sublaminar wires are then passed at each level which is to be fixed. We routinely use two loops of 0.84 mm cold worked Hartshill wire at each level. However in very young patients or in rheumatoid disease we sometimes use just one loop of the same wire which is then split and half taken to each side. We believe that it is important to use the cold worked Hartshill wire rather than heat worked wire from a spool. The reason for this is firstly that we have by our biomechanical studies shown that the cold worked wire is stronger and secondly heat worked wire tends not to retain the shape that the surgeon has bent into it [8].

There is then a tendency in situations where wire passage is difficult for the wire not to follow the course that the surgeon intends.

Once all the wires have been passed the rectangle is threaded onto the wires so that the cephalad end of each loop of wire is passed around the inside of the rectangle except at the upper most level where the caudad end of each loop of wire is passed around the inside of the rectangle. This ensures that the wires lie snuggly in the corners of the rectangle at each end (Figs. 1a and b).

The rectangle is then held flush against the laminae by an assistant using a Hartshill pusher. If at this point in the operation the rectangle does not lie snuggly against the laminae it should be recontoured. The wires are then tightened using a Hartshill jet wire twister and once tight the wires are cut short leaving approximately 1 cm of twist. Once all the wires have been tightened and cut short a secondary twist is incorporated into the wire using a wire holder. The wire is turned in the same clockwise direction that it was turned by the jet twister in order to turn the end of the wire down away from the overlying muscle and at the same time significantly to increase the strength of the wire [8].

Finally the fusion is carried out. This is performed by decorticating the dorsal aspect of the facet joints at each level using a powered burr. The bone

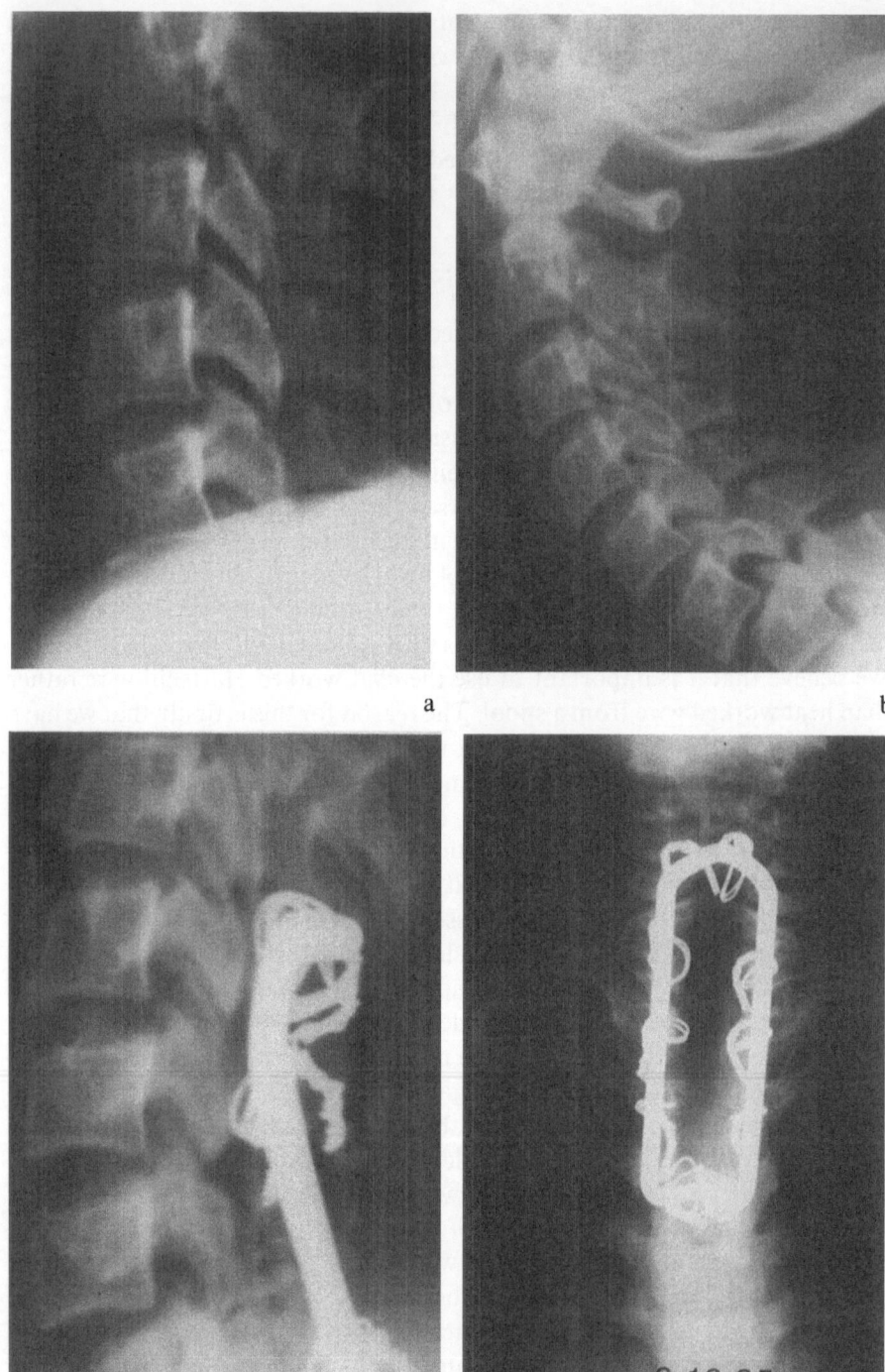

a

b

c

d

graft is then laid on the back of the facet joints lateral to the internal fixation. In routine cases more than adequate bone can be obtained by mincing up the bone removed during the exposure but if there is shortage of bone graft then we use the iliac crest.

The wound is then closed in layers with superficial vacuum drainage.

In routine cases the patient mobilises when comfortable on the second or third day. External support is not essential but the patient usually appreciates a soft collar. Patients are kept off light work for six weeks and heavy work for twelve weeks following their surgery.

Results

Table 1 shows the breakdown of our first 34 cases with a minimum two year follow up where the Hartshill system has been used for the internal fixation of the cervical spine.

The statistics of the patients are shown in Table 2.

The complications are listed in Table 3.

Table 1. *Aetiology*

Trauma	11
Rheumatoid	8
Facet osteoarthritis	7
Tumour	5
Congenital	2
Myelopathy	1
Total	34 patients

Table 2. *Patient Statistics*

Male	13
Female	21
Age range	6–78 years
	(mean 48 years)
Follow up	2–5.5 years

Table 3. *Complications*

Broken wires	2
Infection	2
Neurological	1
CSF leak	1

Fig. 2. a) A patient was involved in a road traffic accident. The patient complained of pain in the cervical spine. A lateral x-ray of the cervical spine was reported as normal. b) Three weeks later because of continuing pain and neurological signs in the upper limbs a full x-ray of the cervical spine was taken and the fracture dislocation of C6 on C7 was discovered. c) A posterior surgical decompression was carried out and a Hartshill rectangle wired into place. It should be noted that because this was a late case with kyphosis no wires were passed at the apex of the kyphosis. The secondary twist in the wires should be noted. d) Posteropative AP x-rays

The only important complication was the neurological one. In a trauma patient there was neurological deterioration by one Frankel grade following surgery but fortunately within three months the patient had regained his pre-operative neurological state and eventually made a full neurological recovery.

In one case of infection the implant had to be removed to resolve the infection but fortunately we were able to wait until his spine was stable.

In neither of the cases where there were broken wires did those wires give rise to any clinical problem.

Case Example

Figures 2a–2d illustrate the use of the Hartshill system in the cervical spine.

The details are given in the caption to the illustrations but one particular additional point needs to be emphasised in this case. Because I was dealing with a kyphosis no sublaminar wires were passed at the apex of the kyphosis. It is potentially dangerous to pass sublaminar wires at the apex of a kyphosis.

Discussion

The Hartshill system is simple to apply and yet provides secure fixation of the cervical spine.

For some cases in the thoracolumbar and lumbar spine we are introducing a pedicle screw device which can be clamped to the rectangle but in the cervical spine we have found no need to use anything other than the standard wires.

Ransford has recently introduced a very useful addition to the Hartshill range for the internal fixation of the occipito-cervical junction (Fig. 3). The Ransford loop is especially useful for the stabilisation of patients with rheumatoid disease of the upper cervical spine.

Fidler is also introducing a useful addition to the Hartshill range (Fig. 4). The Fidler sledge allows secure stabilisation of the relevant segment of the cervical spine whilst at the same time preserving the interspinous ligaments.

Although the Hartshill system is technically simple attention to detail in operative technique is important. Surgeons thinking of using the system are cordially invited to visit our centre or to attend one of our regular instructional hands on courses.

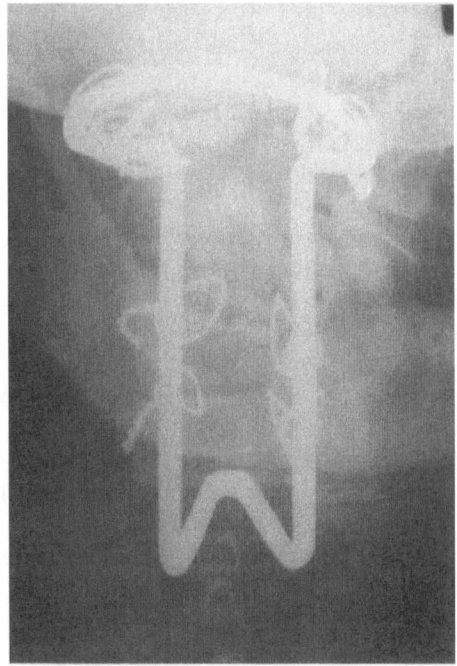

Fig. 3. The Ransford loop for stabilisation of the occipito-cervical junction. It should be noted that the current device that is marketed does not include the roof at the lower end

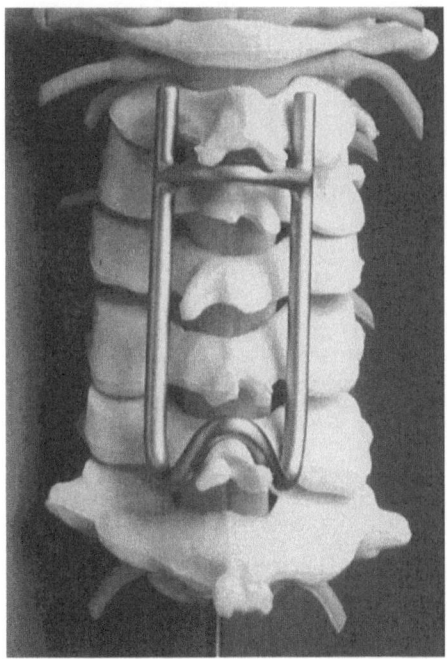

Fig. 4. The Fidler sledge lying on a model cervical spine

References

1. Resina J (1963) Redressment et stabilisation immediate des scolioses par un tuteur metallique. Ass Européenne centre la poliomyelite 1X symposium. Stockholm, Masson et cie, Paris, pp 421–429
2. Dove J (1987) Luque segmental spinal instrumentation: The use of the Hartshill rectangle. Orthopedics 10: No 6
3. Fidler M (1986) Posterior instrumentation of the spine: An experimental comparison of various possible techniques. Spine 11: 367–372
4. Hernandez-Ros A (1965) Codorniu. Nuevas tactica y tecnica operatoria en el tratamiento de las escoliosis. Scritti an a medici in onore di P. del Torto. Saverio Pipola, Napoli, pp 71–79
5. Lange F (1910) Support for the spondylitic spine by means of buried bar attached to the vertebrae. Am J Orthop Surg 8: 344
6. Luque ER (1984) SS1. The state of the Art. Slack 1984: 1–11
7. Luque ER (1974) Anatomy of scoliosis and its correction. Clin Orthop 1974: 105–298
8. Sell P, Crawford RJ, Ali MS, Dove J: The biomechanics of segmental spinal wiring. Submitted for publication to Spine

1.14. The Surgical Treatment of Subluxation of the Lower Cervical Spine

A. Savini, P. Parisini, N. Bettini, and M. Palmisani, Bologna, Italy

Introduction

In our opinion, when today the same meaning given by French Authors to "entorse grave" is attached to anterior subluxation, this then indicates a lesion of the vertebral ligaments without fracture or dislocation. This anterior subluxation corresponds to about 5% [4] of all trauma of the lower cervical spine, in our cases as well as in those of other authors. These relatively rare lesions are becoming increasingly important in orthopaedics as well as in forensic medicine. For this reason we deemed it worthwhile to review, from the clinical and radiological viewpoint, the 16 cases of anterior subluxation which underwent surgery at Rizzoli Orthopaedic Institute from 1977 to 1987.

Materials and Methods

The 16 patients (14 males and 2 females) had an age range from 14–65 years (mean age 30). The cause for the lesions were road accidents in 11 cases, sport related trauma (diving injuries) in 3 cases, a work related accident in 1 case, and accidental trauma in 1 case. The most frequently involved level was C5–C6; the least frequently involved level was C3–C4. We separated recent lesion from old lesions. To do so, we considered a one month interval between the trauma occurrence and the beginning of our treatment as the time reference used to separate the two groups. Out of 16 anterior subluxations, 6 were recent and 10 non recent. In all the 6 recent trauma cases X-ray evaluation showed the signs of anterior subluxations. In 4 cases there were only clinical symptoms of articulation instability (pain, reduced function) whereas in the remaining 2 cases there were also signs of incomplete spinal cord damage. In the latter cases, together with standard radiological tests (X-ray in A-P and lateral projections) we performed C.T. scans and MRI to detect the possibility of spinal cord compression in order to provide an appropriate treatment. These tests demonstrated spinal cord compression

A. Savini et al.

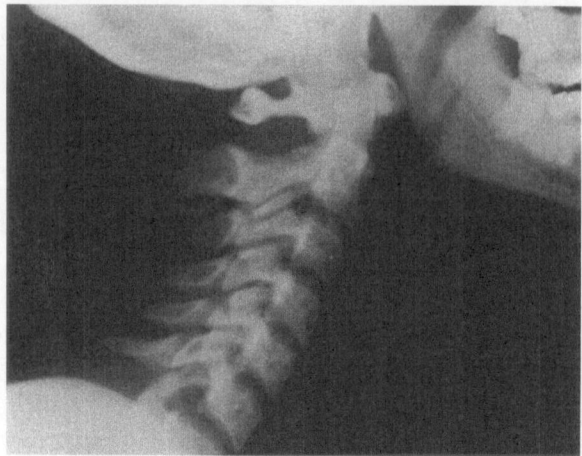

Fig. 1. A 24 year old female with anterior subluxation at the C6–C7 level

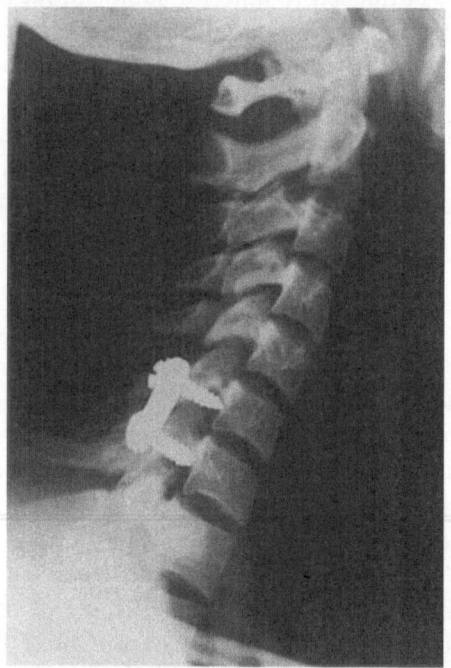

Fig. 2. Same case. Results obtained 1 year after posterior fixation

caused by herniated disk in 1 case, but not in the others. We treated surgically all of the 6 recent lesions. In 5 cases a posterior fixation was performed (Figs. 1 and 2). In the one case with spinal cord compression due to herniated disk we performed decompression anteriorly with anterior fixation. The 10 cases of non-recent trauma were brought to our attention between 30 days

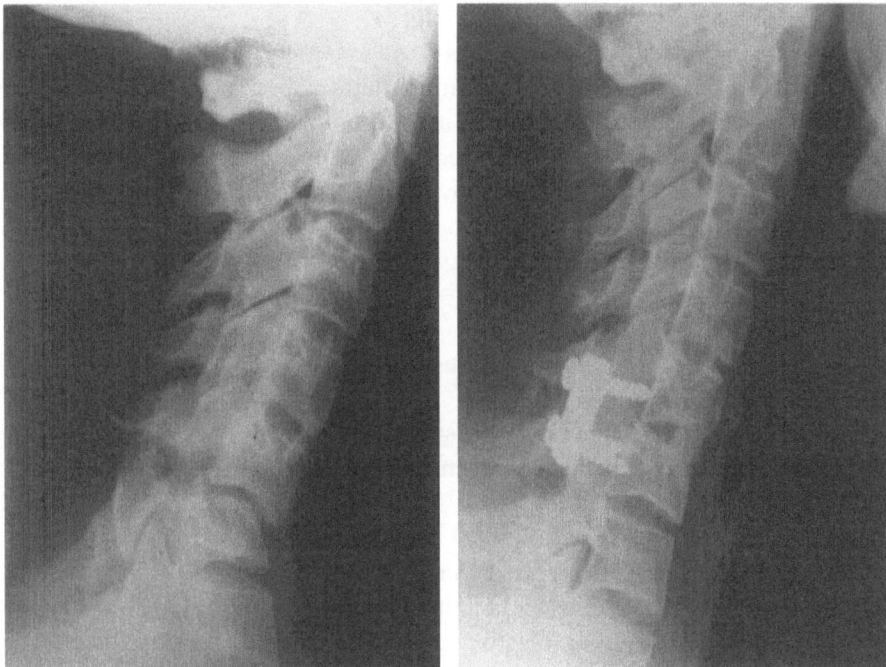

Fig. 3   Fig. 4

Fig. 3. Male aged 22. X-ray 6 months after a road accident demonstrates a fixed deformity with slipping over 30%

Fig. 4. Same case. Result obtained 6 months after anterior fusion release followed by posterior fixation

to 6 months (mean time: 3 months) after the trauma occurrence. In all these cases we observed the clinical signs of joint instability, radicular lesions in 4 cases, and mild pyramidal syndromes in 2 cases. In these 10 cases, on the basis of dynamic X-ray tests only, we detected flexible lesions (2 cases) and fixed lesions (8 cases). These were further divided in relation to sliding: above 30% and below 30%. Moreover, in 6 cases with clinical signs of myelo-radicular damage, C.T. scan and/or MRI were used to exclude possible spinal cord compression. Surgery was performed in all of these 10 cases. In the 2 cases of flexible conditions, after reduction in halo-cast, posterior fixation was performed, with one case followed by anterior fusion. In patients with fixed deformity, 4 cases were treated with anterior release plus posterior synthesis (Figs. 3 and 4) and 4 cases with simple "in situ" fusion. In the cases treated with posterior synthesis with or without fusion, post-surgical immobilization was obtained by a Minerva brace worn for 45–60 days.

In the cases treated with fusion only, immobilization was obtained by means of a Minerva plaster cast until the fusion was achieved.

Results

In all the 6 patients with recent trauma, lesions were stabilized and in the 2 patients with partial cord damage a total neurological recovery was obtained. In all the 10 cases of non-recent trauma, lesion stabilization was obtained and total neurological recovery occurred both in the 4 radicular lesions and in the 2 patients with moderate pyramidal syndromes. In both groups no complications occurred.

Discussion

Anterior subluxations, or "entorse grave" of the French authors, are fairly rare conditions which only recently have been defined from the radiological and clinical point of view [4–6]. Together with a careful physical examination, a thorough radiological evaluation of the lesion is important. In this regard, it must be stressed that the lack of radiologically apparent skeletal lesions is not synonymous with benignity [2, 3, 7]. At 15–30 days from the trauma it is advisable to perform dynamic X-ray tests in all the doubtful cases.

X-ray tests should not follow strict pre-set patterns but should be related to symptoms and to the type of lesion. Thus, for recent lesions with no neurological damage, the 2 standard projections (A-P and lateral), which permit evaluation of the usual signs of instability, are sufficient. On the contrary, the presence of neurological damage requires more tests (C.T. scan and MRI) to investigate the possible presence of spinal cord compression. In nonrecent lesions, together with the standard projections which are useful to determine the slipping ratio, dynamic X-ray tests must be performed to separate fixed and flexible lesions. Also, in non-recent lesions, the presence of neurological signs of medullary damage makes C.T. scan and MRI necessary to detect possible spinal cord compression and to study the morphology of the spinal canal. In our opinion, this careful clinical and radiological approach produces surgical indications, since we, as other authors [5], consider surgical stabilization a necessity for these unstable lesions. Recent lesions without myelo-radicular compression and with or without neurological damage can be treated with posterior fixation only. In these cases we prefer the easier, more stable posterior approach which permits intervention at the site where the lesion is more severe, and at the same time allows a better anatomical reduction of the lesion [1]. However, the presence of spinal cord compression requires an anterior decompression. In non-recent flexible lesions reduction in halo cast is indicated and stabilization can be obtained with posterior fixation. In one case we performed a double approach, which, according to the data obtained so far, we deem to be an overtreatment.

However, in fixed lesions, due to the presence of an abnormal callous formation and in the absence of myelo-radicular compression, if slipping is less
than 30%, the anterior fusion "in situ" alone is sufficient. Conversely, in
lesions with slipping of over 30%, the anterior fusion release must be followed by posterior osteosynthesis. The post surgical immobilization depends
on the presence or absence of posterior synthesis. If posterior synthesis has
been performed, immobilization by Minerva orthopedic brace for 45–60
days is sufficient. Conversely, the presence of anterior arthrodesis alone
makes it necessary to keep the post-surgical immobilization until fusion is
obtained. In conclusion, it is our opinion that anterior subluxations are
lesions whose clinical and radiological aspects must be underlined. In particular, X-ray results if properly obtained, provide relevant therapeutic indications.

References

1. Bombart M, Canevet D, Deckard J (1984) Comparaison sur l'ensemble de la series
   des resultas de la chirurgie par voie anterieure et par voie posterieure. Rev Chir
   Orthop 70:533–537
2. Chesire DJE (1969) The stability of the cervical spine following the conservative
   treatment of fracture and fracture dislocations. Paraplegia 7:193–203
3. Dorr LD, Harvey JP, Nickel VL (1982) Clinical review of the early stability of
   spine injures. Spine 7:545–550
4. Louis R (1979) Entorse grave et hernie discales. Nouv Presse Med 8:1843–1849
5. Louis R, Castera G (1984) Entorses graves du rachis cervical inferieur. Rev Chir
   Orthop 70:527–532
6. Roy Camille R, Saillant G, Berteaux D, Lotart Jacob A, Bisserie M (1977) Entorse
   grave par lesion traumatique du segment mobile rachidien (S.M.R.) de la colonne
   cervicale. J Chir 113:121–130
7. Roy Camille R, Saillant G, Berteaux D, Bisserie M (1978) Entorses graves du
   rachis cervical. Traitment, par voie posterieure. Rev Chir Orthop 64:677–684

1.15. Internal Fixation for the Treatment of Subluxations of the Lower Cervical Spine

C. A. LOGROSCINO and V. F. PALIOTTA, Roma, Italy

Subluxation can occur in the lower cervical spine secondary to hyperflexion or hyperextension injury. Depending on the way the injury occurs, rotational and lateral stresses may also be involved. In the characteristic whiplash injury, there is a combination of hyperflexion and hyperextension stresses in a temporal sequence.

Subluxations can therefore be divided into hyperflexion sprains and hyperextension sprains [5]. Hyperflexion sprains may derive from an indirect injury, due to sudden deceleration for instance, or from a direct injury due to forces acting on the occiput.

The anterior column, formed by vertebral bodies and discs, is subjected to compressive forces, while the posterior columns, formed by facet joints and ligaments are subjected to tensile stresses. The bending movement normally stops when the chin hits the manubrium of the sternum, which thus comes to form the center of rotation of the movement.

First the interspinous ligaments and the ligaments of the facet joints are torn. When the injury is more serious, there is also a fracture of the spinous processes ("clay shoveler's" fracture). Segmental instability may occur, too, when there is an injury to the middle column [3] formed by the posterior longitudinal ligament and the posterior aspect of the bodies and discs. When there is an injury to the posterior part of the disc, in fact, the overlying body tilts forward causing malalignment of the joint facets. In children this mechanism can lead to fractures of the epiphyseal plate.

Owing to the absence of bone and/or joint injuries, standard X-ray examination may not reveal this situation. This is why cervical subluxations often go undiscovered and in at least 30 to 50% of cases the diagnosis occurs later on [2].

Flexion/extension/lateral view dynamic X-rays are thus of basic importance for recognizing the lesion, since they reveal signs that are not shown up by the standard examination. In the case of serious (unstable) sprains, the following signs can generally be picked up by standard X-ray examination with dynamic views:

– Anterior slipping of at least 3 mm of the vertebral body above the lesion.
– Widening of the interspinous space above and below.
– The joint facets do not appear parallel, as they usually are.
– There is a loss of contact amounting to at least 50% between the joint facets.
– The angle of the posterior wall of the vertebrae exceeds 15%.

If at least three of the above five X-ray signs are present, serious instability of the cervical spine due to hyperflexion injury can be diagnosed with certainty [13]. Hyperflexion sprains of the lower cervical spine are substantially characterized by kyphosis.

Hyperextension sprains can be caused by a direct injury (force applied to the face region) or indirect injury (e.g. rapid acceleration).

According to Selecki [12], injuries secondary to hyperextension are at least three times more common than those secondary to hyperflexion. In this case, however, the tensile stresses act on the anterior column while the compressive forces act on the posterior column. The compressed posterior elements, therefore, form a solid barrier that is particularly resistant to compressive forces [13].

Hyperextention sprains are caused by rupture of the anterior longitudinal ligament and by fracture of the anterior portion of the disc. In this case the overlying vertebral body tilts forward.

X-ray signs are very scarce. The intersomatic space can be wider anteriorly than that above and below, and vacuum defects may be observed in the disc. Thickening of the prevertebral soft tissues is sometimes present indicating a possible haematoma.

The diagnosis is based essentially on a dynamic X-ray examination. Posterior dislocation of the body associated with rotation thereof following rupture of the anterior longitudinal ligament can be observed. In more serious cases a small avulsion fracture of the inferior aspect of the vertebral body and separation of the posterior longitudinal ligament may also be present (in 60% of all cases according to Harris) [5].

The spinal cord may be compressed between the lower margin of the overlying vertebra and the posterior arch of the one below [1].

Surgical stabilization is necessary in cases of serious subluxation, namely when there is segmental instability. In fact, torn ligaments do not tend to heal on their own, so immobilization by means of a cast or external orthosis is not sufficient.

Surgical Treatment

Since a lesion of the posterior ligaments occurs in hyperflexion injuries, it is preferable to use a posterior approach. Even in the case of hyperexten-

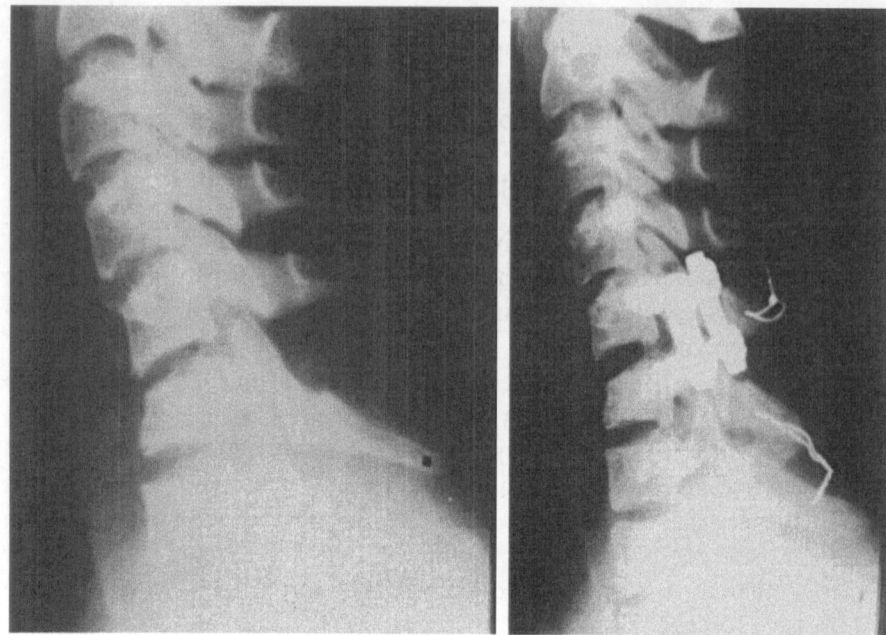

Fig. 1. Female, 16 years old. Subluxation C5–C6. X-ray, lateral view: widening of the interspinous space. Open reduction, internal fixation (Roy-Camille plates) and fusion (Rogers)

sion injuries we prefer to fix the lesion by a posterior approach, since we consider posterior instrumentation to be the most stable.

In the first cases treated we performed a posterior fusion with iliac graft according to Rogers [9]. After the operation the patients are immobilized with halo-cast until the graft has been incorporated; this takes about three months.

Since 1980 we have used metal internal fixation (Roy-Camille plates, Roosen instrumentation) together with the graft. Adoption of internal fixation reduces the time required for immobilization with external orthosis. Moreover, the halo-cast has now been replaced by more comfortable plastic collars.

Sixteen patients affected by subluxation of the lower cervical spine have been treated in this manner. Of these, nine had already been unsuccessfully treated elsewhere (immobilization with Minerva-cast) or had arrived without diagnosis. Most of them were young adults (average age 37 years). The average follow-up is 41 months.

Intense neck pain was present in ten cases, and also initial neurological disturbances (radiculopathy) in six. Most of the patients (eleven) were operated on by using the Roy-Camille plate technique [11]. The method is simple,

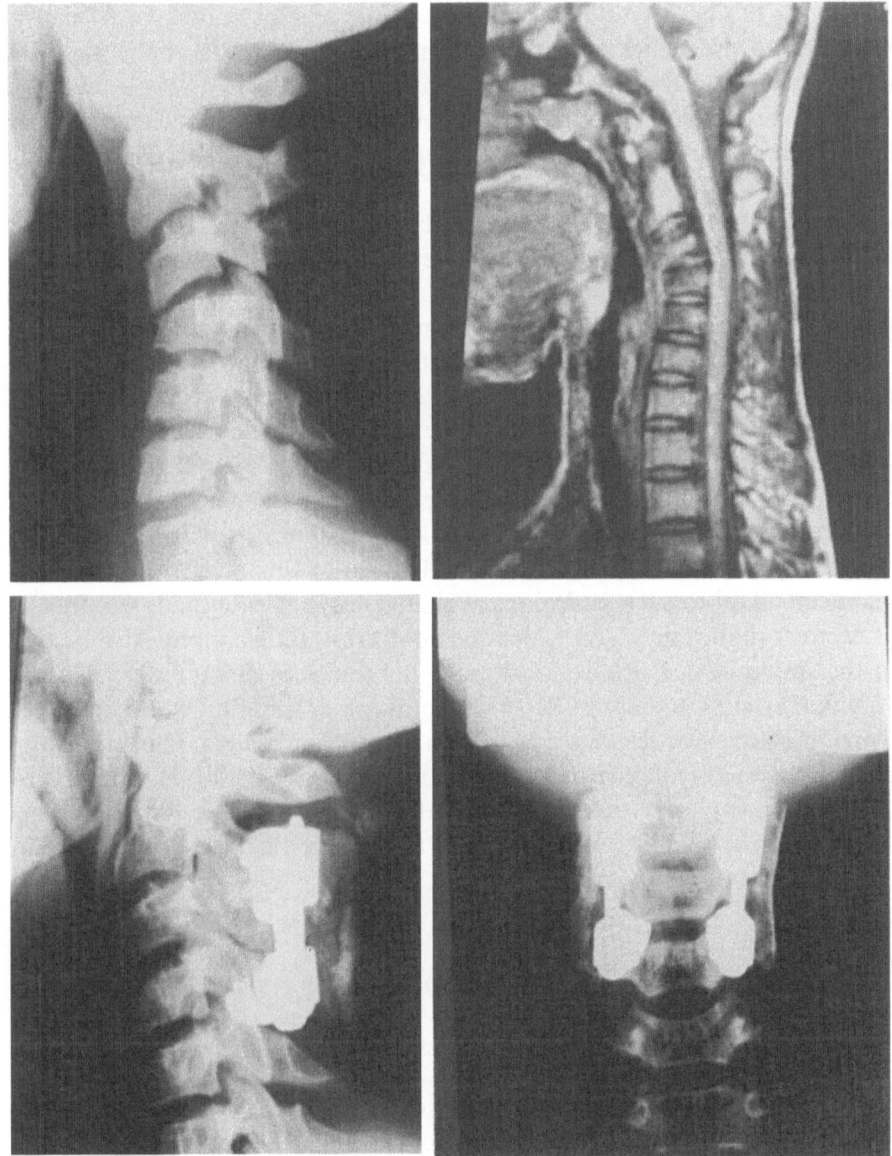

Fig. 2. Male, 14 years old. Subluxation C3–C4. MRI: segmental stenosis of the spinal canal. Open reduction, internal fixation (Roosen) and fusion (Rogers)

reliable and versatile, ensuring good stabilization of the injury and, at the same time, reduction of the subluxation (Fig. 1).

A characteristic of this instrumentation is multisegmental fixation which renders the implant especially solid. The method consists of immobilizing the spinal segment concerned by means of plates and screws applied to articular facets. As the ligamentous lesion may affect several segments, it may be necessary to use plates with three or more holes. An iliac bone graft has always been used together with the fixation.

In all cases fusion of the graft has been observed, together with disappearance of the instability pain, and neurological signs. So far we have witnessed no failure of the instrumentation.

We consider Roy-Camille plates to be particularly suitable for the treatment of hyperextension injuries where the posterior elements have been subjected to compressive forces and the anterior ones to tensile stresses. This type of instrumentation permits fixation in anatomic alignment.

In the last three years we have used (in five cases) a new type of instrumentation which works in compression described by Roosen [10]. This is designed specifically for the upper cervical spine, but it has also given good results when extended to lower cervical spine applications. The instrumentation consists of two hooks and a screw which is applied under compression.

The upper hook is unique; it contains a special inner spring system which renders the instrumentation dynamic. Thanks to this device the metal implant can adapt to such pathological changes as may eventually occur, such as necrosis of the lamina on which the hooks rest, for example. Also because of the spring device, Roosen's instrumentation does not interfere with the vertebral arteries in the transverse vertebral canal. And finally, because of its dynamic characteristics, this type of instrumentation really favours reduction of subluxations secondary to hyperflexion injuries (Fig. 2). It is thus possible to correct completely the kyphosis that is usually present. Since this is a compression system, it can be regarded as the specific means of fixation for the treatment of all kinds of kyphosis.

References

1. Breig A (1978) Adverse mechanical tension in the central nervous system. Almqvist and Wiksell, Stockholm
2. Cheshire DJ (1969) The stability of the cervical spine following the conservative treatment of fractures and fracture-dislocations. Paraplegia 7:193–200
3. Denis F (1983) The three column spine and its significance in the classification of acute thoracolumbar spinal injuries. Spine 8:817–831
4. Forsyth HF (1964) Extension injuries of the cervical spine. J Bone Joint Surg 46A:1792–1797
5. Harris JH, Edeiken-Monroe B, Kopaniki DR (1986) A practical classification of acute cervical spine injuries. Orthop Clin North Am 17:15–30
6. Holdsworth F (1970) Review article: Fractures, dislocations and fracture-dislocations of the spine. J Bone Joint Surg 52A:1534–1551
7. Logroscino CA, Paliotta VF, Aulisa L (1988) Indicazioni all'osteosintesi nelle instabilita' cervicali. Progr Pat Vert 10:57–63

8. MacNab I (1964) Acceleration injuries of the cervical spine. J Bone Joint Surg 46A:1797–1799
9. Rogers WA (1957) Fractures and dislocations of the cervical spine. J Bone Joint Surg 39A:341–376
10. Roosen K, Trauschel A, Grote W (1982) Posterior atlanto-axial fusion: a new compression clamp for laminar osteosynthesis. Arch Orthop Trauma Surg 100:27–31
11. Roy-Camille R, Saillant G, Berteaux D, Bisserie M (1978) Entorses graves du rachis cervical. Traitement par voie posterieure. Rev Chir Orthop 64:677–684
12. Selecki BR, Williams HBL (1970) Injuries to the cervical spine and cord in man. Australian Medical Publishing Company Ltd, New South Wales
13. Senegas J, Vital JM, Barat M, Caille JM, Dabadie P (1987) Traumatismes du rachis cervical. In: Enc Med Chir, S.G.I.M.-Les Martres-de Veyre, Paris, 1825

Cervical Spine II
© by Springer-Verlag 1989

1.16. Results of 14 Cervical Luxations or Subluxations Stabilized with Posterior Louis' Plates

T. PACHE, Lausanne, Switzerland

Between July 1986 and December 1987 11 men and 3 women aged 15 to 69 years (mean 34.7) were operated for a cervical spine luxation or subluxation, more often at C5–C6 levels (7 cases) than C6–C7 and C4–C5. Seven patients were injured from vehicle accidents, 3 in sports accidents (skiing or diving), 2 fell from a tree, 1 fell down the stairs and 1 had an undetermined accident (alcoholism). Three became quadriplegic, 4 presented with motor root lesions and 1 had a medullary contusion. According to the classification of Harris [1], 8 patients presented with a flexion injury (3 bilateral interfacetal dislocations, 2 anterior subluxations, 2 tear-drop fractures and 1 a compression fracture). Six flexion-rotation injuries resulted in unilateral luxations or subluxations. Only 3 were pure ligamentous injuries, the others showed a ligamentous and simultaneous bony lesion (Table 1) discovered during the operation or on radiographs. Twelve lesions were seen on standard radiographs and 2 on functional radiographs. Six sagittal tomograms and 6 axial computed tomograms showed associated fractures but provided little useful information for the operative indication. When the bony lesions did not explain the neurologic lesions, we utilized myelography. It was done for 3 patients and showed no herniated disk. A magnetic resonance performed for a facet fracture with subluxation also did not bring additional information.

Table 1. *Anatomical Lesions*

Isolated ligamentous lesions:	3
Ligamentous and bony lesions:	11
Fracture of the lamina:	7
Fracture of the articular facet:	7
Fracture of the spinous process:	1
Fracture of the pedicle:	1
Fracture of the corpus:	1
Tear-drop fracture:	2

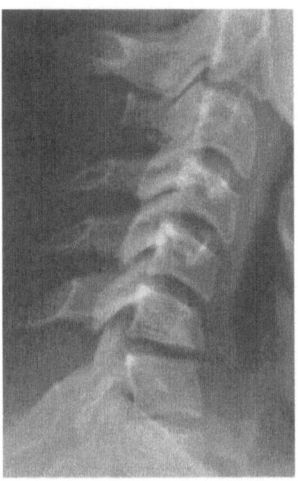   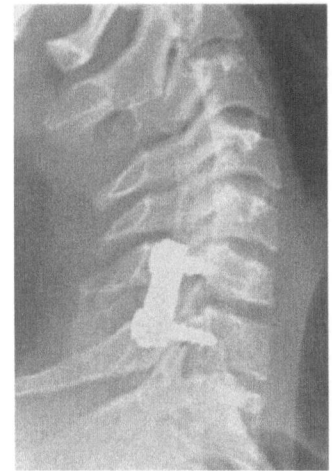

Fig. 1   Fig. 2

Fig. 1. 24-year-old man with medullary contusion. C6–C7 instability 2 months after
the accident

Fig. 2. Same patient as Fig. 1. 2½ months after the operation. A very good result

The radiologic instabilities were analyzed according to the 4 criteria described by Louis [2]. It was interesting to notice that 2 patients presented with
only one positive criterion. There were two unsatisfactory reductions in
minerva plaster. One tear-drop fracture and one pure ligamentous lesion of
a quadriplegic had no positive criterion. When the vertebrae were displaced,
the reduction was accomplished by traction with a Gardner skull clamp for
6 patients and with a Glisson for 1 patient. On an average 2 days were needed
with a traction of 2 to 20 kg to produce reduction. As the patients did not all
arrive at our hospital as an emergency, the mean time between the accident
and the operation was 7 days if no reduction was necessary and 11 days for
the patient who required a reduction. One level was osteosynthesized 6 times
(Figs. 1 and 2) and in 8 cases two levels were fused. This concerned our first
patients or the very unstable lesions. Eight bony grafts between the facets or
laminae were required. One laminectomy, one facettectomy and one
foraminotomy were also done to decompress the nerve. In the cases of very
unstable lesions, 3 required that an additional interspinous wiring be added,
as did a patient who suffered from bilateral locked facets in whom we also
did a laminectomy (Figs. 3 and 4). As a security, we prescribed for 8 weeks
a comfortable rigid molded thermoplast minerva; the quadriplegics had no
minerva prescribed.

    For complications, we had 2 imperfect reductions. These were in 2 pa-
tients operated 3 weeks after the accident and fibrosis hindered the facets' full

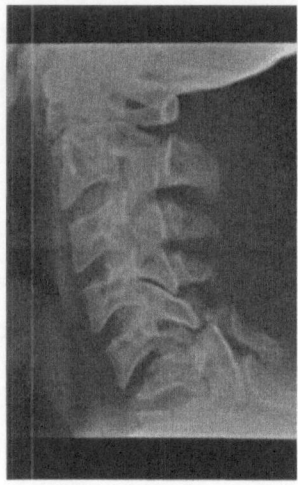
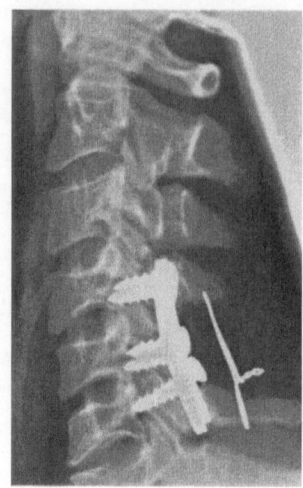

Fig. 3   Fig. 4

Fig. 3. 47-year-old man. C5–C6 bilateral locked facets. C5–C6 left motor root lesion

Fig. 4. Same patient as Fig. 2. 8 months after reduction and laminectomy of C5. Average result

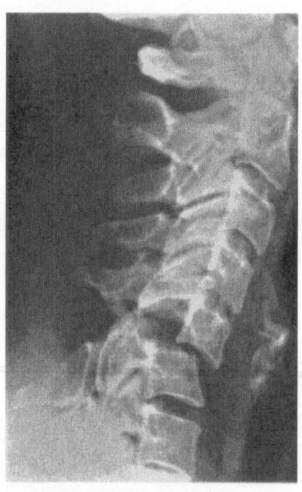

Fig. 5. 50-year-old woman. C5–C6 luxation. No neurologic lesion

reduction. One quadriplegic died of pneumonia and one other suffered from a urinary infection. We had no neurologic or bony complications. The patients stayed at the hospital for a mean time of 3 weeks with the exception of the 2 quadriplegics.

On an average the follow-up of the 13 patients was 10 months. Among the 4 radicular deficits, 2 recovered completely and 2 still showed improve-

Table 2. *Methods of Evaluation*

Very good results

Objective: no neurologic sequelae, except eventually tendinous areflexia or discrete superficial sensitive disturbance; unlimited cervical motion.

Subjective: no pain; recovery of usual professional or sportive activities.

Good results

Objective: discrete neurologic sequelae, not disturbing daily life (work or sport): paresis or light sensitive disturbance; cervical motion little or no limitation.

Subjective: unusual cervical or radicular pain; recovery of usual professional or sportive activities.

Average results

Objective: neurologic sequelae disturbing daily life (important paresis, paralysis, sensation disturbance); limited cervical motion.

Subjective: frequent cervical or radicular pain; definitive partial incapacity of working in the usual profession.

Poor results

Objective: heavy neurologic sequelae disturbing usual daily life; cervical motion very limited.

Subjective: daily pain; definitive total incapacity to working in the usual profession or professional rehabilitation.

---

ment at the last control. The medullary contusion also recovered completely, but the 2 quadriplegics did not recover. On an average the incapacity to work was 4 months and was in direct relation to the neurologic lesions. The evaluation of the results was made taking into account the neurologic or orthopaedic sequelae and also the period of inability to work or participating in sports (Table 2). Seven patients showed a very good and 2 a good result. Two others had an average result; one had a depressive reaction and the other a persistent biradicular deficit which hindered him from working more than 50% of his capacity as a mason. The 2 quadriplegics had a poor result.

A stable posterior osteosynthesis with plates and screws, preceded by skull traction if the vertebrae are displaced and if possible with intubation under local anesthesia, was done on the patient who suffered from bilateral locked facets (Fig. 5). This avoids neurologic complications and produces a good and quick consolidation of the lesion with a comfortable postoperative immobilization. This consolidation is shown 3 months after the instrument's removal on these functional radiographs (Fig. 6).

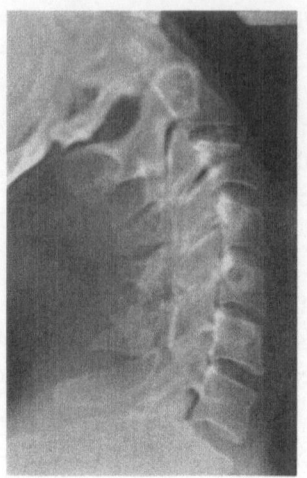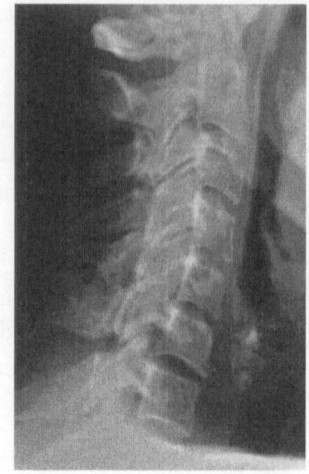

a   b

Fig. 6. Same patient as Fig. 5. Three months after instrument removal. A very good
result. a) Extension, b) flexion

References

1. Harris JH, Edeiken-Monroe B, Kopaniky DR (1986) A practical classification of
   acute cervical spine injuries. Orthop Clin North Am 17:15–30
2. Louis R (1979) Traumatismes du rachis cervical 1. Entorses et hernies discales.
   Nouv Presse Med 8:1843–1849

1.17. Intraoperative and Postoperative Complications of Internal Fixation with AO-plates

A. WEIDNER and S. T. CHIOE, Osnabrück, Federal Republic of Germany

Introduction

Indications for fusion of an intervertebral segment of the cervical spine include managing trauma, tumor, and instability which has been produced by an operative procedure (e.g. spondylectomy). Implanting bone will not produce adequate immediate stability. The cervical spine must still be immobilized after such an operation. Particularly with marked instability as in trauma or spondylectomy, it is often necessary to immobilize the cervical spine with external fixation (halo). This is considerably annoying for the patient. For this reason, procedures have been developed to create sufficient stability intraoperatively so that postoperative immobilization is not needed. Originally used in orthopedic surgery of the extremities, metal implants have been adopted for fixation of the spine. By using metal plates, postoperative immobilization can be avoided. However, this technique has associated with it the following disadvantages. By drilling the holes required for the screws, the esophagus, vessels, dura or even the spinal cord may be damaged; the plates may loosen and cause injury to the esophagus; and implantation of foreign bodies increases the risk of infection.

The goal of this study is to describe the complications occurring in a consecutive series of 116 ventral cervical spine spondylodeses with AO-plates. The follow-up period was greater than 24 months in all cases, so that ventral plate osteosynthesis in the cervical spine could be adequately evaluated. Also, the problem of screw loosening was analysed.

Material and Methods

All patients in this study underwent ventral AO plating by the senior author (AW) in the period from 1983 to 1986. This population consisted of 73 (63%) male and 43 (37%) female patients. The age-group distribution is shown in Table 1. The indications for cervical spine operations were the

Table 1. *Age Groups*

Years	Number
0–19	4
20–29	1
30–39	7
40–49	42
50–59	39
60–69	16
70–79	6
80–89	1
Total	116

Mean: 51 years

Table 2. *Follow-up*

Lost to follow-up	21
2–3 years	55
3–4 years	26
Greater than 4 years	14
Total	116

following: trauma in 17 patients, tumor in 6, rheumatoid arthritis in 3, intraoperative instability due to discectomies in 19, spondylectomies with myelopathy in 57, and postoperative instability (after Cloward fusion) in 14 patients. Corresponding to criteria outlined by White *et al.* [6] the index of instability was 5 points in 23 patients, 6 points in 32, 7 points in 46, 8 points in 12, and 9 points in 3 patients. The average value was 6.48 points. Osteoporosis was present in 5 patients and in an additional 3 patients with rheumatoid arthritis.

Plating across one intervertebral segment was necessary in 43 patients. In 61 patients one vertebral body, in 11 patients two vertebral bodies, and in one patient 4 vertebral bodies were removed. AO plates were used in all ventral plate osteosynthesis [1, 3]. Also spongiosa-screws with a diameter of 3.5 mm were utilized in all cases. In six patients with metastasis bone cement was employed, and in all the remaining 110 cases autologous iliac crest graft was used for fusion. The approach to the cervical spine was usually from the left side. First, the left caudal hole was drilled, then the left rostral, followed by the right caudal, and finally the right rostral hole. Details of the operative technique are in reference 5. All patients received antibiotics preoperatively. Postoperatively, a soft collar was worn for six weeks. X-ray views were obtained intraoperatively, after 6 weeks, and periodically up to 24 months or more after surgery.

Follow-up periods are listed in Table 2. The average follow-up time was 37 months. Follow-up for 95 patients or 82% of the series was greater than 2 years. Follow-up consisted of clinical examination as well as static and dynamic X-ray studies.

Intraoperative Complications

Injury to the esophagus, the vessels, the dura or to the spinal cord and nerves did not occur intraoperatively. In 6 patients, problems developed related to drilling the screws into the vertebral bodies. In 5 patients, the right upper screw (which by our operative technique is the last screw inserted) could not be screwed in place. Because the metal plate was positioned too far to the right at its initial placement, the esophagus could not be retracted far enough to the right. Therefore the right upper screw could not be screwed in place with the desired angle. In 2 of these patients (O.M. and D.A.) we had to remove the screws and the plate after 16 and 21 months.

Postoperative Complications

Analysis of the missing cases is shown in Table 3. A total of 12 patients died. They did not die from complications secondary to the cervical spine operation, and complications associated with their metal plate did not occur. Removal of the implant was indicated in 8 patients within the first 2 years and in 2 patients after two years. The reasons for instrumentation removal are listed in Table 4. In this group 2 patients developed pseudarthrosis. In one patient (Sch.R.), the plate was not positioned in the midline. This was a technical error in which fusion of the upper segment of this two-level stabilization was not achieved. We removed the plate and put in a new plate and graft with a good result. In another patient (B.P.), a fusion could not be obtained. To relieve the patient's pain we removed the plate and performed a dorsal fusion. This patient also had marked osteoporosis. In 2 patients we observed loosening of the screws within the first 6 weeks postoperatively, and to avoid injury to the esophagus, removal of the plate was necessary. In another patient (Q.K.), the plate was not positioned in the midline, so that

Table 3. *Analysis of Missing Cases*

Total number of AO-plates	116
Death	
0–24 months	11
After 24 months	1
Unable to locate	1
Removal of instrumentation	
0–24 months	8
Follow-up	
Greater than 2 yrs	95 (82%)

Table 4. *Reasons for Removal of Instrumentation*

Pseudarthrosis	2
Loosened screws	2
MRI	2
Infection	1
Young age	1
Bad position of the plate	1
Surgery one level above	1
Total	10

the screw was exposed to increased stress which resulted in screw loosening. The plate was removed after 2 months. The spondylodesis had become solid so new internal fixation was not needed. In the other patient (O.M.), the right upper screw could not be inserted. A screw was placed into the bone graft, but it eventually loosened. For reasons of safety the screw was removed after 16 months although further loosening of the screw had not occurred after the 2nd month. The plate had fused tightly to the spine so it could not be removed. In only 4 patients (O.M., Sch.R., B.P. and Q.K.) was removal of screws or plate actually indicated due to loosening of the screws. This corresponds to 3.4% of the total number of cases. Three of these 4 patients were female. One of them had marked osteoporosis. In 2 patients (O.M. and Sch.R.), 4 screws could not be placed in the usually fashion. The angle of the plate-axis to the midline of the cervical vertebrae is an important factor. With O.M. and Q.K. the angle was 8 and 25 degrees respectively. The average angle for all our cases was 5 degrees. The position of the screws was also measured in every case. The sagittal diameter of the vertebral body was divided into thirds. In 80% of the cases, the tip of the screw was positioned within the dorsal third of the vertebral body; in 9% the dorsal vertebral body cortex was perforated. Only 3 screws could not be positioned into or past the middle third. In 2 of 18 patients with loosened screws, removal of the plate was eventually necessary (B.P. and Q.K.).

The operations were performed at a time when routine MRI-studies were not available. In 2 patients, the preoperative diagnosis (myelopathy) was questioned postoperatively when an intramedullary tumor was suspected. To perform an MRI-study, the metal plate was removed in 2 patients, after 17 months (P.E.) and 43 months (W.J.) although neither the screws nor the plate had become loose.

One patient (St.E.) developed a deep infection within the first postoperative week necessitating removal of the plate and application of a halo. This patient's course was otherwise uneventful.

Removal of the plate was performed in 3 patients who did not have observed loosening of the screw or plate. In one patient (D.K.), the plate was removed after 36 months because of his young age (19 years). The second patient (D.A.) developed a pseudarthrosis after a Cloward fusion. After removing the Cloward dowel and after implanting the new bone graft, there was insufficient room for all four screws. Therefore, the plate could only be fixed with two left screws. The plate did not loosen, however, it was removed after 21 months. The third patient (T.K.) required a second operation after 12 months for root compression at the next higher level. During this second procedure the plate was removed. There were no signs of loosening at surgery.

Two plates fractured. One after 24 months (K.A.) and another after 48 months (G.M.). Instability or loosening was not recognizable in the flexion-extension X-rays. On follow-up of one patient (St.R.) fracture of a screw was detected after 37 months, which was without any clinical significance. Four patients developed dysphagia after plating, which did not last longer than 3 months. In the patient in whom a screw had loosened, dysphagia was not noted.

Discussion

Injury to the esophagus, the vessels, the nerves or to the dura had not occurred. The esophagus can be damaged of course in any ventral operation with or without plate fixation [4]. Injuries secondary to loosening of screws can be avoided. The position of the screws should be documented intraoperatively and checked after 6 days and again after 6 weeks. Loosening can be recognized early, and in such cases the implants must be removed. In 10 patients (8.6%), the metal plate or the screws were removed. In one case removal of the plate was indicated because of an infection. Our series does not prove that metal plates produce a higher risk of infection. The eventual removal of a plate does not appear absolutely indicated in the juvenile age group. Though in one adolescent we removed the instrumentation, in the other three patients, who were all younger than 20 years and in whom we left the instruments in, no ill effects resulted. In the case where the plate was removed during a second procedure at the next higher level, the second pathology was not due to the plate or the original operation. The "prophylactic" removal of a plate in poor position in which solid spondylodesis has occurred is not necessary. Incorrectly positioned plates are attributed to poor technique, and their removal in our series was not a consequence of failure of the spondylodesis. A loosening of a plate was not noted. The loosening of screws observed in 4 patients (3.4%) was a consequence of poor operative technique. All 4 screws should always be screwed into the dorsal third of the vertebral body to avoid loosening. Perforation of the vertebral body cortex is not necessary for adequate fixation. The longitudinal axis of the plate should not be angled with respect to the midline of the cervical spine by greater than 5 degrees. By paying attention to these recommendations, any loosening can be prevented or at least minimalized. In 2–4% of all ventral fusions, one must anticipate that the implants will require eventual removal. Usually, the spondylodesis is solid by that time so that external immobilization will not be necessary after removal. One should bear in mind that the halo-system is not without complications and that when employing the halo, sufficient immobilization cannot always be obtained [2, 7].

Based on our study, spondylodesis with the addition of an AO-plate is a safe method if the appropriate operative technique is applied. Marked osteoporosis is a contraindication for internal fixation. In our series all implants were performed in the setting of ventral instability (spondylectomy, tumor, and pseudarthrosis). Therefore our evaluation is applicable to problems associated with ventral instability including trauma. In fact, in none of the 17 trauma cases was loosening of the screw detected. So this method is well suited for traumatic instability as well. The advantage of AO-plate osteosynthesis is that it is a safe method and it produces sufficient stability so that all patients can be mobilized without external fixation therefore making the halo unnecessary. In addition the complication rate is low.

In summary, our results with ventral spondylodesis using AO-plate show that this method can be recommended.

References

1. Correia Martins MA (1987) Anterior cervical fusion – indications and results. In: Kehr P, Weidner A (eds) Cervical spine I. Springer, Wien New York, pp 205–209
2. Garfin StR, Botte MJ, Waters RL, Nickel VL (1986) Complications in the use of the halo fixation device. J Bone Joint Surg 68A:320–325
3. Gassman J, Seligson D (1983) The anterior cervical plate. Spine 8:700
4. Lindsey RW, Clark CR (1988) Esophageal perforation after anterior cervical spine surgery. Paper # 40 Meeting Cervical Spine Research Society 1988, Key Biscayne, Florida, USA
5. Weidner A (1989) Internal fixation with metal plate and screws. In: The cervical spine research society (ed) The cervical spine, 2nd edn. JB Lippincott, Philadelphia, pp 404–421
6. White AA, Southwick WO, Panjabi MM (1976) Clinical instability in the lower cervical spine. A review of past and current concepts. Spine 1:15
7. Whitehill R, Richman JA, Glaser JA (1986) Failure of immobilization of the cervical spine by the halo vest. J Bone Joint Surg 68A:326–332

1.18. Results of Long Term Follow-up of Lower Cervical Spine Fusions in 60 Cases

M. ARAND and O. WOERSDOERFER, Ulm, Federal Republic of Germany

The sometimes passionate controversy of the past years between the advocates of conservative and those of operative therapy of cervical spine injuries has been settled largely in favor of operative treatment. The central issue of this discussion has been the treatment of various forms of instability that can to a high degree be corrected by the development of suitable methods of internal fixation. Another advantage of operative therapy is that operative treatment involving reduction and restoration of the normal form of the spine indirectly causes decompression of neural structures, which makes for favorable conditions for the recovery of neurological secondary injuries.

Material and Methods

Sixty patients with traumatic instabilities of their lower cervical spine were followed-up on average 3.5 (1–9) years after stabilizing interventions. The average age of the patients was 37 years (range 18–81 years).

Twentyseven patients had fracture dislocations, 13 unilateral dislocations, 7 bilateral dislocations, and 13 patients had wedge compression fractures. Fracture dislocations and disco-ligamentous injuries were chiefly limited to the segments C5/C6 and C6/C7, whereas wedge compression fractures mainly affected the mid-section of the cervical spine between C3 and C5.

Multi-level injuries of the spine were observed in only 2 patients. One third of the patients had additional skull injuries or injured extremities.

In 41 patients (68%) accident-related neurological deficits were detected, mainly nerve root compression (45%). Correlation of the type of injury with the nature of neurological damage shows that unilateral and bilateral luxations mainly cause nerve root compressions, whereas compression fractures and fracture dislocations chiefly result in cord damage.

In 31 cases anterior stabilization of the cervical spine was carried out; in 22 cases posterior stabilization. In 7 patients combined antero-posterior stabilization was performed, as these patients suffered from severe instability

Table 1. *Complications of 60 Lower Cervical Spine Fusions*

Operative complications	
Recurrent nerve lesion	5
Neurological deterioration	3
Infection (graft site)	2
Wrong segment fused	1
Jugular vein lesion	1

with an additional anterior vertebral fracture. Anterior spondylodesis was carried out with additional plate fixation in line with the technique of South-wick and Robinson. Posterior stabilization was performed with wires (13 cases), and since 1982 it has been performed with plate fixations according to Roy-Camille [4] or Magerl [1].

The total perioperative complication rate was 20% (Table 1).

Results

Fusion

In 59 patients fusion of the injured segment was achieved after posterior or anterior or combined stabilization. Following posterior spondylodesis there was one case of pseudarthrosis with residual mobility in the fixed segment without any sign of instability.

Reduction

In 48 (80%) of the 60 patients anatomical reconstruction was achieved. Residual malalignment was present in 12 patients. In 7 cases fusion with anterior spondylodesis was carried out in kyphotic position. Four patients showed residual subluxations after incomplete reduction of hemiluxations associated with the anterior approach. In one case an unstable segment with complete tetraplegia was fused in overdistraction. Secondary redislocations after spondylodesis have not been observed.

Implant Loosening

Thirtyfour percent of the implants that at the time of follow-up were still in situ had loosened. Yet in no case did this loosening result in secondary

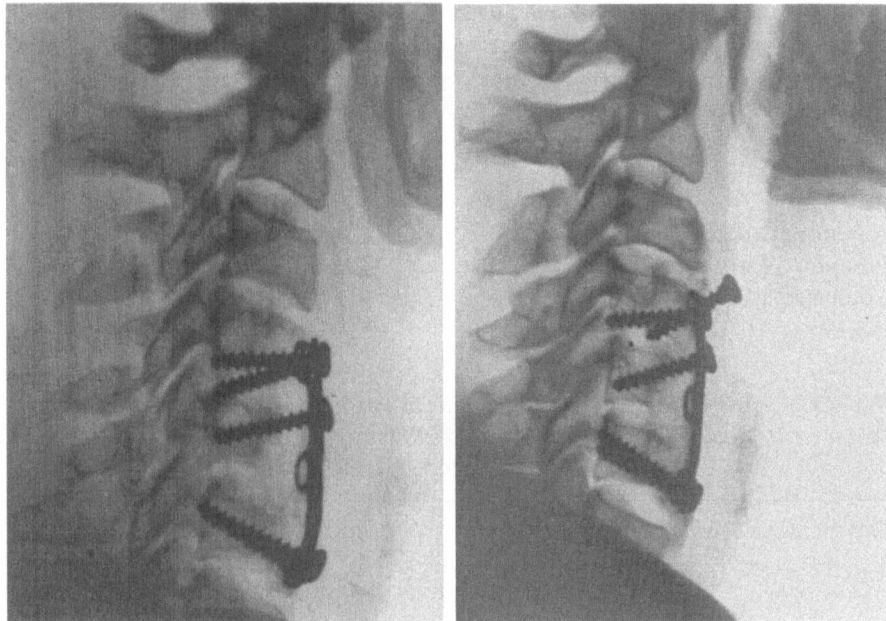

Fig. 1. Screw loosening one year postoperative

dislocation or deficient fusion. In 50% of anterior plate fusions loosening had already occurred after 2–4 weeks. It was mostly the upper screws that loosened by 1–2 thread turns. But this loosening stopped after fusion and stabilization of the segment. In 3 cases more extensive loosening (Fig. 1) was detected, requiring the metal to be removed after completed fusion. There was one case of extensive screw loosening leading to a spontaneous esophageal perforation, which healed without any secondary effects after removal of the metal.

Secondary instabilities or loss of correction were not detected in posterior loosening of implants, which mainly occurred with wire fixations.

Degenerative Formation in Neighboring Segments

The occurrence of degenerative formation in neighboring segments after surgical fusion was investigated with regard to surgical approach and reduction results. 14 of the 60 patients were excluded on account of already existing degenerative formation. Of the remaining 46 patients without preexisting degenerative formation, 21 (46%) showed postoperative degenerative formation. More than half (13) of the degenerative formation occurred after the anterior approach, whereas after the posterior approach it occurred in only 3 of 17 cases (Table 2).

Table 2. *Degenerative Formation in Relation to Surgical Approach in 46 Cases* (14 patients with preexisting degeneration are excluded)

Degenerative formation and approach	(n = 46)	
	no degenerative levels	degenerative levels
Anterior approach	11 (46%)	13 (54%)
Posterior approach	14 (82%)	3 (18%)
Combined approach	–	5 (100%)

Table 3. *Degenerative Formation in Relation to Postoperative Anatomical Reduction of 46 Lower Cervical Spine Spondylodesis* (14 patients with preexisting degeneration are excluded)

Degenerative formation and anatomy	(n = 46)	
	no degenerative levels	degenerative levels
Anatomical reduction	22 (59%)	15 (41%)
Incomplete reduction	3 (33%)	6 (67%)

The cause for this degenerative formation in the neighboring segments is not clear. It is very likely that it is not a genuine degenerative formation in the sense of a disk degeneration with arthrosis, but rather an ossification process of the anterior longitudinal ligament. Mechanical irritation of the anterior longitudinal ligament during surgical preparation and fixing of the plate is likely to be the main cause. Fusions with malalignment are also more likely to lead to changes in the neighboring segments than fusions with anatomical reductions (Table 3).

Neurological Course

Assessment of the neurological findings and the postoperative course was based on the classification by Frankel, with group D being replaced by root lesions.

Sixtyeight percent of patients showed preoperative neurological injuries; this percentage dropped to 46% after surgical decompression and stabilization. At follow-up (mean 3.6 years) 33% showed residual neurological symptoms.

As expected, no patient recovered from complete tetraplegia. Five patients with partial paralysis improved from stage B to stage C; 3 patients

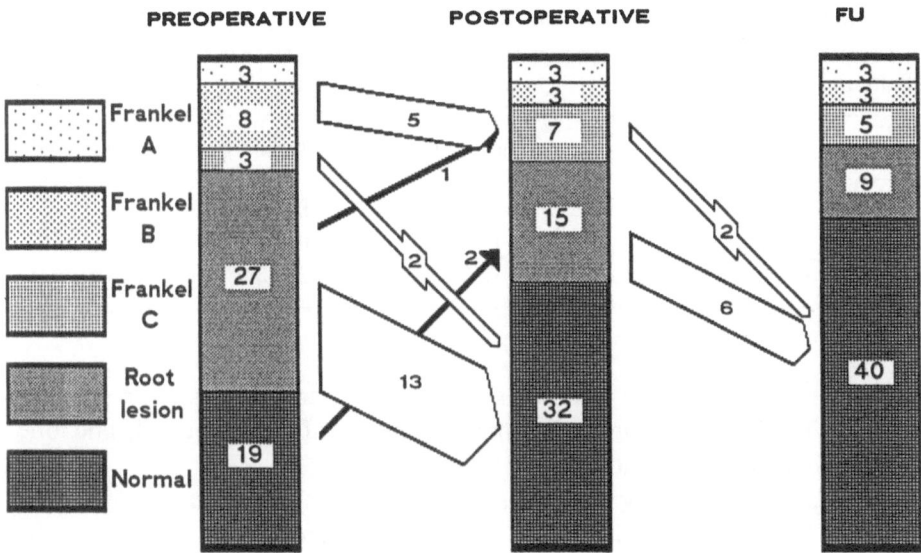

Fig. 2. Preoperative, postoperative and follow-up (FU) neurological findings in 60 patients

showed no changes at all. Two of the 3 patients with partial paralysis stage C recovered completely. Another 2 patients from this group recovered completely in the postoperative interval between operation and follow-up.

Root compressions show the highest rate of recovery. Thirteen of 27 patients improved completely postoperatively. Later on another 6 of the remaining 15 root lesions disappeared completely (Fig. 2).

Pain

Thirtyeight (61%) of the follow-up patients, according to their own statements, were completely pain-free. Twentyone (35%) had recurrent pain in the neck radiating to the shoulder girdle. One third of these patients were under constant medical and drug treatment. One patient suffered from continuous radicular pain.

Correlating the symptoms with the surgical approach (Table 4) shows distinctly that after anterior approach 74% of patients were without pain, compared to 50% after posterior approach.

Mobility of Spine Segments

Based on the superimposition method according to Penning [3] we determined flexion and extension mobility between C2 and C7 in 50 patients, 31

Table 4. *Pain at Follow-up with Respect to Surgical Approach in 60 Cases*

Pain and approach	(n = 60)		
	no pain	moderate pain	severe pain
Anterior approach	23 (74.2%)	8 (25.8%)	–
Posterior approach	11 (50.0%)	10 (45.4%)	1 (4.6%)
Combined approach	4 (57.1%)	3 (42.9%)	–

of which had undergone anterior spondylodesis, and 19 posterior spondylodesis. Thirtysix fixations were monosegmental, 12 bisegmental, and one fusion covered 3 segments.

The average mobility of the fused lower cervical spine was 36.5° ($\pm$12° SD) for flexion, and 17.5° ($\pm$11.3° SD) for extension.

Statistical analyses of mobility (linear regression, stepwise regression, covariance) of the patient's cervical spines produced the following results. There is a statistically significant correlation between total flexion and extension mobility and the age of the patients measured ($p < 0.0001$). Covariance analysis shows a significant dependence of mobility on both the patient's age as well as the length of the fusion ($p < 0.0004$), and for both variables together ($p < 0.0001$).

Taking into account the surgical approach we arrive at a corrected value for the average flexion/extension mobility of the lower cervical spine of 57.2° ($\pm$17.7° SD) after anterior fusion compared to 52.1° ($\pm$14.2° SD) after posterior fusion. The posterior fusions consequently produced a 5° decrease in mobility.

Discussion

With regard to their long-term courses, direct comparison between anterior and posterior stabilization methods for cases of traumatic instabilities of the cervical spine is not possible, as there are different indications for each of these methods. Posterior reduction and stabilization is to be preferred to the anterior method for irreducible locked unilateral or bilateral luxations as well as for fractures of the articular processes, and particularly in the event of root compression symptoms. Reduced discoligamentous injuries, significant vertebral fractures, dislocation of posterior border fragments involving narrowing of the spinal canal, or traumatic dislocation of a disk into the spinal canal are indications for anterior decompression and stabilization.

Long-term follow-up of anterior or posterior stabilization methods nevertheless permit conclusions as to the value of the individual methods regard-

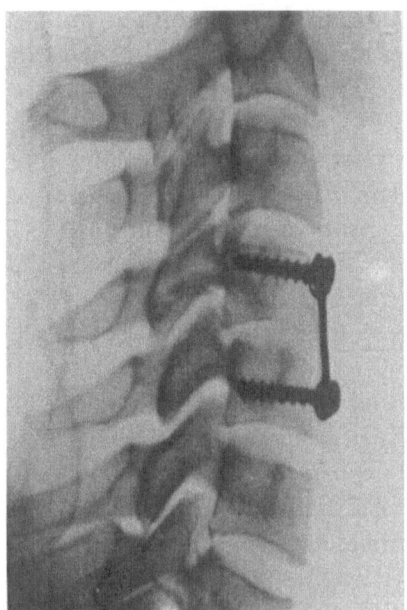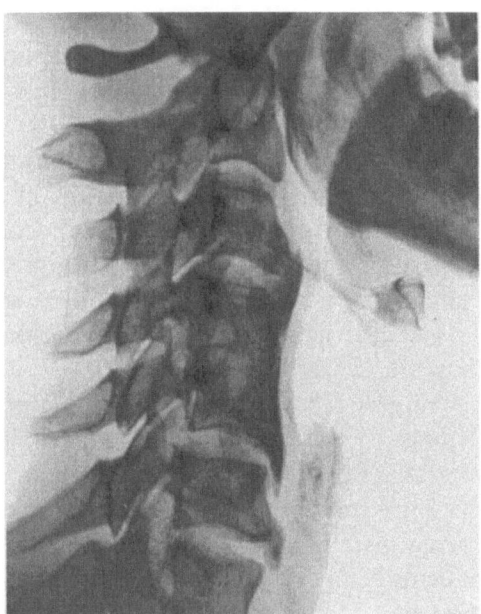

Fig. 3. Degenerative formation three years postoperative

ing permanent stability, neurological improvement, pain, mobility of the spinal segments, and degenerative formation in neighboring segments.

In 60 patients we were able to establish that the occurrence of pseudoarthrosis after anterior fusion with additional plate fixation was an exception. Neither after the anterior nor after the posterior approach with stable fixation were secondary redislocations observed. But after anterior plate fixation loosening of screws was observed in 50% of cases. The undersized, H-plate fixation, which, with complete instability, is located at a biomechanically unfavorable site on the flexion side instead of the tension side of the motion segment is the cause of this anterior loosening of the implant. These clinical observations were supported by biomechanical studies [5].

Plate fixation according to Morscher [2] is more favorably dimensioned, the screws are locked into the plate holes, and this overcomes the disadvantages of other methods allowing reliable anterior stabilization of the unstable spine.

Residual malalignment is caused by inadequate reduction, poor operating technique or choice of the wrong approach.

Anterior fusions of incomplete reductions results mainly in kyphotic fixations. Complete instabilities may result in overdistraction of the spine.

The occurrence of degenerative formation in the neighboring segments after surgical fusions was mainly observed after an anterior procedure. The cause of these degenerative changes is not clear. They are presumably not genuine degenerative processes but ossifications of the anterior longitudinal ligament as a result of mechanical irritation by the implant and damage to the anterior longitudinal ligament and the fibrous ring produced during surgery (Fig. 3).

Analysis of spinal segmental mobility after fusion did not show any significant restriction of movement, in spite of the so-called degenerative formation in neighboring segments. Comparison of mobility of a cervical spine after anterior or posterior fusion shows that mobility depends on the patient's age, the length of the fusion, and the approach.

Cervical spines after posterior fusion are on the average 5° less mobile than after anterior fusions.

Surgery-related scarring of the gliding layers of the cervical muscles and damage to muscle receptors are a possible cause for reduced mobility and increased pain after posterior fusions.

Thirtyfive percent of posttraumatic cervical-spine fusions resulted in recurrent pain in the neck radiating to the shoulder girdle, with only 50% of patients being without pain after the posterior approach, compared to 75% after the anterior approach.

Neurological injuries improved in approximately 50% of cases after surgical decompression and stabilization. As expected, patients did not recover from complete tetraplegia. Patients with root compression symptoms showed the best rate of recovery. There was no significant relationship between neurological recovery and operative approach.

But there were 3 cases of neurological deterioration with the posterior approach; this complication did not occur after anterior decompression and stabilization.

Summary

Long-term results of stabilizing surgery on the cervical spine after traumatic instability show a neurological recovery in approximately 50% of cases, with root compressions showing the best prognosis. The stabilization methods available at present have removed most problems regarding osseous fusion. Whenever indicated, anterior approach and anterior stabilization with rigid plate fixation should be preferred to the posterior procedure.

References

1. Magerl F, Grob D, Seemann P (1987) Stable dorsal fusion of the cervical spine (C2–Th1) using hook plates. In: Kehr P, Weidner A (eds) Cervical spine I. Springer, Wien New York, pp 217–221

2. Morscher E, Sutter F, Jenny H, Olerud S (1986) Die vordere Verplattung der Halswirbelsäule mit dem Hohlschrauben-Plattensystem aus Titanium. Chirurg 57:702
3. Penning L (1968) Functional pathology of the cervical spine. Excerpta medica Foundation, New York
4. Roy-Camille R, Saillant G (1972) Fracture complexes du rachis cervical inferieure. Tetraplegies. Nouv Presse Med 40:2707–2011
5. Ulrich C, Wörsdörfer O, Claes L, Magerl F (1987) Comparative study of the stability of anterior and posterior cervical spine fixation procedures. Arch Orthop Trauma Surg 106:226–231

1.19. Intersomatic Arthrodesis of the Cervical Spine with Autologous Bone Graft

J. M. Vieira, J. J. Reis, and C. T. Freitas, Lisboa, Portugal

Summary

Traumatic pathology of the cervical spine often requires the surgical immobilization of the injured area. Regarding the intersomatic arthrodesis of the cervical spine, two methods are used both alone and jointly. They are the use of a bone graft and the osteosynthesis with implant material. We strongly advise the use of the autologous bone graft alone. In a few and very special cases do we use osteosynthesis material.

Introduction

Cervical spine surgery has improved considerably due to the effort of investigators studying the pathophysiology of lesions and contribution made in the field of biomechanics and biomaterials.

At the same time the "imaging" of the human body provides more and more information, and is helping to fill gaps in our knowledge, thus allowing a better understanding of the post-traumatic pathology.

On the other hand we find that in the vast field of orthopaedic surgery, mechanistic thinking is acquiring a growing importance while the biologic issues are not always considered as they should be.

The attentive observer often finds surgical microworlds from which rise new techniques of immediate psychological impact based upon valid scientific foundation but not always proven valid as the time passes.

Regarding surgery of the cervical spine there is an uprise of several schools, each one with its own technology and directly related, these last years, to the new concepts of biomechanics and new osteosynthesis materials.

All these facts oblige us every now and then to reassess all the work already done so that, with a clear spirit and strong capacity of thinking we may be able to analyse the present situation in order to better estimate the past, understand the present and decide the best course of action for the future.

Material and Methods

A clinical review of 36 patients with recent or old traumatic lesions of the cervical spine was done. All of them received treatment at our university clinic of Orthopaedics, Hospital of Santa Maria, consisting of an anterior intersomatic arthrodesis with autologous bone graft. Our aim was the clinical and radiological evaluation of the bone graft and most of all to evaluate long term functional capacity of the patient.

To the patients presenting with a fracture or fracture-dislocation of the cervical spine we applied skull traction, which was maintained in place for as long as we thought necessary.

In cases of dislocation the initial weight of the skull traction was increased every hour until about 24 kgs. Under the effect of such weight (which is reached in about 12 hours) most of the spine dislocations have a tendency to realign themselves. Whenever this result is not obtained, the patient is submitted to the effect of a muscular relaxant or even a short and light general anesthesia followed with a careful manipulation.

The reduction of the vertebral dislocation was usually obtained, leading to further treatment. In most cases, the vertebrae returned to their normal position.

In all the cases with fracture of the anterior cervical spine or the lateral spine (articular bone masses) we choose the intersomatic anterior arthrodesis. We performed this surgery about one or two weeks after the accident, unless some pressing motive obliged us to operate earlier.

The approaches we made were the anterior one (the most often used) or the lateral one.

Before performing the anterior arthrodesis of the cervical spine (intersomatic) we always removed the injured intervertebral disc. Complete discectomy is performed in order to obtain the local decompression of the medullary canal and to prepare a "bone bed" which is going to ease and speed up the process of bone reconstruction. It was frequent that minor radicular signs and symptoms vanished or become less apparent immediately after surgery.

The bone bed was prepared according to the Cloward technique (circular graft between two vertebral bodies) or in cases of a two-level graft, according to the usual technique.

To keep the graft in place we didn't use plates and screws, except in very particular circumstances. We only used bone grafts taken from the iliac bone, using the Cloward technique and in less frequent cases of a larger arthrodesis (3 vertebras) we took the graft from the upper third of the tibia.

After its placement, the graft may be stable or unstable. In the first case we remove the skull traction one week after surgery and the patient is protected with a Thomas collar. When the graft is unstable the skull traction remains in place for 3 or 4 weeks more and after its removal a Thomas collar is then used.

In the cases presented here the level of the lesions were:

two levels: C2–C3: 1, C3–C4: 1, C4–C5: 7, C5–C6: 13, C6–C7: 9

three levels: C2–C3–C4: 1, C3–C4–C5: 1, C4–C5–C6: 3.

About three months after arthrodesis, all the patients demonstrated a good fusion of the bone graft. There was a new arrangement of the local bone tissue such that by one year after surgery the two vertebral bodies form just one body (Figs. 1–6, 8). Usually the patient completely recovers the complete function of the cervical spine he had before surgery.

In one case it was necessary to reinforce the immobilization of the graft with osteosynthesis material (Fig. 7).

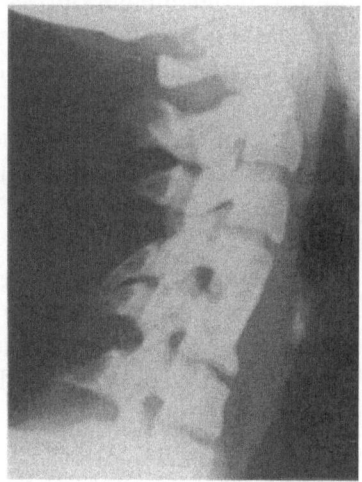

Fig. 1. Fracture-dislocation of C4–C5. Three months after the surgery. (Bone graft)

Fig. 2. a) Fracture-dislocation of C5–C6. b) Unstable bone graft. c) Four months after the surgery; bone fusion

Fig. 3. Fracture-dislocation of C4–C5, operated on 4 months ago (autologous bone graft)

Fig. 4. Fracture-dislocation of C5–C6, treated 10 months ago (autologous bone graft)

Fig. 5. a) Fracture-dislocation of C5–C6. b) One year after the surgery. (Bone graft)

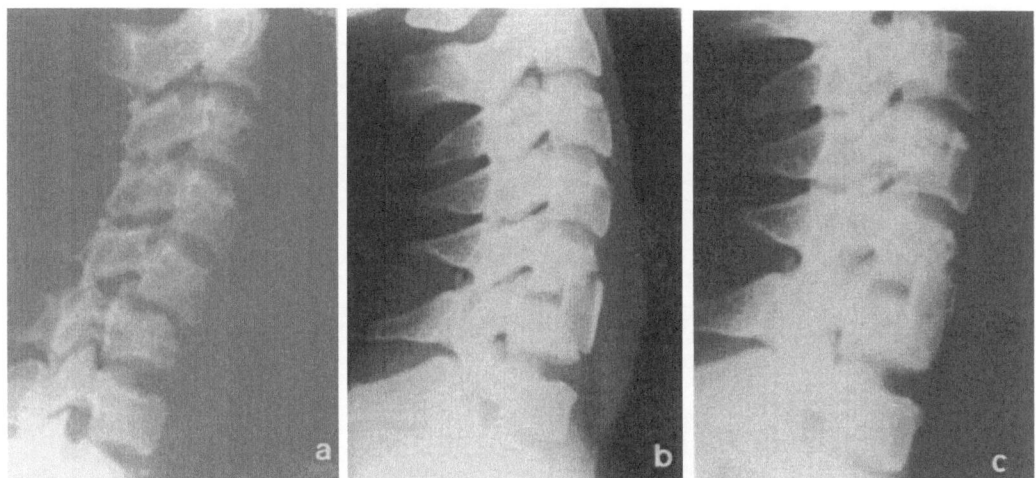

Fig. 2

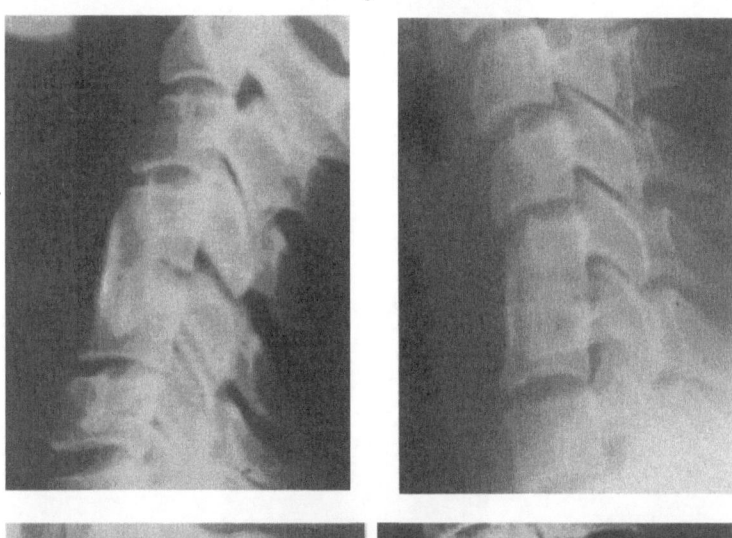

Fig. 3

Fig. 4

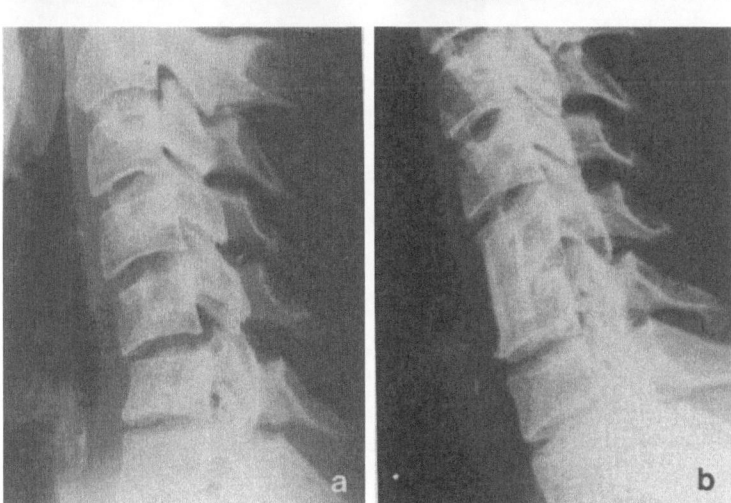

Fig. 5

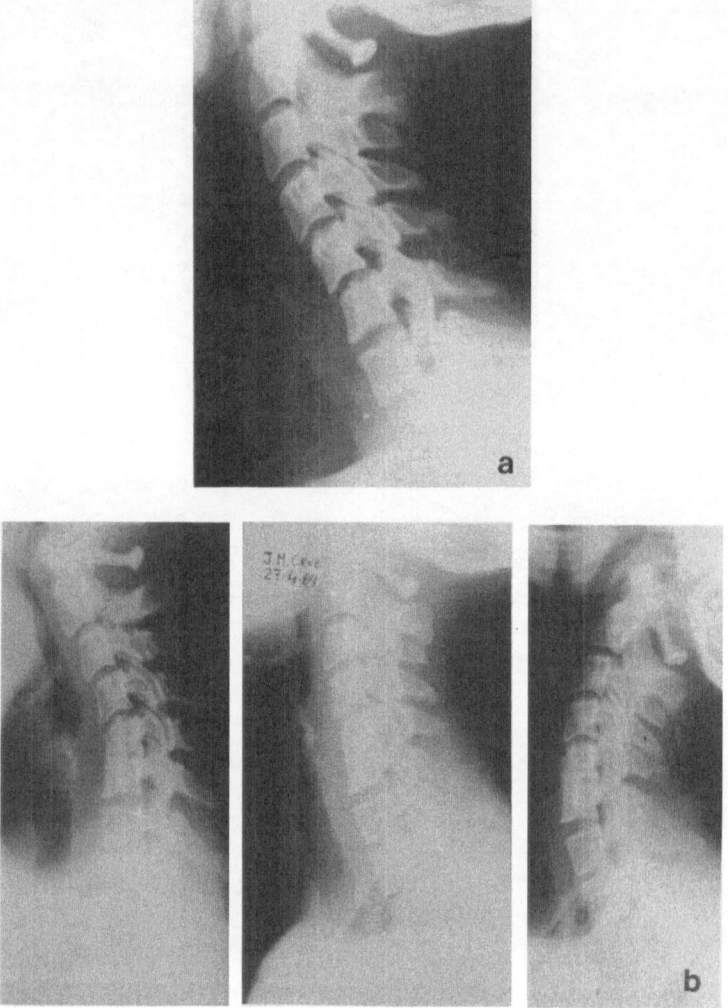

Fig. 6. a) Fracture-dislocation of C5–C6. b) Two years after the surgery. A functional study

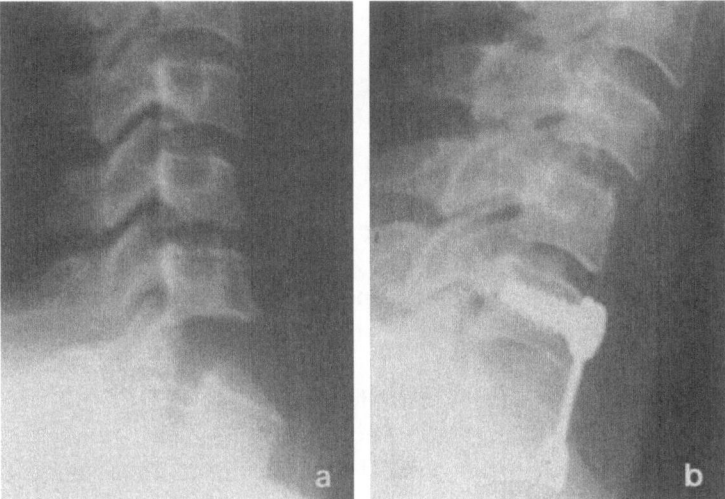

Fig. 7. a) Fracture-dislocation of C6–C7. b) Bone graft and osteosynthesis

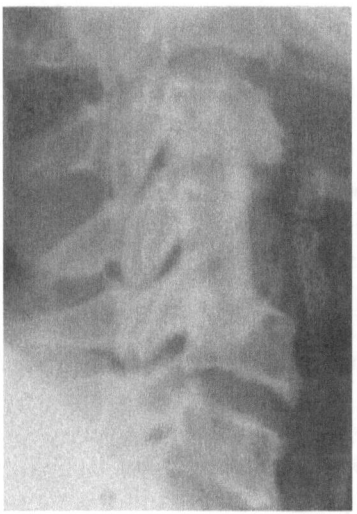

Fig. 8. Traumatic lesion of the cervical spine (sprain-subluxation). Narrow canal. Discectomy and two levels arthrodesis with autologous bone graft was done

Conclusions

A) The anterior intersomatic arthrodesis of the cervical spine with an autologous graft has proved to be a good therapeutic method.

B) There is no reason to discontinue this method or to minimize its value.

C) If justified by particular pathoanatomical or biomechanical circumstances we must then, for security reasons, use osteosynthesis material.

1.20. Diaphragm Pacing in Quadriplegic Patients

H. DE BOECK, W. VINCKEN, and B. CHAM, Brussels, Belgium

Introduction

Severe injuries in the upper cervical spine may result in permanent impairment of diaphragmatic function, so that these patients are dependent on some form of artificial respiration for the rest of their lives.

Diaphragmatic pacing can help these patients by implanting an electronic pacemaker which provides full-time ventilatory support. This system works by the application of repetitive electrical pulses to the phrenic nerve which results in rhythmic contraction of the diaphragm.

The system is a radiofrequency unit which consists of an *external radiofrequency transmitter,* an *antenna* which is taped to the skin of the patient over the subcutaneously implanted *receiver.* The receiver translates the radiowaves from the external transmitter into an electrical current which stimulates the phrenic nerve via the *phrenic nerve electrode.*

Indication – Selection of Patients

Artificial stimulation of the diaphragm is only indicated in a selected group of patients [3, 4, 8]. Candidates for pacing are patients who require chronic ventilatory support because of upper motor neuron respiratory muscle paralysis. This includes quadriplegic patients with complete (C1–C2) or partial (C3–C4–C5) interruption of the motor neurons of the phrenic nerves. Another indication is central hypoventilation. Before proceeding with diaphragmatic pacemaker insertion one must be certain that the patient has a normal or near normal phrenic nerve, diaphragmatic muscle, and lungs.

Therefore, selecting candidates is essential [1, 4, 8]. A patient with a recent spinal cord injury should not be considered as a candidate for pacing until the possible recovery of normal function has been excluded.

The following screening tests should be carried out before implantation of a diaphragm pacemaker:

1. Respiratory center function

2. Lung function
3. Phrenic nerve and diaphragm function which consists of:
3.1. voluntary movement of diaphram observed at fluoroscopy
3.2. test for nerve viability by controlling diaphragm response to percuta-
    neous stimulation of the phrenic nerve in the neck and measurements of
    transdiaphragmatic pressure.

Surgical Procedure

The nerve electrode can be implanted in the cervical or in the thoracic
region. We prefer the thoracic implantation for the following reasons.

Because of variations of the composition and distribution of branches of
the phrenic nerve in the neck, stimulation of the nerve in this region may
result in only partial stimulation of the diaphragm. In the thorax on the
contrary, the phrenic nerve is a single structure which can be easily located.
Pacing in this location results in maximal diaphragmatic stimulation [4].

We prefer an anterior thoracic approach through the third interspace as
this gives a direct exposure to the phrenic nerve. The lung is retracted laterally
and the phrenic nerve is identified under the pleura. The electrode is implanted about 7 to 10 cm above the heart in order to avoid excitation of the heart.
The electrode should be placed near the superior vena cava on the right and
near the aortic arch on the left side. The electrode is placed behind the nerve
and fixed to the surrounding tissue.

A subcutaneous pocket is created through a second incision below the
breast to accommodate *the radio-receiver, the anode* and *the electrode junctions.* The electrode wire and connector attached to the phrenic *nerve electrode* are passed from within the thorax anteriorly into the subcutaneous
pocket where it is connected to the radio-receiver.

After testing the function of the pacemaker the wounds are closed. A
chest tube is left in place for about fourty-eight hours.

The other side is done two weeks after the first procedure. Pacing is
started two weeks after the second operation, meanwhile the patient is of
course still on artificial respiration.

Pacing Schedule

Full-time pacing from the onset is contra-indicated because of risk of
fatigue of the diaphragm, which may result in irreparable damage [2, 7]. The
diaphragm has become very weak in the time between the injury and the
implantation, simply because of disuse; so that it will be very sensitive to
fatigue by electrical stimulation. Initial pacing is started during the day, only

for 1 minute each hour. This is gradually increased by 1 minute each hour until a duration of 15 minutes is attained after about two weeks. Should fatigue occur, which can be observed by a drop in tidal volume compared to the initial tidal volume, then the pacing period should be reduced and the rest period increased. If this is not done, fatigue will irreversibly damage the diaphragm muscle.

After two weeks the duration of pacing can be increased by 5 minutes until a duration of 30 minutes is obtained. This can then be gradually increased alternating with equal periods of rest, until 12 hours of pacing is achieved. Pacing is further increased until a 24 hour period is achieved so that the patient can be completely independent of a mechanical respiratory.

Using this method of pacing minimizes fatigue of the diaphragm, increases the strength and endurance of the diaphragm muscle and permits 24 hours of uninterrupted stimulation of both hemidiaphragms [5, 6].

Case Reports

Case 1

A 23-year old man with paralysis of both hemidiaphragms due to traumatic luxation of the cervical spine at the C3–C4 level required full mechanical ventilatory support. Screening tests with electrodiagnostic studies undertaken one year after the accident showed his phrenic nerve and diaphragm muscles to be in good condition. After a bilateral pacemaker was implanted, positive pressure ventilation was gradually substituted by bilateral diaphragmatic pacing. His postoperative period and respiratory training were without major problems. The only problem was failure of the left receiver, which had to be replaced.

The patient is now independent of mechanical ventilatory support for three years. He lives at home with his family. He manages an electric-powered wheel chair with a chin control switch allowing him independent mobility.

Case 2

A 20-year old patient had a trampoline accident with a C2–C3 luxation and complete quadriplegia and bilateral diaphragmatic paralysis.

A phrenic nerve stimulator was implanted, which after gradually training of his diaphragm muscles provides 24 hours of uninterrupted stimulation. He was independent of his ventilator after 3 months and returned home.

Conclusion

In patients with respiratory paralysis, full-time ventilatory support can be achieved through stimulation of the phrenic nerve which results in rhythmic contraction of the diaphragm. As the quadriplegic patient needs only a relatively small amount of air to meet his basal tidal volume requirements, supplementing mechanical ventilation is not needed. Phrenic nerve pacing is a practical method of supporting ventilation in carefully selected patients. Benefits of phrenic nerve pacing include:
- facilitates return from hospital to home;
- achieves near normal breathing, eating, drinking and speaking;
- pulmonary infections are reduced;
- pacing is totally silent, requires only an apparatus of small size and allows the patient to be more mobile.

References

1. Brouillette RT, Ilbawi MN, Hunt CE (1983) Phrenic nerve pacing in infants and children. A review of experience and report on the usefulness of phrenic nerve stimulation studies. J Ped 102:32–39
2. Ciesielski TE, Fukuda Y, Glenn WWL, Gorfien J, Jefferey K, Hogan JF (1983) Response of the diaphragm muscle to electrical stimulation of the phrenic nerve: a histochemical and ultrastructural study. J Neurosurg 58:92–100
3. Glenn WWL, Gee JBL, Cole DR, Farmer WC, Shaw RK, Beckman CB (1978) Combined central alveolar hypoventilation and upper airway obstruction. Am J Med 64:50–60
4. Glenn WWL, Hogan JF, Phelps ML (1980) Ventilatory support of the quadriplegic patients with respiratory paralysis by diaphragm pacing. Surg Clin North Am 60:1055–1078
5. Glenn WWL, Hogan JF, Loke JSO, Ciesielski TE, Phelps ML, Rowedder R (1984) Ventilatory support by pacing of the conditioned diaphragm in quadriplegia. N Engl J Med 310:1150–1155
6. Gross D, Ladd HW, Riley EY, Macklem PT, Grassino A (1980) The effect of training on strength and endurance of the diaphragm in quadriplegia. Am J Med 68:27–35
7. Oda T, Glenn WWL, Fukuda Y, Hogan JF, Gorfien J (1981) Evaluation of electrical parameters for diaphragm pacing: An experimental study. J Surg Res 30:142–153
8. Yernault JC (1984) Mechanical assistance in chronic respiratory insufficiency due to neuromuscular disease. Bull Eur Physiopath Respir 20:467–470

2. Infection of the Cervical Spine

2.1. Infected Cervical Spine in Five Cases

E. Denaro, Catania, Italy, and P. Kehr, Strasbourg, France

Infections of the cervical spine are rare. Published incidences for cervical infections is 3 to 4% of all infections of the spinal vertebrae. All types of pathogenic microorganisms can cause cervical spine infections but Mycobacterium tuberculosis and the Staphylococcus aureus are the most frequent pathogens found.

We distinguish two types of infections, direct infection and indirect infection. A direct infection occurs secondary to surgical intervention or results from spread of infection from contiguous soft tissue such as the pharynx. Hematologic and lymphatic spreads are the cause of indirect infection.

The clinical presentation may be multifocal and depends upon the virulence of the pathogen as well as the capacity of the patient's immune defenses. The spectrum of spinal infections range from simple spinal pain with functional limitations and fever to complete destruction of several vertebral bodies with neurological signs. These neurological signs may evolve gradually because of progressive compression of the central nervous system by an abscess, or, present suddenly with immediate serious neurologic signs as a consequence of an acute collapse of an infected vertebral body.

It is important to obtain an early etiological diagnosis which can often be accomplished with a needle biopsy either transorally for high cervical lesions from C1 to C3, or via an antero-lateral approach, for lower lesions from C4 to Th1. When needle puncture biopsy is deemed too dangerous, we prefer an open biopsy, which is often more preferable if medullary decompression is required.

Treatment of cervical infections is not standardized. For some cases, simple antibiotic treatment will suffice, where as for other cases, a surgical approach of decompression and stabilization is required. Halo traction, draining of the abscess cavity, resection of the osseous sequestrum, medullary and radicular decompression, reconstruction of the vertebral body(ies) usually using autogenous grafts, are important aspects of surgical treatment.

The following are some examples derived from our experience.

– Case 1 (Denaro): Male patient, age 37 years, suffering from AIDS, first diagnosed two years ago, who complained of a worsening fever and neck pain for which he treated himself with analgesics without any medical advice. The initiation of neurological deficits began gradually but then progressed to tetraplegia which finally led to our consultation. The bacteriological specimen obtained with needle biopsy demonstrated brucellosis, however, this was inconsistent with the radiological appearence which showed excessive bone destruction for this diagnosis. The immunologic deficency associated with AIDS complicated this case. The patient died after some months, in spite of the surgical treatment consisting of decompression, and draining of the abscess.

– Case 2 (Denaro): A young girl, age 26 years, addicted to intravenous heroin for approximatively 4 years. Her symptoms were intense cervical pain associated with a progressive tetraparesis. She was admitted to the neurosurgery department, and a large cervical epidural abscess was diagnosed. She underwent decompressive laminectomy, which resulted in a slight improvement. The bacteriological analysis of the pus indicated Staphylococcus aureus. The persistant neurological deficit and the spinal instability after laminectomy made it necessary for an anterior operative approach to drain the remaining abscess and replace the three destroyed vertebral bodies with an osseous graft and an osteosynthesis with screws and plate. The addition of metallic material was tolerated well and the bony and neurological result has been excellent with a nearly complete recovery of the tetraparesis.

– Case 3 (Denaro): Male patient of 42 years presenting with neck pain and a significant right radiculopathy. The radiographs indicated a narrowing of C4/C5, so the initial diagnosis was soft herniated disc. The patient was treated by his general practitioner, without hospitalization, and with administration of corticosteroids. His symptoms grew worse and a high fever occurred. This led to the patient's hospitalization. The clinical picture at this time was a flaccid tetraparesis, the radiographs showed a complete collapse of the C4/C5 interspace with destruction of the two adjacent vertebral bodies (Fig. 1). Myelography demonstrated a complete block (Fig. 2) and emergency computerized tomography revealed the presence of a large cavity of suppuration invading the vertebral canal and the intervertebral foramen on the right (Fig. 3). This explained the initial finding of a right radiculopathy. The patient was managed with immobilization in a halo, draining of the abscess and needle biopsy, which provided the diagnosis of tuberculosis infection. Surgical management via the anterior approach with medullary decompression and large graft was performed with a good clinical and radiologic result.

– Case 4 (Kehr): Young female patient, age 35 years. The patient presented with a right radiculopathy and motor deficit in the days following a traffic accident in February 1983. The treatment was medical. However, in light of the persistent neurologic signs, discography was performed in March 1984, which revealed a soft herniated disc at C5/C6 (Fig. 5). The discography was followed by a fever of 38°, a sedimentation rate of 16/45 and a leukocytosis

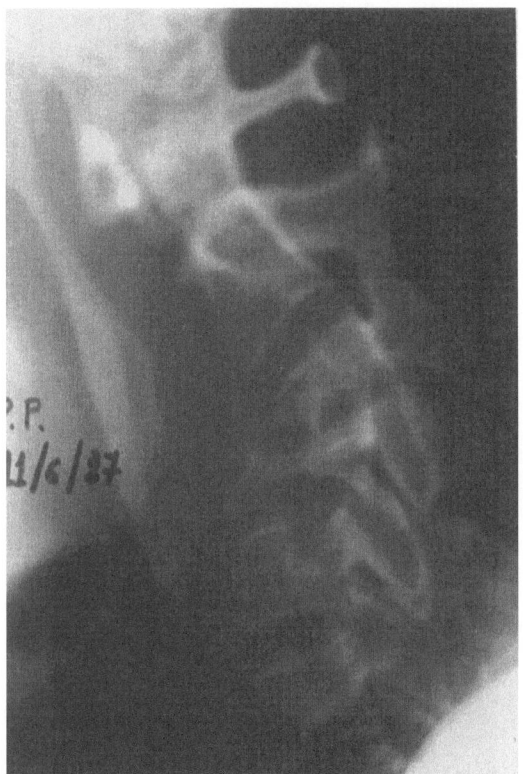

Fig. 1. Case 3: Lateral radiography showing the complete collapse of the C4/C5 disc space

of 11,000. However, the importance of these signs went unrecognized till 1985. In May 1985, we first saw this young woman for a progressive cervical radiculopathy. We managed this surgically with discectomy at C5/C6 by the anterior approach with Robinson graft and without osteosynthesis. The intervention was performed in August 1985. Postoperatively the radiculopathy improved and the patient had an uncomplicated course for three days. On the fourth day, a fever of 38 degrees occurred and the patient complained of difficulty swallowing. The diagnosis of esophageal oedema was made. On the tenth day, pus was expressed from the wound and the sedimentation rate was 70/100. The bacterium from the cultures was Staphylococcus aureus. X-rays indicated an almost complete expulsion of the graft and a serious kyphosis at C5/C6 (Fig. 6). At first, we reoperated from a posterior approach to avoid placing our osteosynthesis for stabilization of the kyphosis in the infected area. Under antibiotic coverage, a posterior osteosynthesis with plates was performed to reduce the kyphosis (Fig. 7). By anterior approach we then removed the graft and placed Gentamycin-impregnated-acrylic beads into the infection site. The patient was placed on long term antibiotic therapy with

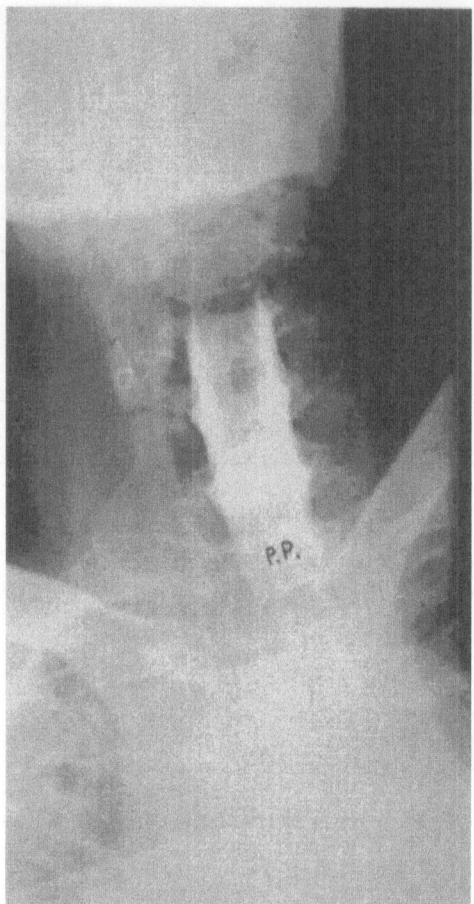

Fig. 2. Case 3: Myelograph with the patient in Trendelenburg position showing the
complete block of the contrast medium at C4/C5

a good result. We removed the posterior instrumentation in December 1988,
because of local posterior pain (Fig. 8). This case represents an iatrogenic
infection, whereby the discectomy awakened a dormant infection caused by
an earlier discography.

– Case 5 (Kehr): Male patient of 75 years, operated in May 1975 by the
anterior approach for management of cervical Pott's disease at C5/C6/C7
which had produced tetraparesis. Of interest in this case is the diagnosis
which had been made by needle biopsy of a left subclavicular cold abscess,
and in the operative management which required ligature of the right vertebral artery. Indeed, with the diagnosis of Pott's disease being certain we went
ahead with surgical management without any further diagnostic examinations. In particular we did not perform vertebral arteriography because there
was no indication that this vessel would be involved in the surgical treatment.

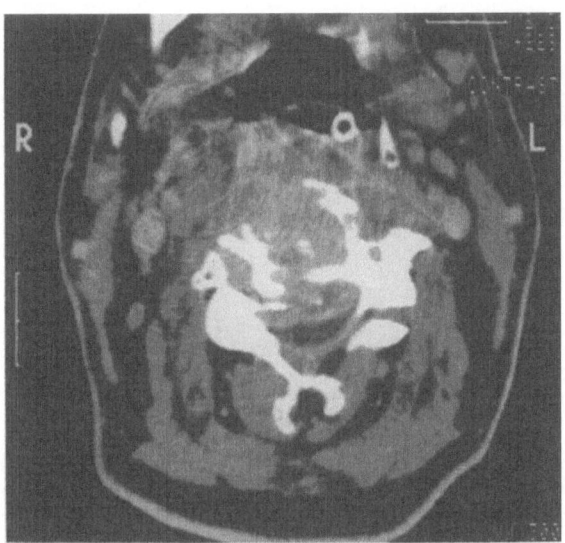

Fig. 3. Case 3: CT axial scan through the C4/C5 disc. The abscess is seen invading the spinal canal anteriorely and with a predominance at the right side

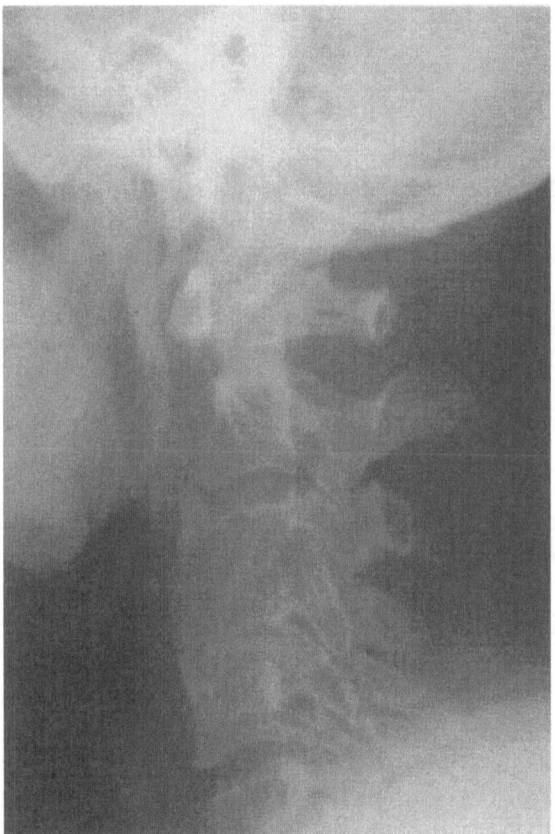

Fig. 4. Case 3: Post-operative lateral radiography showing the good reconstruction after corpectomy of C5 and bone graft between C4–C6

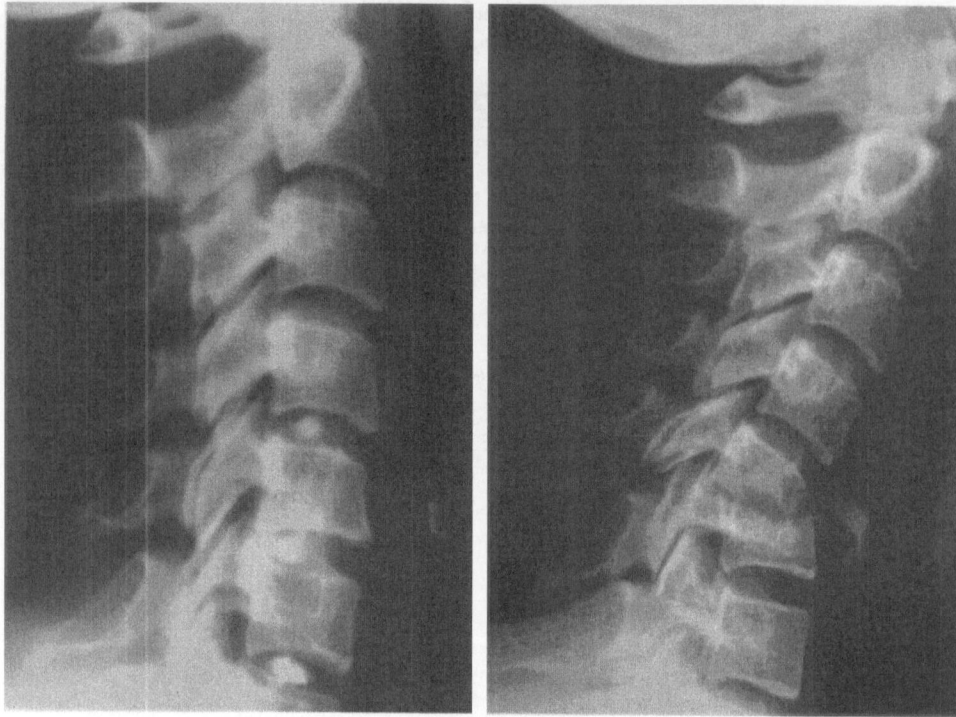

Fig. 5   Fig. 6

Fig. 5. Case 4: The initial discography which was made at another institution showing the disc herniation at C5/C6 which was initially treated medically. The discograph
was followed by subclinical infection after the entry of the pathogen

Fig. 6. Case 4: Lateral radiography showing the expulsion of the graft with the
abscess and the significant cervical kyphosis which had resulted

The patient's neck went into serious kyphosis, secondary to collapse of the
infected vertebral bodies. Our approach to the prevertebral space was from
the right side, the side with the predominant pathology. During this procedure we experienced difficulties. After having ligated the right inferior thyroid artery, we entered the prevertebral muscular plain and fell in a big cavity
filled with caseating necrosis. The right carotid tubercle was no longer palpable, which should have been a warning to us. After the abscess was drained,
we prepared the superior end-plate of T1 using the ronguers and chisel to
prepare the site for the tibial graft that we intended to interpose. Afterwards,
we were about to perform the same technique on the inferior endplate of C4.
In the area we believed to be the midline, a sudden and significant arterial

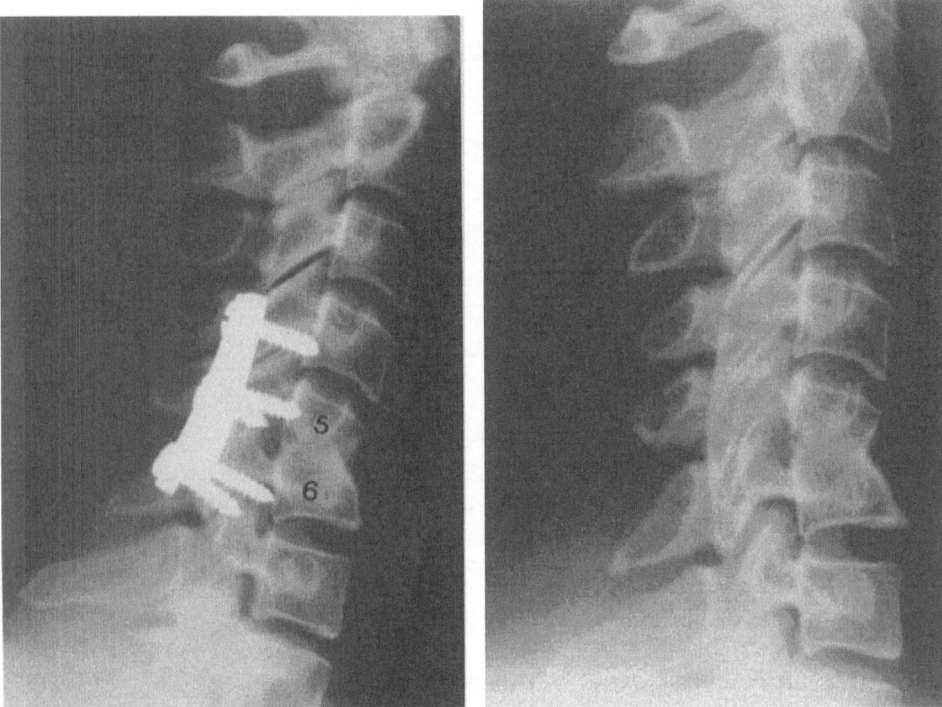

Fig. 7   Fig. 8

Fig. 7. Case 4: Lateral radiograph showing the reduction obtained by the posterior osteosynthesis of C4/C5/C6. Anterior debridement was aided by placing Gentamycin-impregnated-acrylic heads into the infection nidus

Fig. 8. Case 4: Lateral radiograph after removal of the instrumentation three years after its placement. Note the formation of both anterior and posterior osseous bridges between the vertebrae

hemorrhage occurred, due to transection of the right vertebral artery which looped abnormally between the collapsed bodies of C5 and C6 (Fig. 9). The distal end of the vessel retracted into the foramen transversarium of C4. The proximal end was clamped and ligated near the stellate ganglion. A transversectomy of C4 was necessary to expose enough of the distal vessel so that it could be clipped. The operation was otherwise completed as usual. Ligation of the right vertebral artery was well tolerated, and the Pott's disease resolved with regression of the tetraparesis. This case demonstrates the importance of a complete diagnostic assessment in a setting where normal anatomic relations are possibly altered. In future cases of this type we will obtain vertebral arteriography as part of our systematic preoperative evaluation.

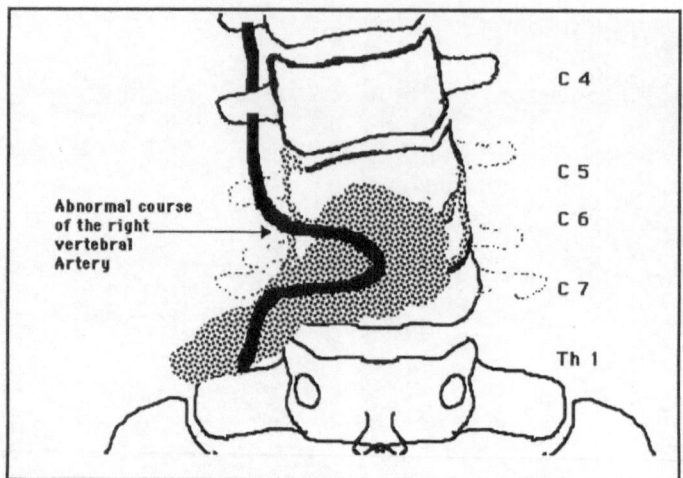

Fig. 9. Case 5: Drawing of the aberrant loop of the vertebral artery in a case of cervical tuberculosis with complete destruction of the vertebral bodies of C5, C6 and C7

Conclusions

These five case reports help to establish the relative rarity of infections of the cervical spine since out of more than thousand interventions on the cervical spine over the past ten years, we have only found these five cases. Even if some cases were overlooked (one or two patients at most), the total incidence remains very low. Our second finding is that the symptomatology at presentation may be misleading, often imitating a radiculopathy secondary to soft disc herniation or an esophageal syndrome. Performing needle biopsy is of great importance when infection is suspected, as well as other examinations including MRI. We found destruction of the vertebral body in all five cases. And in case number one the infection occurred in the setting of immuno-deficiency. The choice of surgical approach depends upon the location of the lesion. Our experience shows that osteosynthesis instrumentation may be placed in or near the area where the abscesses and the destroyed bone have been debrided. What is most important in the cervical spine, is to stabilize the lesion, which an osteosynthesis accomplishes best. This concept is already accepted for infected pseudarthrosis of long bones such as in the leg.

2.2. The Cervical Spine Infected After Surgery

U. RODEGERDTS, D. R. RAO, Bremerhaven, and A. WEIDNER, Osnabrück,
Federal Republic of Germany

Introduction

Complications after anterior cervical spinal surgery are infrequent, and usually due to technical error. Infection is a strikingly rare complication [2, 4], in comparison to infection in the thoracic or lumbar spine. In reviewing the combined cases of our two clinics, we came across four cases of deep infection over the past eight years. Curiously, the cervical spine is infrequently affected even in cases of hematogenous osteomyelitis, with figures ranging from 4–11% of all spinal osteomyelitis [3].

Possible Reasons for Low Incidence

1. The rich vascularity of the cervical spine, with the intraspinal arteries, the vertebral arteries, and the carotid system in close proximity may help keep infection here low.

2. The relatively atraumatic anatomic nature of the anterior cervical spinal surgical approach.

3. In contrast to the peritoneal cavity in the lumbar spine, and the pleura in the thoracic spine, the cervical spine is sheathed by a relatively larger proportion of muscle. In the presence of low grades of intraoperative bacterial contamination, it is possible that this richly vascular muscle plays a more active defensive role.

4. Anterior cervical discectomy is almost routinely augmented by fusion, with the use of bone graft. Disc space surgery in the thoracic and lumbar spine, on the other hand, is not so routinely associated with fusion. It is our belief that the use of bone graft helps keep the incidence of infection low through multiple mechanisms:
– The obliteration, at least partially, of the 'closed space' which would otherwise result from a discectomy alone.

- The early formation of vascular channels through an otherwise avascular disc space.
- The immobilisation which the graft provides may mask or allow resolution in many cases.
- The intention to subsequently use a bone graft necessitates the removal of all disc material and subchondral bone, thus lessening the possibility of an avascular sequestrum.

Factors Which Raise Infection Rate

1. The posterior approach to the cervical spine, possibly because of the large and relatively avascular ligamentum nuchae, consistently gives rise to a higher post operative infection rate, in comparison to the anterior approach.

2. Use of any form of implant, or polymethylmethacrylate, predisposes to local and even subsequent generalized sepsis [1].

3. The neighbouring pharynx and esophagus are a potential source of infection in cervical spinal surgery. The transoral approach to the upper cervical spine is associated with a high infection rate. Perforation of the esophagus by retractors, sharp instruments, or implants similarly increases the chances of infection [1].

4. The prior introduction of bacteria through discography.

Diagnosis

The clinical presentation depends on multiple factors, including the suppression of latent infections by perioperative antibiotics, host resistance, and the virulence of the bacterial contamination.

The mainstay of diagnosis remains clinical suspicion, and findings suggestive of infection or local pressure. Differentiation between the normal postoperative state and early infection is often difficult.

The Erythrocyte Sedimentation Rate (ESR) is usually elevated, but the interpretation here too is complicated by a normal postoperative elevation of the ESR, which may persist for weeks.

A bacteriologic diagnosis is helpful in determining the antibiotic to be used. Blood cultures may reveal the organism. Needle biopsies are usually ineffective, and an open biopsy remains the procedure of choice.

X-rays show an enlarged prevertebral shadow, and in cases presenting late, the radiographs may show a decrease in the disc space, with sclerosis and irregular destruction of the end plates. The implanted bone graft may be partially collapsed, or may have been extruded to lie in the prevertebral space. Radioisotope scans, CT, or Magnetic Resonance imaging may not be of definitive help in the early diagnosis of these infections, but CT and MRI may give a better impression of the spatial extent of the lesion, or the displacement of the graft.

Sequelae of Untreated Infections

1. Spontaneous fusion
2. Neurological deficits
3. Meningitis
4. Vertebral osteomyelitis
5. Increasing deformity
6. Septicemia

Treatment

Because of the varying severity of the clinical manifestation, the often self-healing nature of the disease, and the hesitation to operatively interfere in an area which is likely to be highly friable and adherent to the spinal cord, the cornerstone of treatment of these infections in the lumbar spine has usually been external immobilisation [5].

It is our belief that the essentials of treatment in post operative cervical spinal infection are surgery, antibiotics, and immobilization.

1. Surgery: For abscess drainage, or for the removal of all granulation tissue, and foreign material, and to allow for a better penetration of antibiotics into the infected area. At the same time, the previously inserted bone graft can be assessed, and replaced in cases where it is possibly involved by the infection.

2. Antibiotics: Unless otherwise suggested by culture and sensitivity testing, we have used a combination of Cefazolin and Gentamycin, both administered parenterally for two weeks.

3. Immobilization: In cases where the graft has extruded more than 50%, or is obviously involved by the infection, it is best replaced by a fresh iliac cortico-cancellous graft. Postoperatively, immobilization is continued in an extended plastic cervical collar for 12–24 weeks.

In extensive infection, after surgical debridement and removal of implants, we may be left with an extremely unstable spine. In these cases fusion of the uninvolved anterior or posterior side of the vertebral column, preceded by halo immobilization is advisable.

Brief Case Reports

Case 1. Infection presented on the sixth postoperative day as pus in the wound, after a C4/5 and C5/6 anterior discectomy and fusion, in a 51 year male. The Staphylococcus aureus abscess responded to drainage and antibiotic therapy.

Case 2. Infection presented four weeks after anterior C5/6 discectomy and fusion as minimal wound inflammation. The 65 year male refused surgery then, but subsequently agreed after two months, due to the increasing pain. The inflamed tissue was excised, and a fresh iliac strut graft inserted from C4–C6. Follow up showed an increasing kyphosis, and the patient was operated by us two years later for this angulation, with anterior graft and a plate. Two years after this surgery, the screws used in the internal fixation had broken, but the patient was asymptomatic, and no surgery was immediately planned.

Case 3. On the fourth day after a C5/6 and C6/7 anterior discectomy and fusion, a 38 year football player developed fever. Based on a complete absence of symptoms at the operative site, and chest X-ray changes, a pneumonia was diagnosed then. A blood culture revealed Staphylococcus aureus. The patient responded to antibiotics, and was sent home at two weeks. Five weeks later, he presented as an emergency, with a history of fever over the past few days, severe dyspnea, and a red and swollen operative site. The patient was comfortable immediately after abscess drainage and removal of a sequestered graft fragment, and remains satisfactory (asymptomatic) four years later.

Case 4. A prevertebral Staphylococcus aureus abscess developed three days after discectomy and fusion, augmented by an internal fixation plate, in a 52 year male. The abscess was drained, and the implant removed. Six months later the patient complained of paravertebral pain, and had a mild kyphosis. The patient was subsequently lost to follow up.

References

1. Bohlman HH (1978) Complications of treatment of fractures and dislocations of the cervical spine. In: Epps CH (ed) Complications in orthopaedic surgery. Lippincott, Philadelphia Toronto, pp 611–644
2. Cloward RB (1971) Complications of anterior cervical disc operation and their treatment. Surgery 69:175–182
3. Forsythe M, Rothman RH (1978) New concepts in the diagnosis and treatment of infections of the cervical spine. Orthop Clin North Am 9:1039–1051
4. Robinson RA, Walker AE, Ferlic DC, Wiecking DK (1962) The results of anterior interbody fusion of the cervical spine. J Bone Joint Surg 44A:1569–1587
5. Taylor TFK, Dooley BJ (1978) Antibiotics in the management of postoperative disc space infection. Aust NZ J Surg 48:74–77

Cervical Spine II
© by Springer-Verlag 1989

2.3. The Treatment of Cervical Spine Infections

R. Savini, G. Gargiulo, M. Di Silvestre, Bologna, Italy,
and G. Gualdrini, Cortina, Italy

Infections of the spine represent a rare pathology in highly developed countries. Furthermore cervical spondylitis is even less frequent than thoracic and lumbar spondylitis.

At Istituto Ortopedico Rizzoli in Bologna (Italy) over a period of 20 years (1965–1985) 32 cases only of cervical spondylitis have been observed, 29 deriving from various regions in Italy and 3 from Africa. In most cases (24) the process was tubercular (TBC), in 9 non-specific. The average age was 34 years (5–75) for the TBC cases and 36 years (8–77) for the non-specific cases. In both groups there was predilection for the male sex with a male/female ratio of 3/1. The TBC spondylitis involved the C1–C2 junction (8 cases) as well as the lower cervical spine (16 cases), while the 9 non-specific infections were limited to C3–C7. Among the 25 patients with infections (whether tubercular or non-specific) at C3–C7 level, there was predilection for involvement at 1 or 2 levels, probably due to the earlier diagnosis of the lesion. The clinical picture was characterized in both groups by pain, localized or radiating to the upper limbs, and by fever, particularly in the non-specific group. In 3 patients with TBC there were neurological disorders including progressive paraparesis (in 1 case) and quadriparesis (in 2 patients).

The nature and etiology of the lesion was generally diagnosed on the basis of the patient's history, the clinical and the radiographic picture. One needle biopsy and 2 surgical biopsies were necessary to confirm diagnosis.

Treatment was often conservative (28 cases), with only 5 surgical cases.

In most patients affected with non-specific spondylitis (6 out of 9) the treatment was conservative: an average of 4 to 6 20-day antibiotic Streptomycin treatment cycles were carried out over a period of 4 to 6 months; in all cases, healing was achieved after an average period of 10 months with fusion of the segments affected and with good reconstruction of the cervical lordosis. Surgical treatment was required in 3 patients with non-specific spondylitis due to the severity of the lesion in 1, or to solve a doubt in diagnosis in the other 2 (Fig. 1). All of them obtained a good healing with regression of symptoms.

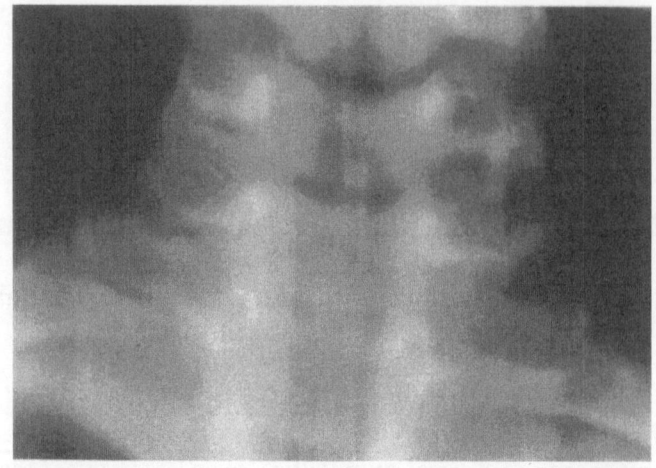

a

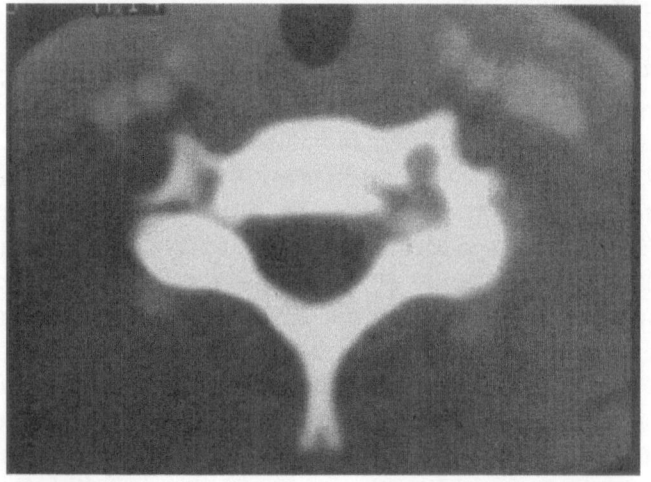

b

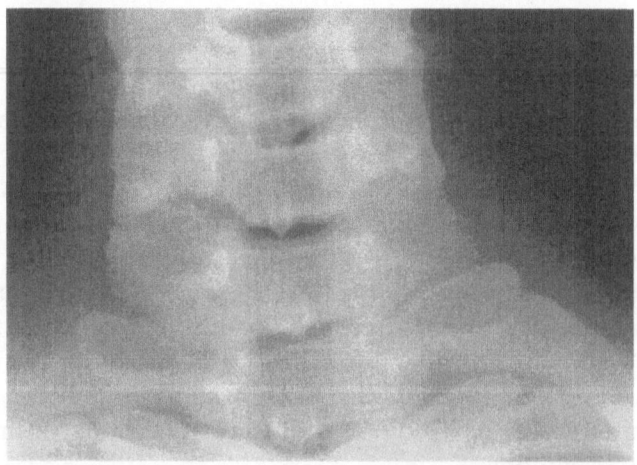

c

All the TBC cases with involvement of C1–C2 junction were submitted to orthopedic treatment with repeated 20-day tuberculostatic cycles and immobilization in bed with a Minerva cast or brace. This led to healing of all cases after an average of 13 cycles and 41 months. In the patients with C3–C7 TBC spondylitis, orthopedic treatment was adopted in 14 cases and always led to healing with no after-effects. Surgical treatment was used in 2 cases, for compromised stability of the spine and for the presence of severe tetraparesis due to spinal cord compression (Fig. 2). In both cases a complete regression of the neurological disturbances and stability of the cervical spine was obtained.

Conclusions

Treatment of pyogenic and tubercular infections has been controversial for a long time [1, 2]. Chemotherapy still remains the fundamental therapy in tubercular and pyogenic infection. Healing is generally successful over time with chemotherapy and immobilization of the cervical spine. Today, early diagnosis permits a prompt conservative treatment, before severe neurological damage or instability of the cervical spine occurs. The surgical indications are limited to particular cases [3]: when there is neurological damage and/or a severe instability of the spine (Fig. 2), if the infection is extended to more than 2 vertebrae, and finally if it is necessary to document infection in a questionable diagnosis (Fig. 1). These cases are frequently the result of late recognition of the disease due to mistaken diagnosis (Fig. 2) or its inadequate treatment.

Surgical treatment permits debridement of the abscess and removal of affected bone, thus allowing the medical treatment to act on healthy tissue. Surgery also permits the reconstruction of the abscess cavity with bone grafts, and the elimination of spinal cord compression. Surgery also prevents respiratory complications and the spread of the infection to the mediastinum. In this way a more rapid recovery is obtained. In severe kyphosis, surgery may be preceded by a gradual correction with a halo-cast which is maintained after the operation until healing is achieved. The anterior approach to the cervical spine between the carotid sheat and the oesophagus is generally preferred as an easier approach to the infection site [1, 3]. The posterior approach should never be used since it is inadequate for radical treatment

---

Fig. 1. Male, 14 years old with cervical pain and with a stiff neck. Note the osteolysis of the pedicle at C6–C7, in the tomography (a) and better documented in CT-scan (b). Open biopsy with a posterior approach was done due to a suspected neoplastic lesion: however, a pyogenic abscess was discovered. Follow-up at 3 years shows good healing and regression of symptoms (c)

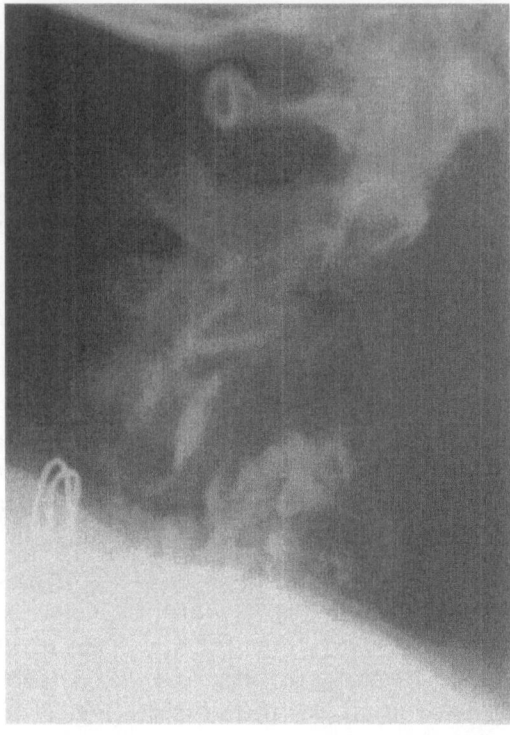

a

Fig. 2. Female, age 51 years with cervical pain for 2 years and progressive quadriparesis for 6 months. Severe osteolysis at C3 and C4. A posterior fusion with wiring
was performed, under the level of the lesion, and radiation therapy for suspected
neoplasia was instituted at another institution (a). Our treatment consisted of: surgical biopsy with debridement of the abscess and anterior fusion (b); the diagnosis was
a specific infection. Minerva cast for 3 months. One year later there was complete
regression of neurologic deficits. After 7 years there was a good clinical and radiographic result (c)

and mechanically unwise, due to the removal of posterior elements which are
frequently the only support for a spine destabilized by infection. The posterior approach is only useful in rare cases in which the infection is limited to
the posterior elements. Surgery may also take place in young patients. We
have in fact observed growth of the bone graft together with the rest of the
cervical spine with no alterations of spinal growth. Surgery must finally be
recommended if it is necessary to solve a doubt in diagnosis and for the
isolation of the etiological agent for appropriate antibiotics. Surgery in also
necessary in cases of negative blood or urine cultures, or when it is impossible
to carry out a CT guided needle biopsy due to the inaccessibility of the site.

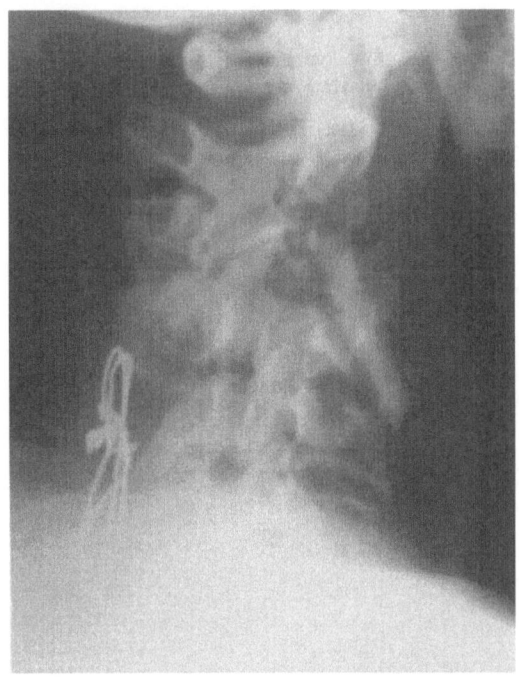

b

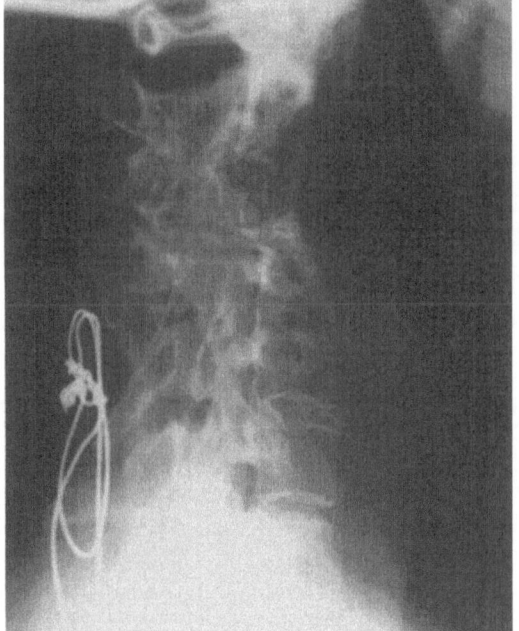

c

References

1. Hodgson AR, Stock FE (1956) Anterior spinal fusion. Br J Surg 44:266
2. Konstam PG, Blesovsky A (1962) The ambulant treatment of spinal tuberculosis. Br J Surg 50:26
3. Savini R, Cervellati S, Di Silvestre M (1984) L'instabilità vertebrale da infezioni. Ital Ortop Trauma 10:153

2.4. Surgery for Tuberculosis of the Cervical Spine with Reduction of Deformity

R. Louis, Marseille, France

Spinal tuberculosis is a disease now rarely encountered in the industrialized countries. The cases that do arise are usually seen in emigrants from developing countries. It is therefore useful to review our experience with our collegues who have very little experience in Europe. We report our extensive experience in this field based on 325 case histories of Pott's disease treated at Dakar during a five year tour of duty (1966–1971). In the context of two surgically treated cases of tuberculosis of the cervical spine we review the principles, methods and results involved in the surgical treatment of 52 cases of severe spinal tuberculosis.

Our work is a continuation of that of Hodgson, who advocates the direct anterior approach to the vertebral bodies infected with tuberculosis. Our contribution has been to demonstrate how to reduce the kyphoses before surgical fixation by pre- or perioperative reduction by means of spinal traction to restore the lordosis. Such reduction often functions as an emergency method to help reverse an associated neurological lesion.

Material and Methods

The first case is that of a 6 year old girl with a 16 month history of progressive spinal tuberculosis. When she was referred to us, she had a flaccid quadriplegia with a kyphotic deformity of 80° from C2 to C5. Head traction was applied with a sling and a weight of 5 kg and the appropriate antibiotics were given as well as a small dose of corticosteroids. After 10 days of traction, signs of recovery soon appeared and the child was operated via a right anterior pre-sternocleidomastoid approach.

Traction was continued throughout the surgery. The exploration revealed enormous loss of substance of the vertebral axis. The infected bone was excised down to the dura mater. The vertebral bodies were reconstructed with iliac grafts inserted between the odontoid apophysis and the vertebral body of C5.

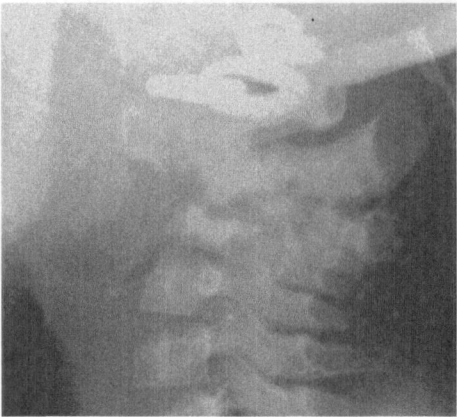

Fig. 1. Pott's disease at C2–C4, 80° angulation, flaccid paraplegia, in a girl 6 years old

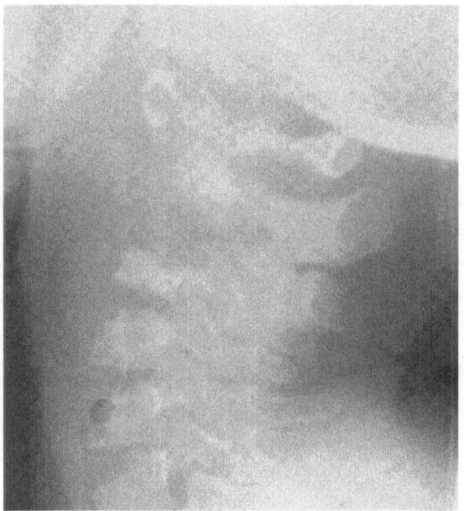

Fig. 2. Vertebral appearance after traction to restore lordosis, resulting in reduction of deformity with demonstration of loss of substance and commencement of neurological recovery

The child was kept in bed for two weeks and then, when neurological recovery was complete, a plastic minerva jacket was applied. Consolidation of the infectious focus was obtained after four months. Reduction of the deformity was complete, as was the neurological recovery. At three year follow-up the patient was neurologically intact, free of infection, and was without spinal deformity. The second patient was a young African woman, age 20 years, with spinal tuberculosis from C6 to T1 of 10 months duration

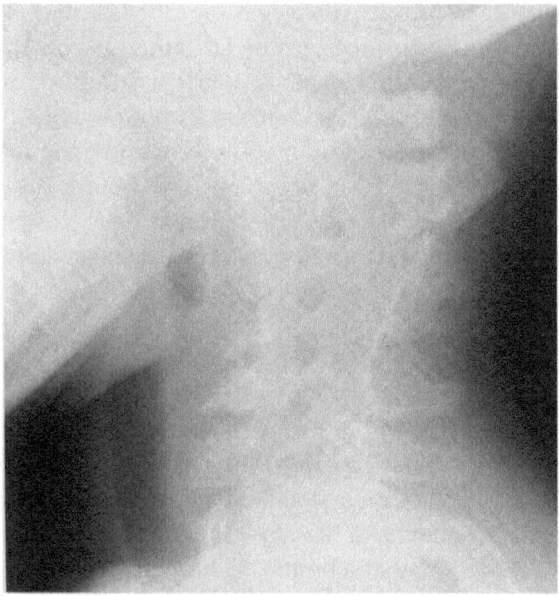

Fig. 3. Definitive result after reduction and fusion of C1–C5 with iliac bone grafts.
Complete neurological recovery was obtained

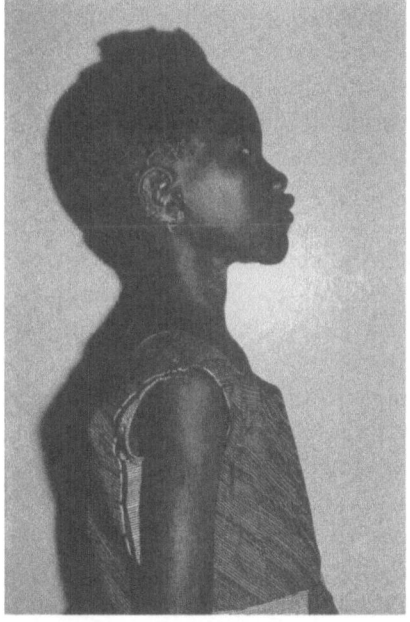

Fig. 4. Picture of the child one year later

and a kyphosis of 25° without paraplegia. Specific antibiotic treatment was given and surgery was performed via the left anterior route. The procedure included excision of the lesion, reduction under traction to restore the lordosis, reconstruction of the anterior vertebral column with iliac grafts and application of external plaster stabilization. She remained in the plaster for 6 months. Bony consolidation was complete, with total restoration of spinal structure. Seen again four years after treatment, the patient was without infection, neurologically intact and without progressive spinal deformity.

Discussion

Our definition of severe Pott's disease is that which presents with destruction of more than two vertebral bodies, with a kyphosis at the infectious focus exceeding 30°, and very often associated neurological complications. Although the current treatment of this disease is normally not surgical, apart from aspiration of an abscess or biopsy, a surgical procedure is indicated in severe cases in order to restore structure and accelerate neurological recovery. To Hodgson's classical method of excision of the diseased bone by the direct anterior approach, we have added complete reduction of the deformity using spinal traction to restore the lordosis. In fact, we have shown that the kyphosis of spinal tuberculosis, if it has not fused, can be reduced similar to a recent fracture of the spine provided the posterior articulations are not involved.

Reduction is accomplished subjecting by the spine to three forces. Two opposed axial forces of 5 to 10 kg, or sometimes up to 15 kg in the adult, in addition to one force at a right angle to the other two is applied to the apex of the kyphosis. The vertebral bodies can then be reduced using the posterior articulations as a hinge upon which the vertebral bodies can be aligned. The next step is to excise the infected bone, to decompress the anterior aspect of the vertebral canal and the dura mater, and finally to restore bony continuity by means of large fibular bone grafts lined if necessary with iliac bone grafts. We have shown in the laboratory that the reduction of a kyphotic deformity by applying two axial forces requires forces of 5 to 10 times greater than those employed in the method of reduction by three forces (two axial and a posterior force at a right angle to these). We have employed this technique in the acute setting to reduce a serious kyphosis and/or to decompress the spinal cord. The patients were fixed in a scoliosis reduction frame, similar to that for recent fractures of the spine. And then reduction was obtained gradually under radiographic control and without anaesthesia. Plaster fixation was then applied together with chemotherapy and antibiotics.

The value of this method is the immediate interruption of the vicious circle of compressive ulceration due to the osteolytic foci and the immediate decompression of the vertebral canal from the tuberculous abscess made worse by the kyphosis. The goal of reducing the tuberculous focus in the active stage is therefore threefold. 1) orthopaedic: structural restoration of the spine with elimination of the kyphotic deformity, 2) neurological: eliminating the angulation of the spinal canal and the compression of the anterior aspect of the neuromeningeal structures by the tuberculous abscess which act as a mass and which is made worse by the angular kyphosis and 3) the cosmetic result, especially in children, of eliminating the kyphosis in these patients.

However, we have found it necessary to operate on children in two stages. We first restore structure using an anterior approach with reconstitution of the spinal column with bone grafts. This is insufficient to arrest the kyphotic mechanism because of subsequent asymmetric growth. In these cases a second posterior approach is required to fuse the laminae posteriorly with grafting at the same level as the anterior fusion to achieve definitive stabilization of the initial correction.

Results

In 52 cases of severe vertebral tuberculosis operated at Dakar, there were two deaths. One due to a complication associated with blood transfusion and one due to an anaesthetic accident. The average reduction of the kyphoses after the period of consolidation was 66.5%, whereas the immediate postoperative reduction was 89.5%, indicating a mean loss of reduction of 15% during the months preceding consolidation. From the neurological aspect, 29% of patients showed neurological complications. There was complete or partial recovery in 86.5% and no neurological recovery in only one case. In all our cases, consolidation had occurred within a 2 year follow-up period.

Conclusion

Tuberculosis of the cervical spine sometimes presents in a severe form with angular kyphosis and a neurological syndrome. The employment of preoperative and/or postoperative reduction by vertebral traction aimed at restoring lordosis is the best means of restoring the structure of the spine, decompressing the neuromeningeal structures, and restoring near-normal appearances and dynamics. Reduction produces a loss of substance in the vertebral bodies which requires repair by the insertion of autogenous bone grafts.

References

1. Hodgson AR, Stock FE (1956) Greffe vertébrale antérieure; rapport préliminaire sur le traitement radical du mal de Pott et de la paraplégie pothique. Br J Surg 44:267
2. Hodgson AR, Stock FE (1960) Anterior spine fusion for the treatment of tuberculosis of the spine: the operative findings and results of treatment in the first one hundred cases. J Bone Joint Surg 42:295–310
3. Hodgson AR, Stock FE, Fang HS (1960) Anterior spinal fusion. The operative approach and pathological finding in 412 patients with Pott's disease of the spine. Br J Surg 48:172–178
4. Louis R, Conty CR, Pouye I (1969) Traitement chirurgical du mal de Pott chez l'Africain de l'ouest avec correction des gibbosités. Sicot, XIᵉ congrès, Mexico, pp 720–738
5. Louis R (1971) Ostéotomies vertébrales par voie antérieure. Rev Chir Orthop 57 [Suppl] 1:163–174

Cervical Spine II
© by Springer-Verlag 1989

2.5. Suboccipital Pott's Disease – Report of Two Cases

D. R. Ramon, A. Sanjuan, P. Fernandez de Retana, S. Garcia,
and J. M. Segur, Barcelona, Spain

Introduction

Currently osteoarticular tuberculosis [5, 8, 10] remains the most frequently observed extrapulmonary form of tuberculosis [10]. The spine is involved in 50 to 60% of the cases of osteoarticular tuberculosis, most commonly of the dorsolumbar level [2, 3]. Cervical Pott's disease is an uncommon localization (1 – 10% of the cases with spinal involvement) and its appearance in the suboccipital region is even rarer (0 – 4.8%), although its consequences are much more serious [1, 4, 6, 12].

The aim of this paper is to present two cases of suboccipital Pott's disease.

Clinical Cases

Case 1

A 21 year old male patient born in Pakistan, presented with a tender mobile mass, located in the left latero-cervical region which limited the extension and rotation of the neck. The mass had evolved over a four month period and no relevant previous medical history was recorded. It was associated with generalized myalgias.

Pharyngoscopy revealed a mass bulging on the left side of the pharynx. Both X-ray examination of the cervical spine and computerized axial tomography showed a lytic lesion in C2, protrusion of the odontoid into the foramen magnum, displacement of the esophagus by a mass located in the prevertebral space, and lateral deviation of the spinal cord by involvement of the epidural space (Figs. 1 a, b).

Tuberculous etiology was suspected but could not be confirmed; clinical examination, Mantoux test and chest X-ray were negative. Specific chemotherapy was started and a surgical procedure was performed through

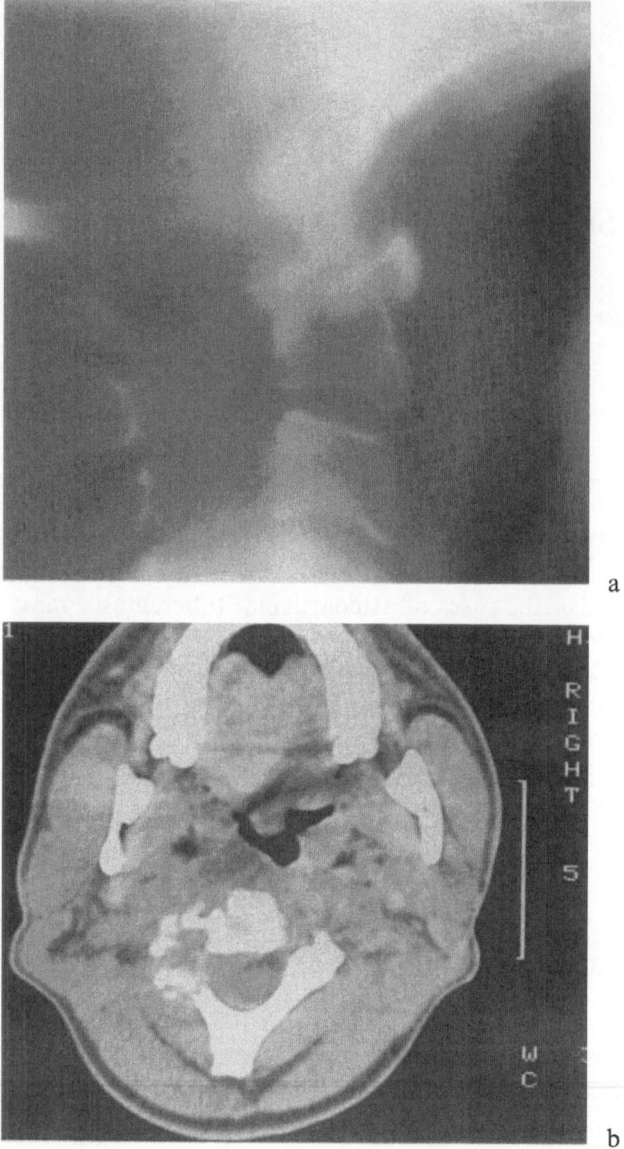

a

b

Fig. 1. Case 1. X-ray (a) and axial computed tomography of C1–C2

a posterior incision which disclosed an eroded left lamina of the axis and an
apparently well encapsulated pseudotumoral mass from which a yellowish
fluid was obtained. Cultures yielded no bacterial growth. Pathological examination revealed the presence of caseous granulomas compatible with tuberculosis.

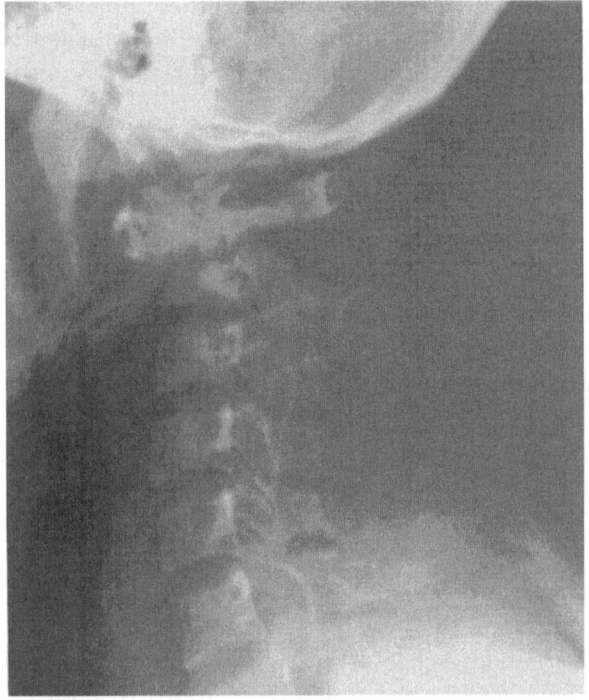

a

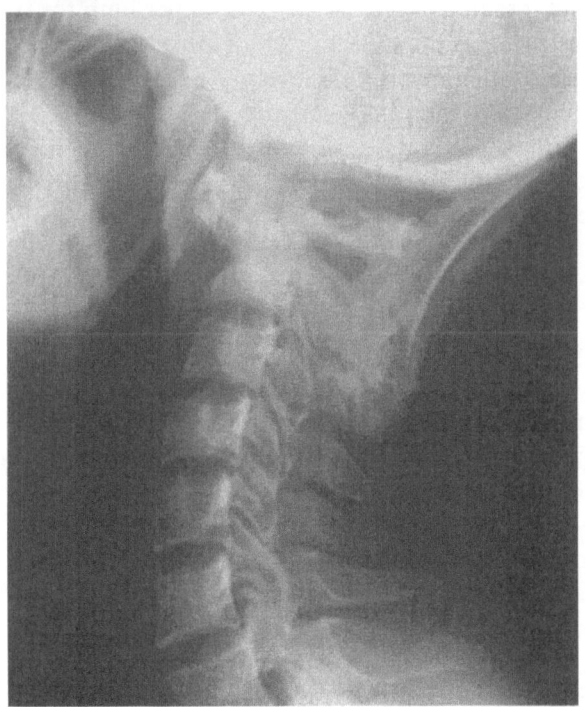

b

Fig. 2. Case 2. X-ray before (a) and after the occipito-atlanto-axial arthrodesis (b)

External fixation of the cervical spine with a Minerva plaster cast was performed. One and a half years after surgery the patient was found to be asymptomatic and X-ray examination showed signs of consolidation.

Case 2

A 26 year old male patient from Gambia had been complaining of cervical pain and a stiff neck for over a period of four months. Family medical history revealed his brother had pulmonary tuberculosis. A 5 × 6 cm fluctuant indolent mass was palpable at the low anterior aspect of the right chest wall. X-ray and tomography of the cervical spine showed a lytic lesion in the C2 vertebral body associated with an osteoporotic odontoid and a retropharyngeal soft-tissue abscess. Bone scintigraphy showed a hyperactive lesion of the right chest wall. Caseous material was obtained by puncture of the mass. Bacteriological cultures were positive for Mycobacterium tuberculosis.

Upon confirmation of the diagnosis the prevertebral space was drained by transoral puncture, the cervical spine was immobilized by a Minerva plaster cast and standard chemotherapy was started. The patient was readmitted in the emergency ward thirty days after discharge complaining of paresthesias and loss of strength in his right upper limb for two days. X-ray and tomograms revealed the existence of atlantoaxial subluxation associated with an increase of the prevertebral space (Fig. 2a). Skull traction was performed. Neurological symptoms disappeared shortly thereafter. An occipito-atlanto-axial arthrodesis was performed 24 days later. The patient was asymptomatic 6 months after operation. X-ray examination showed consolidation of the arthrodesis (Fig. 2b).

Discussion

In recents years, the evolution of tuberculosis has undergone a transformation in terms of its incidence and the age in which it appears. The incidence in the developed countries has increased with the influx of immigrants from Afro-Asian countries [5, 7, 9]. On the other hand we observed that while Pott's disease was formely associated with infancy, adults between the 2nd and 5th decades are more frequently affected at present [2, 5, 7].

The clinical picture includes the painful syndrome associated with cervical rigidity and symptoms of compression of the respiratory and alimentary tracts related to the presence of a prevertebral mass.

The severity of suboccipital Pott's disease is enhanced with the presence of neurological symptoms.

Characteristically Pott's disease is plurivertebral and plurifocal. It may involve different levels of the cervical spine and extravertebral space. It is necessary to confirm the diagnosis by complementary studies. The tuberculin allergy test is generally positive in patients suffering from Pott's disease. A negative result may be observed in 14–25% of cases and therefore does not exclude the disease. Direct surgical penetration into the vertebral focus is necessary sometimes to reach a definitive diagnosis. The culture of the material obtained is not positive in all of the patients [8, 9]. Pathological study needs to be performed to confirm the suspected etiology.

Chemotherapy has radically transformed the prognosis of this disease. Surgical treatment is restricted nowadays and it is still a matter of controversy among different authors. While some consider it necessary to perform debridement and fusion, others show excellent results with chemotherapy alone. Chemotherapy is generally used at present, while surgery is restricted to certain forms difficult to diagnose, and for complicated cases (neurological complications or resistance to medical treatment).

References

1. Chahal AS, Jyoti SP (1980) The radical treatment of tuberculosis of the spine. Int Orthoped 4:93–99
2. Dowd CHF, Sartoris DJ, Haghighi P, Resnick D (1986) Case report 344. Skeletal Radiol 15:65–68
3. Fang D, Leong JCY, Fang HSY (1983) Tuberculosis of the upper cervical spine. J Bone Joint Surg 65-B(1):47–50
4. Lifeso RM, FRCS, Weaver PH, Harder EM (1985) Tuberculous spondylitis in adults. J Bone Joint Surg 67-A(9):1405–1413
5. Lifeso R (1987) Atlanto-axial tuberculosis in adults. J Bone Joint Surg 69-B(2):183–187
6. Magnet JL, Thierry A, Couaillier JF, Tavernier C, Strauss J (1984) Ostéite tuberculeuse de l'atlas. A propos d'une observation. Rev Rheum 51(5):273–275
7. Morvan G, Martini N, Massare C, Nahum H (1983) La tuberculose du rachis cervical. Etude radiologique à propos d'une série multicentrique de 53 cases. Rev Chir Orthop [Suppl] II, 70:76–80
8. Neal SL, Kearns MJ, Harris JP (1986) Manifestations of Pott's disease in the head and neck. Laring 96:494–497
9. Scott JE, Taor WS (1982) The changing pattern of joint tuberculosis. J Bone Joint Surg 64-B:250
10. Simon L, Blotman F (1978) Le mal de Pott. Spondylodiscitis tuberculeuses. In: Encyclopédie Medico-Chirurgicale. Editions Techniques, Paris, pp A-10
11. Tuli SM (1974) Tuberculosis of the craniovertebral region. Clin Orthop 104:209–212
12. Wang LK (1981) Peroral focal debridement for treatment of tuberculosis of the atlas and axis. Chin J Orthop 1:207

Cervical Spine II
© by Springer-Verlag 1989

2.6. Osteomyelitis of the Cervical Spine: Surgical Series

J. E. O. Hughes, G. V. DiGiacinto, and N. Sundaresan, New York, N.Y.,
U.S.A.

Drug Related Cervical Osteomyelitis

With the increase in drug abuse, infectious complications associated with
it have become common in neurosurgical practice [1]. Over the past seven
years, we have surgically managed 60 cases of osteomyelitis of the spine in
two teaching hospitals of Columbia University, Harlem Hospital Center, a
682 bed general hospital which serves the Harlem community, and St. Lukes-
Roosevelt Hospital Center, a 1300 bed community hospital serving the upper
west side of Manhattan. At both hospitals, we take care of many intravenous
drug abusers. In this surgical series there have been 17 cervical, 16 thoracic,
and 27 lumbar cases. A total of 63 surgical procedures have been performed.
All operations have been carried out anteriorly except in 5 cases when the
pre-op diagnosis of osteomyelitis had not been known and in one case when
a posterior occiput to C_2 fusion was performed.

Clinical Picture

This report is restricted to the 17 cases of cervical osteomyelitis. The
patients (13 male, 4 female) ranged in age from 24 to 76. Four were in their
30's, four in their 40's and six in their 60's. All but three patients were drug
abusers. The levels involved were C_1: one case; C_3-C_4: three cases; C_4-C_5:
one case; C_5-C_6: two cases; C_6-C_7: four cases; and C_7-T_1: four cases. One
patient had two levels involved, C_5-C_6 and C_6-C_7 and one patient had three
levels involved, C_4-C_5, C_5-C_6 and C_6-C_7.

Eleven patients presented with at least one month of neck pain. Three
patients denied significant neck pain. (All of our thoracic and lumbar patients had severe back pain.) One patient had three weeks of cervical pain,
two patients two weeks and one patient three weeks of neck pain. Eleven
patients presented with root pain. Nine patients had symptoms of cord
compression.

Only five patients had no neurological deficit. Eleven of seventeen patients had significant arm and/or hand weakness. There was usually bilateral involvement. Seven patients had myelopathy. Six patients were quadriparetic. Five of these patients could not walk.

The classic presentation was a middle aged intravenous drug abuser with one to two months of severe neck pain, two to three weeks of arm pain and a recent onset of bilateral upper extremity weakness who had just started having trouble walking. Bladder involvement was rare. As noted above this symptom complex would then evolve into quadriparesis.

Radiographic Studies

Only seven of the seventeen patients had bony changes diagnostic of infection (destruction of at least one cortical end plate). The other ten patients had misleading bony changes. However, sixteen patients had evidence of soft tissue swelling (anterior displacement of the pharyngeal air shadow). Most patients had presented earlier in the emergency room complaining of neck pain. The anterior swelling on the plain spine films was frequently missed and the patient was sent on his way without the pain medicine they requested. This is the earliest sign of infection, occurring prior to bony changes in most cases.

Lateral tomograms originally gave us the earliest indication of destruction of the anterior cortical plate. CT scans have been positive for infection in the last seven cases. Three of these patients had non-diagnostic plain X-rays. Both CT and MRI of the patient with osteomyelitis of the odontoid were thought to show neoplasm.

The only other MRI (C_4-C_5) was not truly diagnostic.

However, we don't have enough experience to predict the usefulness of the MRI. We recently had a L_2 epidural abcess that we interpreted incorrectly as an intramedullary tumor by MRI.

We will continue to see nondiagnostic studies in these patients as the patients who have classic X-ray findings will get correct medical treatment and won't come to surgery. It has long been our experience in neurosurgically treating patients with pyogenic osteomyelitis and Pott's disease that these patients have not been diagnosed early enough to avoid neurologic compromise.

Surgical Pathology

The most important thing to remember about the surgical pathology is that it frequently is not very impressive or diagnostic [3, 9]. One patient operated on by one of the authors with extensive experience in spine tumor surgery was thought to have a negative exploration until the path and culture reports came back positive. Two other patients had only a slight watery exudate when the disc was incised. A total of six more patients had a definite thin watery exudate. Gross pus was very rare in our series. Only one of the cervical patients had definite pus. The anterior soft tissue mass seen on X-ray is swollen prevertebral fascia and muscle not a pyogenic abscess.

Eleven of seventeen patients had a greater than 50% destruction of at least one vertebral body.

It's known that white cells stimulated by pyogenic bone infections contain a proteolytic enzyme which dissolves the disc [13]. Tuberculosis does not stimulate this response. In operated Potts disease, the disc usually appears normal. We were therefore originally surprised to find normal appearing disc in six cases. In only three patients had the disc been dissolved. In eight patients the involved disc was mascerated but only partially dissolved. In all cases the posterior longitudinal ligament was thickened and bound down to proliferative epidural granulation tissue. In some cases this granulation tissue was quite thick extending a level or two above or below the center of the osteomyelitis as seen on myelogram.

Bacteriology

As in most other series Staph. aureus was the most common organism [10, 12]. Four patients had Staph. aureus cultured from the wound. Three of these patients had blood cultures positive for S. aureus. Three patients with negative surgical cultures had S. aureus in the blood. Another patient had gram positive organisms on smear but negative wound and blood cultures. Another patient had been treated for S. aureus endocarditis 2 months prior to treatment of the cervical osteomyelitis. This means nine out of seventeen patients probably were infected with Staph. aureus. Two surgical specimens grew out Pseudomonas aerugines and one E. coli. In five patients, a particular organism was not implicated.

Surgical Approach

All cases were explored anteriorly if the diagnosis was suspected. The affected disc is removed along with destroyed bone. This must be done all the way through the posterior longitudinal ligament to the dura. There were fifteen patients explored anteriorly. Three patients had a laminectomy initially. One of these patients eventually was drained anteriorly. These three patients did not have diagnostic X-ray changes suggesting bone destruction, were deteriorating neurologically and received emergency laminectomies.

Nothing was found other than epidural granulation tissue. Bony changes in the vertebral bodies were confirmed on post-op X-rays (Tomos and CT).

Three patients had excision of the affected disc and 24 hour drainage without fusion. Three patients had bone chips placed in the excised disc space. Eight patients had a block of iliac bone used for the fusion when an extensive portion of the body or more than one body was removed. Any bone that was felt to be abnormal was excised. There were three early complications. Two patients had to be reexplored because the block of bone became dislodged. One of these patients detached her Halo and the other had no postoperative Halo tongs. The most serious complication was a patient who became transiently quadriplegic in the postoperative period when a retained posterior portion of the C_6 vertebra fractured compressing the cord. This would not have happened if we had gone back to the dura originally or had the patient in tongs postoperatively. Fortunately, emergency reoperation the night of surgery reversed the quadriplegia.

One patient with osteomyelitic destruction of the odontoid was electively fused posteriorly after initial anterior diagnostic debridement.

One patient with osteomyelitis at C_7-T_1 decompressed in the middle of the night by the senior author was thought to have metastatic cancer once again emphasizing how the findings can be misleading. I proceeded to bridge C_7-T_2 with two Steinman pins and then fashioned an acrylic vertebra. The disc appeared normal and there was no pus or watery exudate. The vertebral body had been replaced by granulation tissue thought to be tumor. As it was in the middle of the night we did not call the pathologist in for a frozen section. Fortunately, there has been an eight month follow up without signs of infection. Eight patients with significant bone excision and iliac grafts were treated with halos postoperatively. All seventeen patients fused but three patients developed poor alignment. One patient developed a 30° gibbus at C_3-C_4 because she kept loosening her Halo. Two patients with cervical thoracic lesions were poorly aligned postoperatively. They both developed significant lateral angulation at C_7-T_1 requiring reoperation anteriorly. This was due to trouble getting good X-rays of the cervical-thoracic level with the patients in a Halo. We now tend to keep these patients in bed in pulley traction for a few weeks before attaching the Halo vest. One of these two patients had developed flexor spasms in his lower extremities after initial improvement from his first operation. This was relieved by the second operation. His case (C_4-C_7) became further complicated when he developed a 30° forward angulation at C_3-C_4 when the refused to keep the Halo on.

One of these 17 patients died three weeks postoperatively when he developed a new sepsis unrelated to his cervical fusion.

All patients improved significantly after operation. The severe neck pain is characteristically gone the day after decompression. Neurologic deficit of recent onset (cord and root) usually clears rapidly. Even profound deficits improve. If there is unacceptable plateauing of the patients neurological status we restudy the patient and don't hesitate to do more decompression if the cord is still compressed. We did this in four patients, two patients who developed C_7-T_1 angulation and another C_7-T_1 patient in whom initial laminectomy was nondiagnostic. The fourth patient demonstrates the importance of reevaluating a poor result.

This 46 year old intravenous drug abuser with two months of severe neck pain developed profound weakness in both upper extremities but had normal leg function. He could just flex and extend his left forearm and close his left hand. He could close his right hand but otherwise his right upper extremity was functionless. X-rays revealed marked changes of osteomyelitis. At surgery C_6 was 60% destroyed, C_5 and C_7 were 20% gone. There was no C_5-C_6 or C_6-C_7 disc found. The C_4-C_5 and C_7-T_1 discs were normal. The C_6 and C_7 bodies were excised as was the lower half of C_5. There was a lot of proliferative granulation tissue in the ventral epidural space surrounding the roots greatest on the right side. Bone grafts were placed from C_5-T_1. Within four days there was marked improvement in both upper extremities. A Halo was maintained on ten pounds pulley traction. However, at four weeks both upper extremities were again almost plegic and both legs quite weak for the first time. A myelogram with CT revealed no cord compression from C_5-T_1. However, there was a large ventral epidural defect from C_1-C_5 centered on C_3 which now showed bony destruction.

At reexploration the anterior border of C_3 was eroded and the C_2-C_3 and C_3-C_4 discs were partially destroyed. The bony fusion from C_5-T_1 was already solid. A groove was drilled from C_2-C_5 widened posteriorly, decompressing the cord which was compressed by thick epidural granulation tissue. There was immediate improvement in all four extremities. Unfortunately, he became septic at 3 weeks from aspiration pneumonia and died. The neck was healing well.

All but one patient, who is still convalescing, regained independent ambulation and use of at least one upper extremity. Two patients had poor function of one upper extremity. This excludes the patient who died but he should have been a good neurological result.

Our present series is a continuation of the series of 12 patients from Harlem Hospital reported by Dr. Henry Messer in 1976 [11]. In his cases operative fusion was not deemed necessary. Five of his patients had root involvement but none had cord compression. We did more extensive bony debridement completely uncovering the cord. Our patients may have fused spontaneously without bony grafting as did all of Dr. Messer's patients. This is illustrated in the following case.

This 48 year old IVDA developed severe neck pain while recovering from a total laryngectomy and left radical neck resection. He developed a pharyngeal cutaneous fistula which was unsuccessfully repaired twice, the last time with a delto-pectoral flap. Staph. sepsis was treated for four weeks. His sputum grew out acid fast bacterium and abnormal T-cell function was noted suggesting AIDS. He refused HIV testing. He was also being treated with insulin for diabetes. When first seen he had moderate weakness of both legs and profound weakness of both upper extremities. Myelogram revealed a block at C_4. There were bony changes consistent with osteomyelitis.

With difficulty, we explored the spine through the right neck which was bound down by radiation changes. We were limited by the large pharyngeal cutaneous fistula. The C_3 vertebra was destroyed. A groove was drilled and widened posteriorly uncovering the cord from C_2-C_4. Again there was no pus, only thick granulation tissue. We had already opened the scarred right jugular vein when we got into what we thought was the lower end of the pharynx. Because of this we were reluctant to perform a fusion.

There was immediate postoperative neurological improvement. He was kept in bed with Gardner Wells Tongs. He had fused spontaneously and was neurologically clear within four weeks.

Discussion and Conclusion

Spinal osteomyelitis is increasingly associated with increased intravenous drug abuse. Garcia and Grantham [5] in their review of the records of the Presbyterian Hospital in New York City only found 40 cases over a 25 year period from 1935–1960. Only ten of these were operated upon.

The surgical pathology is similar to that found in our lumbar and thoracic cases. When laminectomy is done because the preop diagnosis is incorrect the surgeon may "find nothing" or mistake granulation tissue for tumor. Frank pus is very rare. Usually only thin water exudate is encountered. The "para spinal abscess" seen on X-ray is really swollen soft tissue. Bone destruction runs the gamut from more destruction seen at surgery than expected on X-ray to just erosion of the cortical end plate. Frequently normal or a partially digested disc is found. These cases ended up in published series of spinal epidural abscesses [1, 2]. During this period where we've operated on 60 cases of spinal osteomyelitis we have only encountered two patients who have had free pus in the epidural space (both lumbar) without any evidence of osteomyelitis. Emphasizing the term epidural abscess in these bony spinal infections is of more than semantic or academic concerns. It leads to laminectomy which is the operation described in these series. It is the wrong operation when the pathology is anterior.

Our surgical indications in spinal osteomyelitis include:

1. Neurological deterioration
2. Failure to respond to organism specific antibiotic treatment

3. Persistent severe pain
4. Increasing vertebral body destruction with or without gibbus
5. Vertebral body destruction of greater than 50%
   Operative treatment consists of:
1. Drain abscess (usually just serous fluid in disc space) and obtain culture
2. Remove all foreign body – undissolved disc and sequestered bone
3. Decompress dura
4. Fuse except in rare cases where after decompression only narrowed disc
   space has been drained

The results have been quite good. Spinal pain is almost always relieved soon after decompression. Most of these patients are drug addicts used to complaining constantly of pain. Their narcotic requirement drops dramatically. All patients should improve neurologically. If they don't improve, plateau at an unacceptable level, or experience late deterioration, the patient should be restudied and reoperated if cord or root compression persists. Severe neurological deficit is not a contra-indication to surgery. We have one thoracic case who had complete loss of cord function for seven months who made a complete functional recovery. Many authors have stated that vascular compromise of the blood supply to the cord plays an important role in the sometimes devastating neurological deficit seen in spinal infections. We have not been convinced that any of our cases suffered cord infarction due to arteritis. Our experience confirms the eloquent experiments on cord compression in rabbits with epidural pus done by Feldenzer [4]. In their model, neurologic deficit was due to compression not vasculitis.

Post operative stabilization with Halo is very important in cervical cases. Our postoperative complications were due to inadequate external stabilization until fusion took place. We allow lumbar cases to ambulate as soon as they are pain free – they do anyway. Thoracic cases ambulate early in fitted thoraco lumbar polyethylene clam shell braces, cervical cases required Halos for two to three months until fusion is solid.

Osteomyelitis at C_7-T_1 presents a particular problem because inadequate lateral X-rays delay diagnosis and can make following alignment postoperatively a problem.

References

1. Baker AS, Ojemann RG, Swartz MN *et al* (1975) Spinal epidural abscess. N Engl J Med 293:463–468
2. Browder J, Myers R (1937) Infections of the spinal epidural space: an aspect of vertebral osteomyelitis. Am J Surg 37:4–26
3. Digby JM, Kersly JB (1979) Pyogenic non-tuberculous spinal infection: an analysis of thirty cases. JBJS 61-B:47–55

4. Feldenzer JA, McKeenen PE, Schoberg DR *et al* (1988) The pathogenesis of spinal epidural abcess: microangiographic studies in an experimental model. J Neurosurg 69:110–114

5. Garcia A, Grantham SA (1960) Hematogenous pyogenic vertebral osteomyelitis. JBJS 42-A:429

6. Hancock DO (1973) A study of 49 patients with acute spinal extradural abcess. Paraplegia 10:285–288

7. Holzman RS, Bishko F (1971) Osteomyelitis in heroine addicts. Ann Intern Med 75:693–696

8. Hulme A, Dott NM (1954) Spinal epidural abscess. Br Med J 1:64–68

9. Kemp HBS, Jackson JW, Jeremiah JD (1973) Pyogenic infections occurring primarily in invertebral discs. JBJS 55-B:698–714

10. LaRocca H (1982) Spinal sepsis. In: Rothman RH, Simeone FA (eds) The spine. WB Saunders, Philadelphia, pp 757–774

11. Messer HD, Litvinoff J (1976) Chondro-osteomyelitis of the cervical spine frequently associated with parenteral drug use. Arch Neurol 33:571–576

12. Stone DB, Bonfiglio M (1963) Pyogenic vertebral osteomyelitis, a diagnostic pitfall for the internist. Arch Int Med 112:491–500

13. Sullivan R, McCaslin FE (1960) Further studies on experimental spondylitis and intercorporeal fusion of the spine. JBJS 42-A:1339–1348

3. Degenerative Lesions and Management

Degenerative Lesions and Management

Cervical Spine II
© by Springer-Verlag 1989

3.1. Complications of Cervical Laminectomy, How to Avoid Them, Diagnosis and Treatment

J. A. Epstein and Nancy E. Epstein, Stony Brook, New York, U.S.A.

In this paper the complications of cervical laminectomy in both the seated position and in the prone position will be discussed. Emphasis will be placed on the performance of laminectomy for decompression of the spinal cord and nerve roots secondary to spinal stenosis and spondyloarthrosis.

Accuracy of diagnosis is paramount as is the proper selection of patients. Every effort must be made to exclude the possibility of motor neuron disease which closely resembles the symptoms seen in patients with spondylostenosis who present with a motor dominant myeloradiculopathy. A complete history and neurological evaluation supplemented with electromyography and sensory evoked potentials (providing evidence of nuchal delay) will exclude motor neuron disease. Among the deterrents in patient selection is a history of alcoholism or diabetes since both are associated with myelopathy, radiculopathy, and peripheral neuropathy. Such individuals also have difficulty in wound healing, and have little resistance to infection. Patients who are depressed, without motivation and without family support cannot cooperate properly in postoperative rehabilitation, and invariably, the procedure ends in failure. Verbiest pointed out that individuals with the acute onset of symptoms and with rapid deterioration should not be operated upon in this state. Preferably, they must be placed in a cervical collar or in tongs and given high dose steroids for several days until their neurological status stabilizes [10].

Patients with cervical kyphosis are best operated upon through an anterior approach by means of vertebrectomy and strut fusion since the cord will not migrate dorsally after laminectomy. Before and following laminectomy, it is mandatory that the cervical lordotic curve be preserved so that displacement of the cord away from ventral osteophytes can be maintained.

Complications of surgery in either the prone or the seated position very often relate to the presence of pulmonary obstructive disease with hypertension resulting in excessive bleeding from epidural veins. Such blood loss is difficult to control and if not replaced rapidly enough will result in ultimate failure of perfusion.

We prefer to use the sitting position for cervical laminectomy and have done so for the past 30 years. Despite various reports in the literature citing unacceptable risks [4], we have found that the advantages of this position far outweigh those provided by the prone position [3]. The surgeon has optimal exposure at eye level with a relatively dry field, since blood drains away and bleeding is simpler to control. Diaphragmatic excursion and ventilation occurs without difficulty. The anesthesiologist has better access to the airway with a lower airway pressure and better cardiopulmonary function. The elastic bandaging of legs prevents pooling and venostasis, maintains blood volume and also increases the venous pressure slightly. In combination with judicious fluid volume loading and slow positioning of the patient this reduces the deleterious effects of the seated position that may relate to hypotension. The arms are supported to avoid traction injury to the brachial plexus. By means of controlled ventilation and muscle relaxation, unplanned movement does not occur preventing unexpected deep inspiration with aspiration of air through open venous channels. The neutral position of the head is mandatory. This avoids kinking of the endotracheal tube, improves the venous drainage from the brain, and prevents stretching and angulation of the cord against spurs in the floor of the canal that occurs with the head in the flexed position. It also prevents narrowing of the canal that occurs when the cervical spine is placed in hyperextension, minimizing the effects of dorsal intrusion of infolded yellow ligaments.

Infiltration of the paravertebral muscles with a local anesthetic and epinephrine, will reduce the amount of general anesthesia required and preserves the patient's compensatory vital mechanisms. The patient therefore awakens more quickly from anesthesia. Also, light levels of anesthesia result in less peripheral vasodilatation and myocardial depression. Cord compression can be readily identified by sudden bradycardia and a decrease in sympathetic activity. Instrumentation of the spinal cord and nerve roots can be recognized quickly by a rise in blood pressure and heart rate. Cardiovascular hypertension is better tolerated and better treated when minimal amounts of anesthetic agents are used since all gas anesthetics are potent myocardial depressants as well as peripheral vasodilators.

The prone position is especially useful if the cervical spine is unstable and must be maintained in traction or in a halo. Again, the neutral position and avoidance of pressure point ischemia is mandatory with special reference to the orbital area. Torsion must be avoided since both the vertebral and carotid circulation are treatened with the occurrence of ischemia, thrombosis and embolism. The prone position has one major defect, namely pressure against the abdomen and thoracic structures with increased intraabdominal and thoracic airway pressures and vena caval compression. In the morbidly obese patient with a short neck, this position is poorly tolerated and it should, therefore, be avoided [4]. The arms should be abduced no greater than 90 degrees to reduce stretching of the brachial plexus by the head of the humerus. This position also reduces traction on the nerve roots and it is useful in both the prone and the seated position.

Venous air embolism has been reported when using the prone position with the head elevated 30 degrees, the most common posture assumed. It rarely occurs when the head is maintained in a neutral posture horizontal with the trunk.

Because of the minimal exposure, a central venous line is rarely required for a simple laminotomy and foraminotomy [4]. For the more complicated procedures, a central venous line is placed in the atrium or the superior vena cava and may be used to aspirate a collection of air. It may actually be impossible to aspirate sufficient air even with the central venous line in a proper position, and much valuable time may be wasted during an episode of air embolism. More important, the Doppler device can immediately alert the anesthesiologist to the presence of air when even minimal amounts enter the atrium so that corrective measures can be taken before there is any deleterious effect on vital function. However, the Doppler does not determine the volume of air.

In the past, air embolism has been noted to occur in as many as 25% of patients operated upon in the seated position, and in 10% in the prone position [6]. Now, with the use of the Doppler, this percentage has dropped to as low as 6% [9]. The major problems occur when the posterior fossa is being explored because the stiff venous sinuses in this area remain patent when opened, permitting ready aspiration of air. Certainly, in the presence of a low central venous pressure and careless surgical technique, the incidence of air embolism will increase. A considerable amount of air must be aspirated before clinical symptoms occur, this is in the vicinity of 35–50 ml. Air enters the venous system and is carried to the right side of the heart into the pulmonary circulation. Here it accumulates in the right ventricle resulting in pulmonary hypertension and right ventricular collapse. Blockage of the pulmonary vessels is further complicated by neurogenic reflexes. The foramen ovale of the heart may be patent in 20–30% of patients [7]. In the presence of an increase of pressure in the right atrium, air passage occurs through the septum secundum in the fossa ovalis forcing air into the left atrium. Cerebrovascular complications follow with cardiovascular collapse, acute heart failure, severe hypoxia and infarction of the brain. It is important to note that nitrous oxide is 34 times more soluble in blood than nitrogen and when released, can augment the amount of air in the right side of the heart to a severe degree. It is for this reason that nitrous oxide anesthesia must be turned off immediately, and 100% oxygen substituted.

With the use of the end tidal carbon dioxide monitor, the decrease in alveolar carbon dioxide due to obstruction of blood flow and the presence of air in the pulmonary circulation provides an additional warning sign of embolism. Also, the esophageal stethoscope is more sensitive than a precordial stethoscope but again, when changes were discerned, the major problem has already occurred.

When the Doppler defines even tiny amounts of air, the alerted surgeon takes immediate precautionary measures such as flooding the field with saline, and the use of sponges or gelfoam to close off open vascular channels. Gentle jugular compression can also help detect an open venous channel by back flow so that it can be closed promptly. Positional changes can also be used to fix the bolus of air by moving the patient into the left lateral position. This maintains the air in the right atrium or ventricle and prevents flow into the pulmonary circulation. Also, the patient's head may be lowered below the heart.

Patients who have a myelopathy may respond adversely to the use of succinylcholine with a potential hazard of acute hyperkalemia secondary to denervation hypersensitivity. Controlled ventilation maintains the intrathoracic pressure above zero mm. of mercury, and proper fluid loading prior to induction of anesthesia maintains blood volume so that the systemic venous pressure is supported.

Insofar as medication is concerned, vasoconstrictive drugs employed to maintain perfusion are neosynephrine or ephedrine given intravenously. Closed chest massage may help break up an air lock in the right ventricle. PEEP can be used to 8–10 cm to increase the venous pressure and to prevent ingress of air, but it is not used routinely since it will cause increased venous bleeding during the procedure.

Awake nasal intubation is considered if there is a limited range of cervical mobility, if the patient appears to have a difficult airway, or if the patient is morbidly obese. Hyperextension movements must be avoided since the spinal canal narrows sharply and may result in cord compression with quadriplegia. Preoperative medication combines the use of a sedative with an antianxiety drug as well as a narcotic and an antisialagogue such as beladonna derivatives. Vistaril, 50–100 mgs intramuscularly is an excellent antianxiety drug as well as a potent antiemetic and will potentiate the effects of narcotics.

It is mandatory to maintain perfusion of the spinal cord with the patient in either position, perhaps more so when seated, since infarction may occur if the cord is in a stenotic canal under tension or compression. A radial arterial line is used for continuous blood pressure monitoring and blood gas sampling with the transducer placed at the level of the operative field. The right internal jugular vein is the ideal site for the position of a central venous catheter, and it is the most direct route to the right atrium. A Swan Ganz catheter may be employed under specific medical circumstances especially where cardiac disease and pulmonary disease complicate management. A central venous line allows for rapid infusion and administration of vasoactive drugs should the need suddenly arise. The Doppler must be placed over the precordium where it can detect air at approximately 0.05 cc per kg per minute. This is supplemented with the use of end tidal CO_2 monitor. When a drop in the end tidal CO_2 occurs, hemodynamic alterations with a drop in blood pressure and sudden arrthymias are often too late to correct.

In the seated position, the legs are elevated to facilitate venous return. The pin hole sites of the 3 pin head holder are plugged with vaseline or lubricating jelly to prevent air entering the venous circulation. Fluid loading is extremely important, and the patient is given between 500–1000 cc of lactated Ringer's solution intravenously to increase and to maintain central venous pressure prior to slowly sitting the patient up.

We prefer to maintain the patient under a light general anesthetic since the patient will awaken quickly postoperatively, allowing immediate evaluation before being transferred to the recovery room. With light anesthesia, blood pressure will be more readily maintained at normal levels since the bodies homeostatic mechanisms will be preserved. Also, less peripheral vasodilatation and myocardial depression occurs. Cardiovascular hypotension is better tolerated and more readily treated since the patient has a minimal amount of inhalation anesthetic in his system. All gas anesthetics such as halothane, ethrane, and forane are potent myocardial depressants as well as peripheral vasodilators.

With the patient under anesthesia, complete muscle relaxation occurs and the neck can be manipulated in unnatural positions with resultant injury to the spinal cord.

Controversy exists over the use of PEEP. The fear of elevating the pulmonary pressure to help control air embolism is that the right atrial pressure will increase, and exceed the left atrial pressure, resulting in air crossing through the septum resulting in parodoxical emboli to the brain, heart or kidneys. This rarely occurs, however, one must be alerted to this possibility. For this reason PEEP is not used routinely.

Causes of excessive bleeding from epidural veins relate to the presence of coagulation factor deficiencies and defective fibrin formation and, therefore, preoperative PT and PTT studies are mandatory. Bleeding and clotting times should be obtained in all patients who have been on nonsteroidal anti-inflammatory drugs for any extended period. This is especially important when an individual has been on aspirin, the most noxious agent in this category. Resulting platelet dysfunction must be evaluated by appropriate bleeding and clotting times. Chronic pulmonary hypertension and pulmonary obstructive disease should be treated preoperatively and increased intraabdominal and intrathoracic pressure should be avoided.

To control bleeding, one must only use bipolar coagulation within the spinal canal. Oxycel* cotton soaked in thrombin and/or peroxide is very

---

* Oxidized cellulose.

helpful when placed in the lateral gutters to control oozing from epidural veins, one of the main sources of air embolism. The use of surgicel* is indicated only on a temporary basis since it swells, and if left in situ can compress and injure a nerve root.

The most common cause of quadriplegia when the patient awakens from anesthesia aside from severe surgical trauma, is anoxia and infarction of the spinal cord because of vascular compromise and impaired perfusion. Certainly, inadvertent trauma to the spinal cord makes it mandatory that surgical technique be as perfect as possible. Intraoperative dexamethasone has a protective effect in this regard [1]. Monoplegia can occur following injury to the fifth nerve root. It is uniquely vulnerable possibly because of adherence to osteophytes during dissection, and possibly because of its longer course. It is also located in the most mobile area of the cervical spine, with more prominent degenerative changes. The patient usually awakens with a paralysis of the deltoid. With time, the majority of these lesions heal without deficit.

In order to prevent postoperative subluxation, the major portions of the facets must be preserved and no more than the medial ¼ need be removed or undercut in order to perform a proper foraminal decompression [8]. Also, denervation and necrosis of the paraspinal muscles can occur with prolonged use of self retaining retractors. With the loss of the support of the paraspinal muscles, kyphosis results. It is also helpful to maintain the muscular attachments to the spinous process of C2 which is the main anchor in this area and helps preserve the lordotic curve. Postoperatively, isometric exercises and appropriate physical therapy will help maintain proper posture in this regard [3].

Despite the emphasis placed in this paper on air embolism, it rarely occurs. It is overrated as a primary concern during surgery if the above precautions, especially the use of a Doppler device, are used. Certainly, the advantages of the seated position by far outweigh any presented in the prone position. The uniquely dry field helps dissection of nerve roots in the foraminal entry zones and prevents injury to the motor root which is often separated from the sensory root above it and is very poorly covered with epineurium [3]. Any attempt to remove osteophytes in the prone position is almost invariably a failure since one cannot get the proper dry field exposure and visualization needed. Under such circumstances, simple foraminal decompression can well provide an excellent result if properly performed. Only those osteophytes that are critically situated need be removed. Since dorsal migration of the cord occurs in the presence of maintained cervical lordosis, laminectomy makes it unnecessary to remove ventrally situated osteophytes crossing the midline. This procedure is indicated where multiple levels of the spine are involved, with the anterior approach being reserved where essential-

---

* Oxidized regenerated cellulose.

ly a single level or at most 2 levels are compromised. Again, the presence of stenosis will affect judgement in this regard [3].

The use of dexamethazone intravenously at the time of induction of anesthesia (10 mgm) and given in decreasing doses for 4 to 7 days helps preserve homeostatic mechanisms and reduces incisional pain considerably, contributing to a benign postoperative course [3].

Instability, postoperatively, is not a factor of concern if the technique described is followed closely [3]. This has finally been reported in the orthopaedic literature by Matjasko [4].

Cephazolin is the prophylactic antibiotic of choice to be used perioperatively. It is cost effective with limited toxicity and has a longer half-life of 2 hours as compared to other first generation cephalosporins [2].

Just as there exists a great difference between rhetoric, effort, and achievement, there is a yet greater difference between the ease of making a decision to operate on a patient as compared to the difficulties encountered in deciding not to operate. Difficult as it is, the latter remains by far the best way to stay out of trouble.

Alternative methods of treatment are available and should be employed in high risk individuals or in patients in whom the diagnosis is in doubt [3].

Acknowledgements

The authors wish to express their appreciation to Dr. Dominick Nardi for his kind assistance and advice regarding anesthetic management.

The authors wish to express their appreciation to Ms. Shery Lynn Grimm for her assistance in the preparation of this manuscript.

References

1. Braughler JM, Hall ED (1985) Current application of "high-dose" steroid therapy for CNS injury. J Neurosurg 62:806–810
2. Dempsey R, Rapp RP, Young B (1988) Prophylactic parenteral antibiotics in clean neurosurgical procedures: A Review. J Neurosurg 69:52–57
3. Epstein JA, Janin Y (1983) Management of cervical spondylotic myelopathy by the posterior approach. In: The cervical spine, 1st Edition. JB Lippincott Co., Philadelphia, pp 402–410
4. Matjasko J, Petrozza P (1985) Anesthesia and surgery in the seated position. Analysis of 554 cases. Neurosurgery 17:695–702
5. Mikawa Y, Shikata J, Yamamuro T (1987) Spinal deformity and instability after multilevel cervical laminectomy. Spine 12:6–11
6. Miller RD, Alfery DD, Shapiro HM (1981) Neurosurgical anesthesia and intracranial hypertension. In: Anesthesia, Vol 2. Churchill Livingstone, New York, pp 1118–1121

7. Perkins-Pearson NK, Marchell WK, Bedford RF (1982) Arterial pressure in the seated position: Implications for paradoxical air embolism. Anesthesiology 57:493–497
8. Raynor RB, Pugh J, Shapiro I (1985) Cervical facetectomy and its effect on spine strength. J Neurosurg 63:278–282
9. Standefer JM, Bay JW (1984) The sitting position in neurosurgery: A retrospective analysis of 388 cases. Neurosurgery 14(6):649–658
10. Verbiest H (1973) The management of cervical spondylosis. Clin Neurosurg 20:262–294

3.2. Laminectomy Versus Open-door Laminoplasty for Cervical Spondylotic Radiculomyelopathy and OPLL

N. NAKANO, T. NAKANO, Sapporo, Japan, and K. NAKANO, Hakodate, Japan

Introduction

Laminectomy has been performed in cervical spondylotic radiculomyelo-pathy and ossification of the posterior longitudinal ligament (OPLL), but wide laminectomies could result in laminectomy membrane formation and spinal deformity several years after the operation. Since 1978, the authors have used a simple open-door laminoplasty method (Fig. 1). Retrospective study was done to determine if there was any difference in the results of laminectomy or laminoplasty.

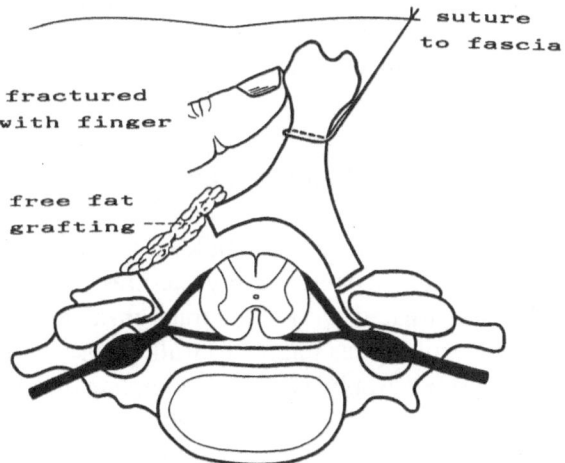

Fig. 1. Surgical technique of Nakano laminoplasty. (Reprint from Nakano N (1988) Clinic of the Cervical Spine. In print in Japanese, Nankodo, Tokyo)

Materials and Methods

Laminectomy was performed on 14 patients and followed up with an average of 10 years and 8 months. The age distribution at operation was 46 years to 74 years and the average was 59.2 years. Laminoplasty was done on 95 patients and followed up with an average of 4 years and 6 months. Age distribution at operation was 32 years to 75 years, and the average was 55.0 years. The air drill was used for laminoplasty but not for laminectomy. Most of the patients were out of bed by two weeks in the laminectomy group and by three days in the laminoplasty group after the operation. Results were evaluated by the Japanese Orthopaedic Association scoring system with a total normal sum of 17 points. A percentage improvement score was also obtained.

Results

The operative time for laminectomy was 100 minutes to 255 minutes and the average was 169.2 minutes. Blood loss was 111 ml to 562 ml, and the average was 343.3 ml in the laminectomy group. The operative time for laminoplasty was 80 minutes to 240 minutes, and the average was 151.0 minutes. Blood loss was 200 ml to 1307 ml, and the average was 505.0 ml in the laminoplasty group.

Overall results of laminectomy were as follows. Pre-operative score was 7.0 and post-operative score was 15.3. And overall results of laminoplasty was pre-operative score of 7.0 and post-operative score of 15.0. Percentage improvement in laminectomy was 81.1%, and in laminoplasty it was 81.4%.

Illustrative Cases

Case 1: Y.M., A sixty-seven year old male had numbness in all fingers of both hands and a gait disturbance. X-ray pictures revealed OPLL in the cervical spine. He was treated with skull traction at another hospital but symptoms worsened until he was unable to walk or use chopsticks. He then visited this hospital. Myelography showed a complete defect from C3 to C6. Laminectomy was done from C3 to C6. Twelve hours after the operation, motion of his fingers had improved and numbness of both hands were gone. He has no difficulty in daily activity 12 years after the operation, and post operative flexion-extension films shows no instability. Clinical score results improved from 2 points to 15 points.

Case 2: T.M., A sixty-two year old male had numbness in both hands, including all fingers. The condition worsened until he had difficulty using chopsticks, and he was unable to walk. He was brought by ambulance. An

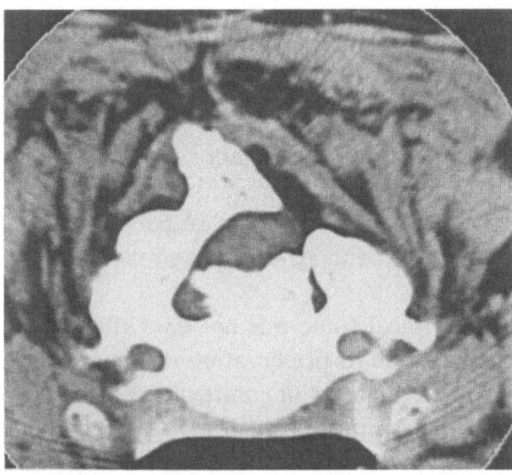

Fig. 2. Case 2. In a CT 9 years after surgery, the anterior dura seems to be compressed, however, clinical results improved from 5 to 15 points

axial tomogram revealed OPLL and myodil myelography showed a filling defect from C3 to C6. Laminoplasty was performed from C3 to C6. Postoperative CT scan showed that ossification still occupied a large portion of the spinal canal, but clinical results improved from 5 points to 15 points over a nine year period (Fig. 2).

Discussion

In cervical spondylotic radiculomyelopathy and OPLL, it has been said that wide laminectomies could be a cause of laminectomy membrane formation and spinal deformity several years after the operation. Recently various methods of laminoplasty have been performed in Japan with an attempt to avoid these complications, however, the technique of these methods takes a long time and introduces some operative difficulties.

Since 1978, we have done a simple open-door laminoplasty, and satisfactory results were obtained. Results of the laminectomy were also almost the same as the results of the laminoplasty.

Laminoplasty, which creates a small enlargement of the spinal canal, also brought improvement. Therefore, improvement may not be due to the degree of enlargement of the spinal canal, but due to improvement in circulation to the spinal cord and nerve roots.

No instability was found in both groups, which might be related to avoiding damage to the facets. However, good results were obtained. The spinous process of the cervical spine is important for attaching the muscles.

These have to be removed in laminectomy but not in laminoplasty. This is an advantage for laminoplasty because it maintains the cervical muscles in function.

Summary

Laminectomy had been performed on 15 patients and since 1978, open-door laminoplasty on 95 patients had been used in cervical radiculomyelopathy and OPLL.

Instability of the cervical spine was not seen after the operation in both groups, which might be due to preservation of the facets.

After laminoplasty, even a small enlargement of the spinal canal results in improvement. Therefore, improvement may not only be due to the degree of enlargement of the spinal canal, but may also relate to improvement in circulation of the spinal cord and nerve root.

There was no significant difference in the results of these two procedures but the operative time was shorter and earlier ambulation was associated with laminoplasty.

3.3. Spondylosis of the Cervical Spine: Formation of Osteophytes

L. Ceciliani, L. Pedrotti, F. Benazzo, and U. E. Pazzaglia, Pavia, Italy

Degenerative arthritis can arise in any of the articulating parts of the cervical spine. Thus the disks, the interapophyseal and the uncovertebral joints may all be involved in the degenerative process in which an initial structural lesion of the intervertebral disk causes a reduction in disk thickness and overloading of the uncal and interapophyseal articulations with the formation of osteophytes.

Posterior osteophytes are clinically important because they reduce the diameter of the vertebral canal while anterior osteophytes are often the first radiographic sign observed.

Anterior osteophytes grow in a forward direction while posterior osteophytes develop vertically. The pathogenesis of osthephyte development is correlated with the particular mechanics of the cervical spine. In flexion and extension each vertebra slides and rotates with respect to the underlying vertebra. The particular characteristics of this movement are determined by the geometrical configuration of the vertebrae and by the extendability, elasticity and compressability of the ligaments and disks.

Relative moment occurs at the disks and at the articular facets. During flexion the disk space assumes a wedge shape with its base facing posteriorly.

In the normal cervical spine the weight of the head is counterbalanced by contraction of the posterior cervical muscles. The load placed on the disks is proportional to the degree of flexion and extension.

During flexion forces develop in the vertical and horizontal directions (K and S) whose resultant vector is directed antero-inferiorly (Fig. 1). Anterior osteophytes grow in this very same direction and their development enlarges the anterior surface area of the vertebral border which causes a better weight distribution.

Posteriorly, however, the resultant vector is vertical and corresponds exactly with the topographic orientation of posterior osteophytes. Here osteophytes grow one next to another often covering the superior border of the annulus fibrosus.

In order to study the histology of osteophytes we obtained 137 intervertebral disks from 20 cadavers ranging in age from 53 to 97 years. The

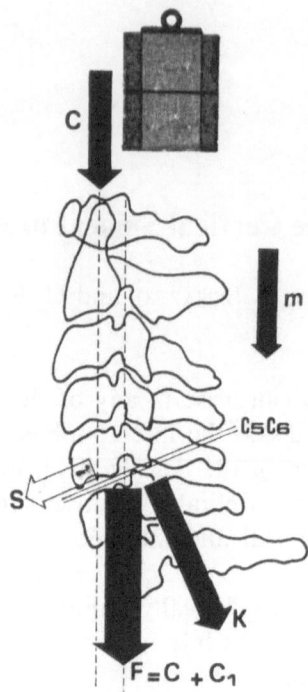

Fig. 1. Diagram of the weight distribution in the cervical spine

specimens were cut in the horizontal (transdiscal and somatic), coronal and median sagittal planes. We examined the following structures: the interverte-bral disks, the anterior and posterior edges of the vertebral bodies and the anterior and posterior longitudinal ligaments.

The ribbon-like anterior longitudinal ligament adheres to the anterior portion of the vertebral bodies forming the interdisk ligamentous space of Policard which contains potentially osteogenic cells.

The anterior longitudinal ligament is thicker over the concave anterior face of the vertebral body from which it is slightly detached.

The posterior logitudinal ligament is not ribbon-like and is less adherent than the anterior longitudinal ligament to the vertebral body. Degeneration of the nucleus pulposus and the annulus fibrosus begins with an alteration in the distribution of proteoglycans in the pericellular areas. This brings about a reduction in the quantity of proteoglycans in the nucleus and a resultant progressive loss in water content. Fissures of the nucleus appear early and precedes the formation of osteophytes. These fissures can be concentric or radial and in the latter case they favor the migration of fragments of the nucleus pulposus (Figs. 2 a, b).

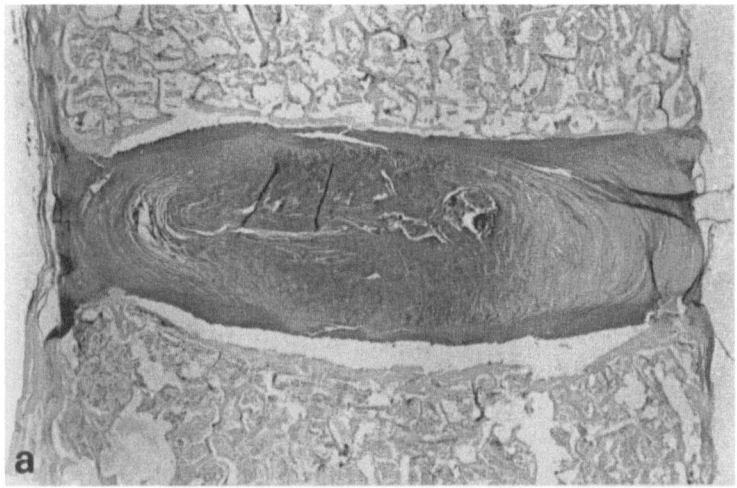

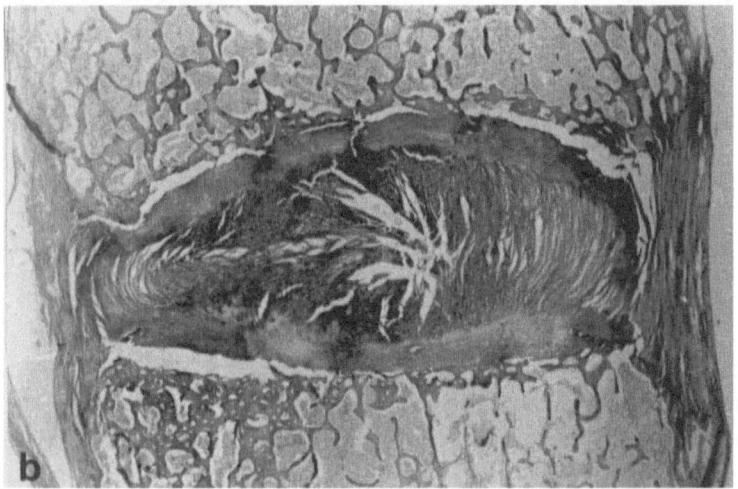

Fig. 2a, b. Haematoxylin-eosin (original magnification 1.5×). Progression of fissures in the intervertebral disk

It seems that lesions appear first in the nucleus and then in the annulus.
As degeneration progresses the nucleus loses its homogeneity and it becomes
difficult to distinguish between it and the annulus.

Anterior osteophytes grow as degeneration progresses but posterior osteophytes show no correlation to the degree of degeneration.

Histologically, anterolateral osteophytes are characterized by lamellar
bone trabeculae which delineate the medullary space exactly like that of the
vertebral body. The anterior longitudinal ligament is lifted by and covers
anterolateral osteophytes and there is a constant relationship with anteriorly

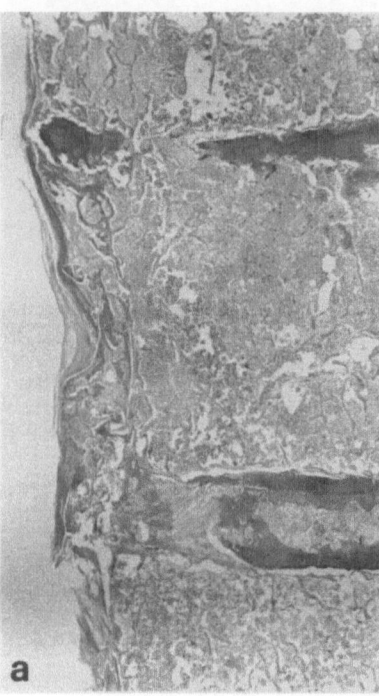
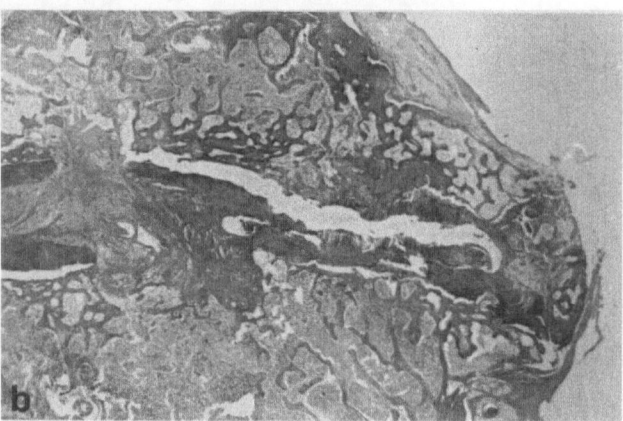

Fig. 3. Haematoxylin-eosin (original magnification 1.8 ×). a) Structure of the anterior osteophytes and their relationship with the discal material. b) Posterior osteophytes with hypertrophy of the posterior margin

or laterally herniated disks. Where there are older osteophytes the disk appears fragmented due to progressive internal ossification.

Anterior disk protrusion causes widening of the interdisk ligamentous space of Policard. The latter is bordered by vertebral periosteum and the anterior longitudinal ligament anteriorly and by the vertebral body and the most external lamella of the annulus posteriorly.

The space of Policard is easily widened anteriorly and laterally due to the presence of loose connective tissue containing potentially osteogenic cells. This tissue is the equivalent of the germinal layer present in all periosteal tissues. A mechanical stimulus such as anterolateral disk protrusion can reactivate the osteogenic cells. The newly formed bone tissue fills a space between the protruded disk posteriorly or medially and the longitudinal ligament anterolaterally. Posterior osteophytes are smaller and represent the hypertrophy of the posterior margin which may be seen radiographically as a doubling of the vertebral wall. They never assume the same form or dimension of anterior osteophytes because they lack the loose interdisk ligamentous space with osteogenic potential. Their position however inables them to narrow the anteroposterior diameter of the vertebral canal (Figs. 3a, b).

There is no cause–effect relationship between the pathoanatomic and radiographic pictures and the clinical picture unless the osteophytes are located in particular anatomic areas or come into contact with nervous or vascular structures.

References

1. Boni M (1966) Considerazioni anatomo-patologiche e cliniche sulle protrusioni del disco nel rachide cervicale. Estratto dagli Atti del LI Congresso della Società Italiana di Ortopedia e Traumatologia – Catania, ottobre 1966
2. Boni M, Ceciliani L, Pazzaglia UE (1983) Fisiopatologia della colonna cervicale nei rapporti tra senescenza e artrosi. Estratto dagli Atti del Convegno di aggiornamento su "La patologia del rachide cervicale". Napoli 27–28 maggio 1983
3. Ceciliani L, Pazzaglia UE, Mora R (1983) Artrosi del rachide. Patologia. Relazione al 3° Corso di aggiornamento sulla radiodiagnostica dello scheletro. Reggio Calabria, 14–15 aprile 1983
4. Eyring E (1968) The biochemistry and physiology of the intervertebral discs. Clin Orthop 67:16–28

3.4. Cervical Osteochondrosis – and a Possible Etiologic Basis in Lower Spinal Deformity

D. R. Rao and U. Rodegerdts, Bremerhaven,
Federal Republic of Germany

Introduction

Cervical osteochondrosis occurs in three components of the intervertebral joint – 1. the anterior disc related structures, 2. the posterolateral uncovertebral articulation, and 3. the posterior facet joints. It is generally accepted that the degenerative pathology in these three areas is a linked process, and that disc malfunction is the triggering event that sets off the entire chain.

The currently accepted etiology of this disc malfunction in degenerative or idiopathic cervical osteochondrosis is that of a biochemical process, probably related to aging. The mucopolysaccharides in the nucleus pulposus are replaced by alternative mucopolysaccharides which do not have the same water absorption characteristics. Simultaneously, elastic fibres of the annulus are replaced by a greater proportion of collagen. Both these changes cause the disc to gradually loose its turgor, and by altering the smooth roller mechanism of disc motion result in the changes of cervical osteochondrosis.

The purpose of this paper is to present a hypothesis for the etiology of cervical osteochondrosis, based on mechanical functions, not just of the involved level, but of the entire structural form of the spine, and to present a radiological observation which supports this hypothesis.

Biomechanical Review

Let us first review a few basic principles cogent to our hypothesis:

1. *Spinal attitude:* In the coronal plane, the normal adult spine is a completely straight column, or may have a mild right thoracic curve. This normal posture maintains the head in line with the centre of gravity of the trunk, and requires practically no muscular activity for its maintenance, as evident by electromyogram studies. The minute there is a lateral deviation of a part of the spinal column, muscles on the opposing side of the spine come

into play, and bring about a compensatory tilt in the opposite direction, in an attempt to restore the neutral position in line with the centre of gravity. This is very similar to the simple principle of moments (Force [F] 1 × Distance [D] 1 = F2 × D2) that we are used to, with three modifications:

1.1 The tendency and ability to compensate for these spinal deviations is much less in the thoracic spine, owing to its multiple ligamentous and bony restraints, and because of its moment of inertia. Deviations from the normal straight attitude in the lower spine are therefore more likely to be compensated for in the cervical spine.

1.2 The lateral deviation [D] that may arise and require compensation, as well as the compensatory lateral tilt, are never purely coronal plane deviations, but involve a more complex element of sagittal and axial rotation, the phenomenon we call 'coupling'.

1.3 The increased muscle force [F] that brings about the compensatory tilt causes an increased pressure at the intervertebral joints that it spans, interfering with the normal physiology of disc nutrition in these areas.

2. *Disc anatomy:* The multilaminar annulus fibre anatomy is such that axial rotation in either direction is likely to immediately tense one set of fibres. It has been estimated [1] that while an average of 16° rotation is required to produce complete failure of the disc, definite changes occur even in the range of 3°–4°, probably in the form of altered adherence between individual fibres, and possible permanent deformation of the fibres.

3. *Coupling:* This interrelationship of motion axes is greatest in the cervical and lumbar spine, and often involves rotations in two planes combined with lateral bending. Compensatory tilts of the cervical spine would therefore involve not only lateral bending, but also an axial rotation, a rotation we have already seen is probably the most injurious force at the disc level.

4. *Disc nutrion:* The nutrition of the disc after the second decade relies on diffusion between the nucleus and the vertebral body. This diffusion is dependent on a) the colloidal absorption powers of the nucleus mucopolysaccharides, and b) alternating compression and relaxation of the disc resulting from surrounding muscle contractions pressing against the turgor of the disc. Changes in either this muscle contraction, or the annulus integrity which is responsible for the disc turgor, are therefore likely to interfere with this mode of disc nutrition.

So we now have a situation in which:

- Deviations in coronal posture of the lower spine necessitate compensatory movements in the cervical spine to maintain the centre of gravity.
- The lateral deviations which may occur are more complex and involve rotations in other planes.
- These rotational stresses are capable of microscopic disc injury even at low levels.

– The altered muscular forces that come into play when there is a deviation from spinal posture hamper disc nutrition.

Radiological Review

It was with this hypothesis, and with our observation on radiographs that cervical osteochondrosis was commonly associated with lower spinal deformity, that we reviewed more than 150 patients who had presented with the complaint of neck pain in our outpatient clinic over the past one and a half years. Of these patients with neck pain, we included only those patients who
– had no evidence of disorders other than degenerative cervical osteochondrosis, such as previous cervical spinal trauma, congenital anomalies, tumours, infections, generalised inflammatory disorders
– had anteroposterior (AP) and lateral X-rays of the whole spine, taken routinely, in addition to AP, lateral and flexion-extension views of the cervical spine.

The final number of patients included in this radiological review was 64, with 34 women and 30 men. The age distribution ranged from 19–74 years, with a peak in the middle ages.

In this radiological study, the evidence of cervical osteochondrosis that was used was the presence of anterior or posterior osteophytes, and a decrease in disc space. Anterior osteophytes were present in differing grades of severity in 52 of the 64 patients, while posterior osteophytes were likewise present in 59 of these patients. A disc space decrease was present at one or more levels in 38 of the patients.

On reviewing X-rays of the whole spine, some mean values were obtained:
Thoracic kyphosis 35.7°
Lumbar lordosis 40.4°
Sacral inclination 39.1°

The range of normal values in these cases is however extremely variable, and it is difficult to determine correlations if we want to study the effect of deviations in these values on other parts of the spine. Our study restricted itself to alterations in the anteroposterior view of the spine.

In the AP view of the whole spine, we were surprised to find that of these 64 patients who complained of neck pain, there were 52 patients who had a scoliotic lower spine. The curves in 10 of these patients could be considered normal – a mild right thoracic curve.

In the remaining 42 patients, the scoliotic deviation was uniformly spread out over the differing age groups, and ranged in amount from 4°–32°, with the maximum (23) having curves of between 6°–10°. There was a slight preponderance of left sided curves – 26 left and 16 right. A leg length discrepancy (mean 8.8 mm) was found in 34 of these patients, with an equal distribution of shorter left and right sides. There was no correlation of the side of the scoliosis to the side of the shorter leg length. The curves were distributed fairly evenly over the thoraco-lumbar spine. Nine of these patients, almost all with a larger curve, had a secondary curve, which ranged from 5°–27°.

Conclusion

It is thus clear that a large number of these patients who came to us with the complaints and findings of a typical cervical osteochondrosis, also had mechanical deformities in the lower spine. A direct cause and effect relationship is difficult to establish at this moment, but will hopefully be a subject for research over the next few years. The review of a few well established biomechanical principles, and the results of our radiological review have however prompted us to start thinking of the mechanical interrelationships of the entire spine as a unit, not just in severe scoliosis or kyphosis, or ankylosing spondylitis, but also in the evaluation of the so called 'degenerative spine'.

Reference

1. Farfan HF, Gracetovsky S (1984) The nature of instability. Spine 9:714–719

Cervical Spine II
© by Springer-Verlag 1989

3.5. Pre- and Post-operative Evaluation in Patients Affected by Spondylotic Myelopathy

U. Borromeo, P. Cherubino, and V. Cosi, Pavia, Italy

Introduction

The clinical status of patients with spondylotic myelopathies and their surgical outcomes can be evaluated by considering certain clinical parameters such as strength, sensitivity, gait and pain. The aim of this study is to examine the characteristics of somatosensory evoked potentials (S.E.P.) before and after cervical spine surgery for spondylotic myelopathy and to see if any correlation exists between S.E.P. recordings and clinical status, according to previously published data [1, 2].

Materials and Methods

Somatosensory evoked potentials were measured in 13 patients who were operated on for spondylotic myelopathy (11) or herniated cervical disk (2). Surgery consisted of the Cloward operation in 9 cases and multiple subtotal somatectomy in 4 (see Table 1). The patient group consisted of 2 females and 11 males whose ages ranged from 36 to 75 years of age (average age 56). The most common complaint had been of cervical spinal pain which radiated to the arms and was accompanied by paraesthesia and weakness. 7 patients had had difficulty in gait due to lack of lower limb strength. Matsukado's classification (1976) [3] was used to divide patients according to their level of disability (see Table 2). In the course of this study all 4 limbs were stimulated but here we take into consideration only the data relative to the median nerve. S.E.P.s were measured 5–15 days before and 6–8 months after surgery by stimulating the right and left median nerves with rectangular electrical pulses of 0.1 ms duration, 3.3/sec frequency and of sufficient intensity to cause slight contraction of the opponens twitch. E.E.G. signals were recorded using surface electrodes at Erb's point and at the cervical (Cv7) and cortical (C3–C4) levels with a linked-ear reference and analyzed with the Nicolet Pathfinder II system (bandwidth: 15–3000 Hz; double analysis time

Table 1. *Patient's Data*

Patient	Sex	Age	Diagnosis	Operation	Levels
C.M.	F	61	S.M.	CL.	C4−C5, C5−C6
C.N.	M	73	S.M.	CL.	C4−C5, C5−C6
D.M.A.	M	69	S.M.	M.S.S.	C4−C7
F.G.	M	54	S.M.	CL.	C5−C6, C6−C7
M.G.	M	75	S.M.	CL.	C3−C4, C5−C6
M.C.	F	45	S.M.	M.S.S.	C4−C7
M.O.	M	63	S.M.	M.S.S.	C3−C6
P.V.	M	36	H.D.	CL.	C5−C6, C6−C7
P.P.	M	65	S.M.	CL.	C4−C5
S.P.	M	37	H.D.	CL.	C5−C6
S.R.	M	59	S.M.	CL.	C4−C5
T.A.	M	51	S.M.	M.S.S.	C4−C7
Z.L.	M	50	S.M.	CL.	C4−C5, C5−C6

S.M.: spondylotic myelopathy; H.D.: herniated cervical disk; CL.: Cloward operation; M.S.S.: multiple subtotal somatectomy.

Table 2. *Matsukado's Classification* [3]

Patient	Diagnosis	Disability group	
		Preoperative	Postoperative
C.M.	S.M.	3	2
C.N.	S.M.	3	2
D.M.A.	S.M.	4	3
F.G.	S.M.	3	2
M.G.	S.M.	4	3
M.C.	S.M.	3	1
M.O.	S.M.	3	2
P.V.	H.D.	2	1
P.P.	S.M.	3	3
S.P.	H.D.	2	1
S.R.	S.M.	3	1
T.A.	S.M.	3	2
Z.L.	S.M.	3	2

1: Normal working and social lives; 2: Reduced activity; 3: Confined to the house; 4: Confined to bed.
S.M.: Spondylotic myelopathy; H.D.: herniated disk.

of 100 and 30 ms; 2 averages of 500–1000 artifact-free peaks). In this study the latencies of the waveforms at Erb's point (E.P.), at the cervical level (N13) and at the cortical level (N19) as well as the interpeak intervals E.P.–N13, E.P.–N19 and N13–N19 were recorded and compared with data obtained from 20 normal age matched subjects. Post-operative S.E.P. changes were tested using analysis of variance for repeated measurements.

Results

Pre-operative S.E.P.

Normal latency was observed at Erb's point in all limbs examined. The cervical recordings however were unsuccessful in 6/26 trials of 3 subjects. The cortical response was recorded in every case and the N19 peak was delayed in 8 recordings (3 bilaterally). The interpeak interval E.P.–N19 was significantly increased in 12 recordings (5 bilaterally) while the E.P.–N13 and N13–N19 interpeaks were pathologically increased in 6/20 and 3/20 recordings in 4 and 2 subjects respectively. In 2 of 5 patients with absolute latencies and interpeaks intervals within the normal range there were significant left and right asymmetries of N13 and N13–N19 in 1 case and E.P.–N13 and N13–N19 in the other. Thus the median nerve S.E.P. recordings were completely normal in only 3/13 patients.

Post-operative Potentials

No abnormalities in recordings at Erb's point were observed. A previously absent prolonged bilateral cervical response appeared in 2 patients. In 2 other subjects there was a normalization of the N13 latency. Cervical potentials were recorded in all but one patient. A significantly reduced latency in the cortical response was observed in 3 recordings in 2 subjects, but in no case was there a pathological increase in previously normal N19. In 2 subjects the interpeak N19 returned to within the normal range. 4 abnormal E.P.–N13 interpeaks were recorded in cervical waveforms that had been previously absent (Figs. 1–3). In 2 cases there was normalization of the interpeak. E.P.–N13 was pathologically increased in only one recording (Figs. 4–6). The recalculated interpeaks were normal bilaterally in one patient and unilaterally in another subject. A significant reduction in latency was observed in one case and a significant increase was observed in a second case (see Table 3).

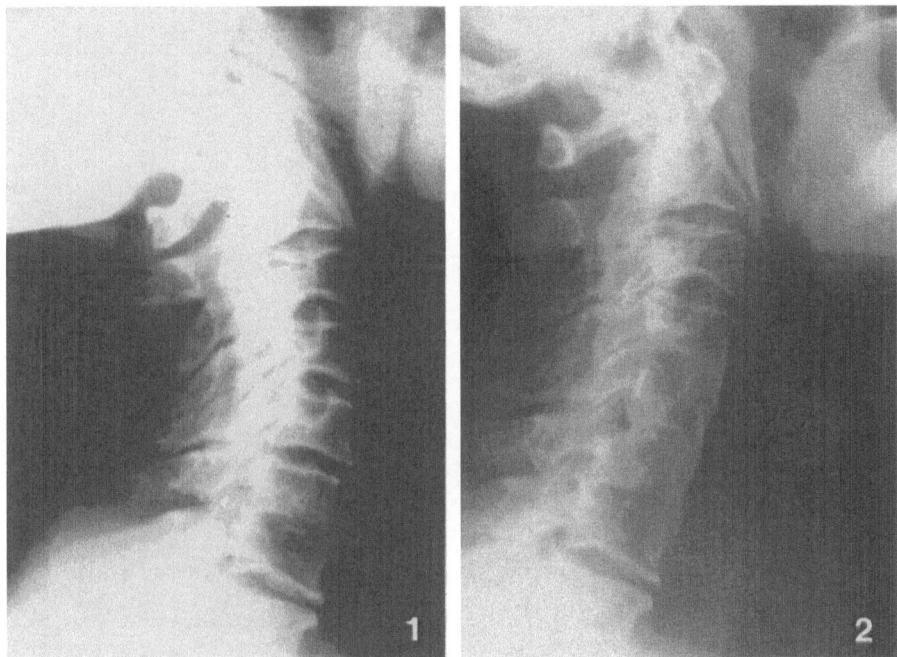

Fig. 1. S.R., a 73 year old male, began experiencing paraesthesias and sensory deficits of the upper limbs about 2 years ago which was followed by paraesthesias of the lower limbs and difficulty with gait

Fig. 2. After the S.E.P. recording a M.S.S. of C4–C6 was performed and at the last examination the patient reported improvement in gait and sensation

Table 3. *Recordings of S.E.P. pre- and postoperative*

| | EP | | | N13 | | | N19 | | |
	Abs	Del	Nor	Abs	Del	Nor	Abs	Del	Nor
Pre	0	0	26	6	2	18	0	8	18
Post	0	0	26	2	2	22	0	5	21

| | EP–19 | | | EP–N13 | | | N13–N19 | | |
	Abs	Del	Nor	Abs	Del	Nor	Abs	Del	Nor
Pre	0	12	14	6	6	14	6	3	17
Post	0	10	16	2	9	15	2	3	21

Abs: absent; Del: delayed; Nor: normal.

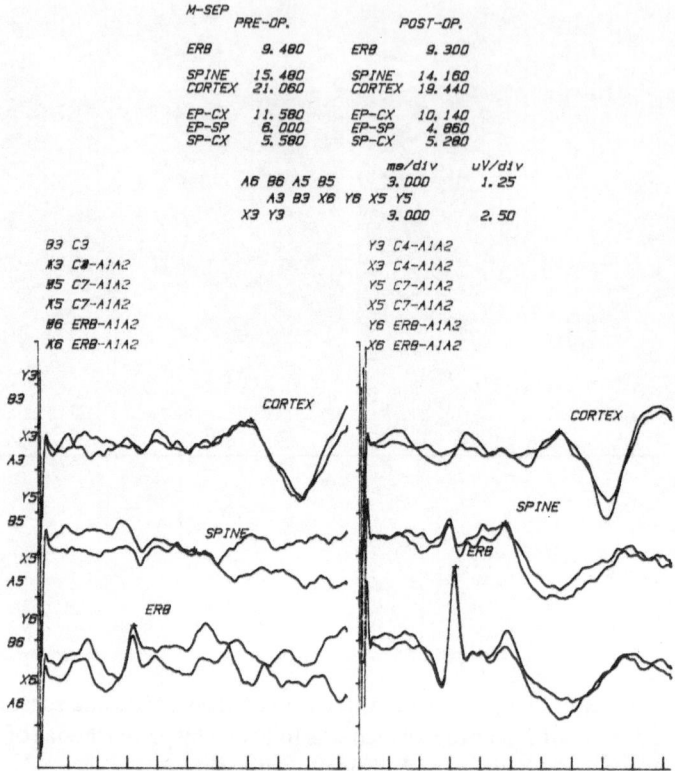

Fig. 3. The post-op. S.E.P. recording showed a remarkable improvement in identifiability of peaks from the cervical response with respect to the pre-op. recording

Fig. 4. P.P., a 65 year old male, began loosing strength in his right arm in 1964 and 3 years ago started complaining of hypoaesthesia of both hands and marked loss of strength in his left leg

Fig. 5. After recording the patient's S.E.P. pattern he underwent surgery for decompression of C4–C5 using the Cloward technique

Fig. 6. The latest follow-up examination revealed a slight improvement in the patient's clinical conditions. The post-op. S.E.P. recording was essentially unvaried with respect to the pre-op. recording

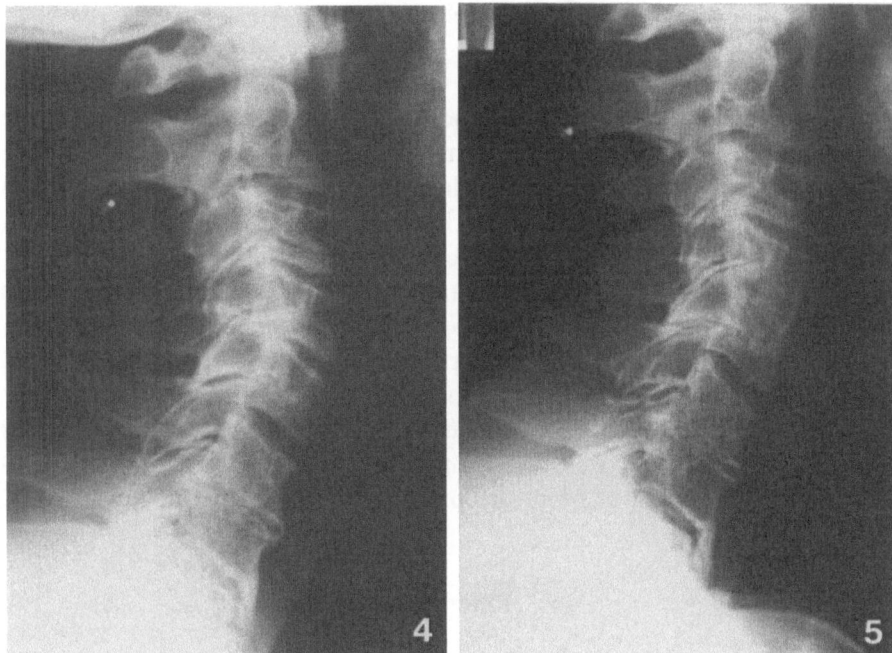

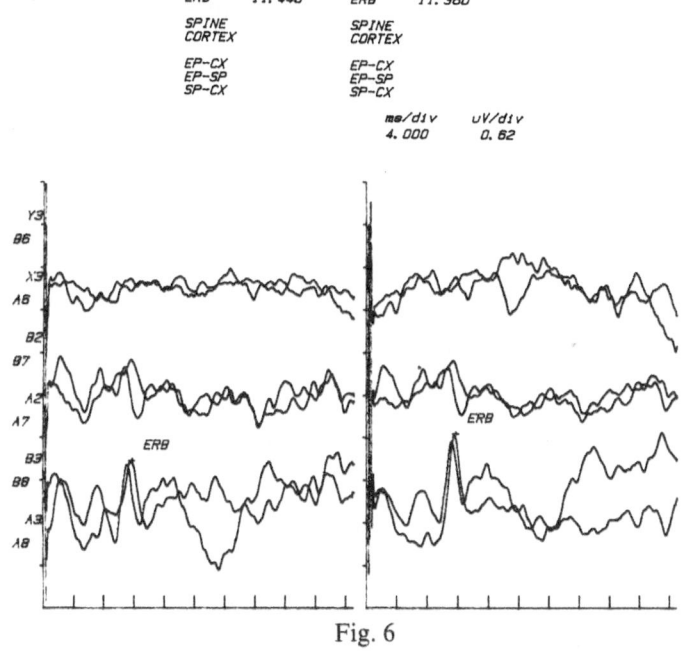

Fig. 6

Conclusion

Although our results contain only the most relevant parameters, we can draw some conclusions. Notwithstanding S.E.P. recordings investigate the sensitive routes, they have been extensively used in diagnosing and staging spondylotic myelopathy. Therefore, they can be applied in surveying clinical results of operated patients. In our series we found no statistically significant differences in any of the parameters considered.

There was however a trend toward improvement in S.E.P. recordings shown by a greater number of post-operative peaks in some patients and a reduction in latency in others. The improvement of each recording paralleled the patient's clinical improvement. Conversely, patients who remained clinically unchanged, showed no change in S.E.P. patterns. S.E.P. patterns recording therefore is a useful instrument for the objective long term evaluation of patients operated on for decompression in spondylotic myelopathy.

References

1. Siivola J, Sulg I, Heiskari M (1981) Somatosensory evoked potentials in diagnosis of cervical spondylosis and herniated disc. Electroencephalogr Clin Neurophysiol 52:276–282
2. Yannikas C, Shahani BT, Young RR (1986) Short latency somatosensory evoked potentials from radial, median, ulnar and peroneal nerve stimulation in the assessment of cervical spondylosis. Arch Neurol 43:1264–1271
3. Matsukado Y, Yoshida M, Goya T, Shimosi K (1976) Classification of cervical spondylosis or disc protrusion by preoperative evoked spinal electrogram. J Neurosurg 44:435–441

Cervical Spine II
© by Springer-Verlag 1989

3.6. Cervical Myelopathy Secondary to Lower Cervical Spondylosis in Down's Patients

T. S. Whitecloud, III, P. M. Olive, and J. T. Bennett,
New Orleans, LA, U.S.A.

The incidence of cervical myelopathy in Down's syndrome patients secondary to abnormalities of the upper cervical spine have been well documented [3]. However, this study indicates that lower cervical spondylosis may prove to be more significant than upper cervical abnormalities as a causative factor of cervical spondylotic myelopathy in this group of patients.

Materials and Methods

One hundred thirteen Down's syndrome patients were evaluated clinically and radiographically at the Pinecrest State School. All patients with atlanto-axial instability defined by a fixed interval of 5 mm or by 4 mm of motion were excluded from the study group [1]. Eight patients (7%) were found to have atlanto-axial instability and were eliminated leaving 105 patients in the study. The ages ranged from 21 to 50 years with a mean age of 35. There were 69 males (65.7%) and 36 females (34.3%).

All patients were examined for signs of cervical myelopathy. Gait, activity level, deep tendon reflexes, ankle clonus, and Babinski signs were evaluated and noted. Flexion and extension lateral radiographs of the cervical spine of each patient were obtained. The radiographs were evaluated for anterior osteophytes, posterior osteophytes, abnormal disc space narrowing, sagittal plane translation, sagittal plane rotation, spinal stenosis, and congenital anomalies.

Spinal stenosis was defined as any interval between the posterior aspect of the vertebral body and its corresponding spinolaminar line less than 13 mm [12].

Abnormal sagittal plane translation and sagittal plane rotation were defined as greater than 3.5 mm and 11° respectively [11].

Results

One patient had congenital spinal stenosis. The sagittal diameter between C3 and C6 was 12.5 mm. The patient was hyper-reflexic, had bilateral sustained ankle clonus, and could not ambulate without assistance.

Three patients were found to have Klippel-Feil syndrome. The most common radiographic abnormality was the presence of anterior osteophytes which occurred in 59 patients (56.2%). Chi-square analysis using 2 by 2 multi-way frequency tables demonstrated that there was no significant correlation between the presence of anterior osteophytes and any abnormal physical finding.

Forty-eight patients (45.7%) had posterior osteophytes. When present, 88% had two or more levels involved.

Abnormal disc space narrowing occurred in 54 patients (51.4%). Nineteen of these patients (35.2%) had narrowing at two or more levels. Narrowing was highly associated ($p < 0.0001$) with the presence of both anterior and posterior osteophytes.

Excessive sagittal plane translation and rotation were present in six (5.7%) and one (0.95%) patients respectively. They did not significantly correlate with any abnormal physical finding.

Ataxia was present in 7 patients (6.7%). One hundred percent of patients with ataxia also had either hyper-reflexia or clonus. Six of the 7 had abnormal radiographs: 5 had disc space narrowing and osteophyte formation while 1 had spinal stenosis.

Hyper-reflexia was the most common abnormal physical finding. It was present in 36 patients (34.3%) and was found to significantly correlate with the presence of posterior osteophytes and disc space narrowing ($p < 0.0075$).

Ankle clonus occurred in 18 patients (17.1%). It was highly associated with hyper-reflexia ($p < 0.0001$).

A summary of the overall results is shown in Table 1.

Table 1. *Comparison of Radiographic Signs of Lower Cervical Spondylosis with Physical Findings Consistent with Cervical Myelopathy*

Age	Signs of spondylosis	Hyper-reflexia or clonus	Hyper-reflexia or clonus and signs of spondylosis	Hyper-reflexia or clonus and no signs of spondylosis
21–30 (39 pts.)	30 (76.9%)	10 (25.6%)	3 (20.5%)	2 (5.1%)
31–40 (41 pts.)	26 (63.4%)	14 (34.1%)	13 (32%)	1 (2.4%)
41–50 (17 pts.)	7 (41%)	5 (29.4%)	4 (23%)	1 (5.8%)
51–58 (8 pts.)	3 (37.5%)	3 (37.5%)	3 (37.5%)	0 (0%)
21–58 (105 pts.)	66 (62.8%)	32 (30.5%)	28 (26.7%)	4 (3.8%)

Discussion

The objective of this study was to evaluate the prevalence of lower cervical spondylosis in adult Down's syndrome patients and to correlate this with physical findings consistent with cervical myelopathy.

Friedenberg and Miller [8] reported on the prevalence of cervical spondylosis in the normal population in a comparative study of symptomatic and asymptomatic patients. They showed that 25% of asymptomatic patients will have radiographic signs of cervical spondylosis by age 40 and 75% of patients will have them by age 60.

In our study group, 70% of the patients had radiographic evidence of cervical spondylosis by age 40. This age group consisted of 80% of the patients studied.

Fidone [6] also reported an increased instance of degenerative changes in cervical spines of 41 Down's patients. Although his study group was small, he found that 50% of patients in their 30's and 100% of patients over 40 had signs of spondylosis characterized by osteophytes, subarticular sclerosis, cystic changes or disc space narrowing. This increased prevalence of lower cervical spondylosis is probably secondary to excessive amounts of motion within the spinal segments due to inherent ligamentous laxity. Other well recognized abnormalities in Down patients due to ligamentous laxity include patellar subluxation, dislocation of the hip, pes planus, and atlanto-axial subluxation [3–5]. Cervical spondylosis and myelopathy have also been associated with the excessive motion that occurs in patients with athetoid cerebral palsy [1, 8].

Anterior osteophytes, the most common radiographic abnormality, did not correlate with any abnormal physical finding while disc space narrowing and posterior osteophyte formation were highly associated with the findings of hyper-reflexia and clonus. The production of osteophytic outgrowths is probably secondary to disc degeneration (anterior and posterior osteophytes were highly associated with disc space narrowing) but only the posterior exostoses are in close proximity to the neural elements and thus have the potential to impinge upon them.

Cervical myelography demonstrated spinal cord compression from a posterior osteophyte in our first case example that stimulated this study. Bailey and Casamajor also demonstrated spinal cord compression by posterior osteophytes in 1911 [2]. The contributions of Pallis, Jones, and Spillane [10] and Nurick [9] also suggest that cervical myelopathy can result from narrowing of the sagittal diameter of the spinal cord from posterior osteophyte formation.

Conclusions

It is concluded that adults with Down's syndrome have an increased prevalence of spondylosis in the lower cervical spine and this occurs at an earlier age than the normal population. They may be predisposed toward developing cervical myelopathy, however, longitudinal studies would be needed to confirm this.

A detailed physical examination is difficult to obtain due to the patient's inability to fully cooperate.

Lower cervical spondylosis leading to myelopathy may be a greater risk than atlanto-axial instability in adults with Down's syndrome.

Physicians that deal with Down's syndrome patients should be aware of these findings in addition to the well known abnormalities of the upper cervical spine. It is recommended that these patients be followed with a yearly neurologic evaluation, and if the physical findings are consistent with cervical myelopathy, appropriate radiographic studies should be obtained.

References

1. Anderson WW, Wise BL, Itabashi HH, Jones M (1962) Cervical spondylosis in patients with athetosis. Neurology 12:410–412
2. Bailey P, Casamajor L (1911) Osteoarthritis of the spine as a cause of compression of the spinal cord and its roots. J Nerv Ment Dis 39:588
3. Burke SW, French HG, Roberts JM, Johnston CE, Whitecloud TS, Edmunds JO (1985) Chronic atlanto-axial instability in Down syndrome. J Bone Joint Surg 67A:1356–1360
4. Cope R, Olson S (1987) Abnormalities of the cervical spine in Down's syndrome: Diagnosis, risks, and review of the literature, with particular reference to the Special Olympics. South Med J 80:33–36
5. Dzentitis AJ (1966) Spontaneous atlanto-axial dislocation in a mongoloid child with spinal cord compression. Case report. J Neurosurg 25:458–460
6. Fidone GS (1986) Degenerative cervical arthritis and Down's syndrome. N Engl J Med 314:320
7. Friedenberg ZB, Miller WT (1963) Degenerative disc disease of the cervical spine. A comparative study of asymptomatic and symptomatic patients. J Bone Joint Surg 45-A:1171–1178
8. Fuj T, Yonenobu K, Fujiwara K, Yamashita K, Ebara S, Ono K, Okada K (1987) Cervical radiculopathy or myelopathy secondary to athetoid cerebral palsy. J Bone Joint Surg 69-A:815–821
9. Nurick S (1972) The pathogenesis of the spinal cord disorder associated with cervical spondylosis. Brain 95:87–100
10. Pallis C, Jones AM, Spillane JD (1954) Cervical spondylosis. Brain 77:274–289
11. White AA, Southwick WD, Panjabi MM (1976) Clinical instability in the lower cervical spine. A review of past and current concepts. Spine 1:15–27
12. Yates A (1983) Computed tomographic evaluation of cervical pain syndromes. In: Genant HK (ed) Spine Update 1984. University of California Press, San Francisco, pp 291, 307

3.7. Long Term Clinical and Radiographic Evaluation of Cervical Herniated Disks Operated by Cloward's Technique

P. CHERUBINO, L. CECILIANI, F. BENAZZO, and U. BORROMEO, Pavia, Italy

Introduction

One can expect that fusion of one or more cervical spinal segments leads to a subsequent functional overloading of the disks above and below the fusion with the possible creation of new compressions [1]. To verify this hypothesis we examined clinically and radiographically a series of patients who had been operated on for cervical decompression using the Cloward technique [2, 3]. Particular attention was paid to the presence of radiographic changes in the disk spaces directly above and below the fused cervical segment(s).

Patients and Methods

Data relative to the studied patients is shown in Tables 1–3.

Table 1. *Patient's Data*

No.	Sex	Age at surgery	Present age	Follow-up (year)
37	25 M	45.49	56.97	11.5
	12 F	(16–67)	(25–80)	(7–16)

Table 2. *Disk Level Distribution*

Levels	No.	%
C3–C4	3	5.17
C4–C5	10	17.24
C5–C6	28	48.27
C6–C7	17	29.31

Table 3. *Level of Surgergy*

Operations	No.
C3–C4, C4–C5	2
C3–C4, C4–C5, C5–C6	1
C4–C5, C5–C6	4
C4–C5, C5–C6, C6–C7	3
C5–C6	13
C5–C6, C6–C7	7
C6–C7	7

The preoperative diagnosis were: spondylotic myelopathy in 4 cases; disk herniation in 6 cases; spondylotic radiculopathy in 17 cases; fracture-luxation in 9 cases; and tumor in 1 case.

Anteroposterior and lateral radiographs of the cervical spine and CT-scans were taken for each patient. All patients were clinically evaluated with particular attention to the superior and inferior limb strength, sensation and gait, on duration and severity of symptoms prior to surgery, and on the eventual reappearance of any type of cervical or peripheral symptoms. Nurick's scale was employed for the clinical evaluation of the patient's pre- and postsurgical conditions.

The radiographic evaluation consisted of measuring the height, in mm of the adjacent disks at their midpoint, the dimensions of any osteophytes present, the protrusion in mm of the uncus, and the diameter of the vertebral canal at its narrowest point.

Results

According to Nurick's scale, 29 cases were rated as improved, 6 unchanged and 2 worse. Five of the cases rated as unchanged by Nurick's scale with follow up ranging from 9 to 12 years experienced a worsening of symptoms beginning 3–4 years before being examined for this study. They had therefore enjoyed a long period of well being, and they also would have rated better in a hypothetical former evaluation. The percentage of patients rated as improved was therefore 78%, a figure which agrees with practically all the literature data presented on this topic.

From the radiographic point of view the mean thickness of the disks above the fused segment was 5.70 mm (range 2–8 mm). The mean thickness of the underlying disks was 5.25 mm (range 2 to 10 mm). We must take into account a radiographic magnification of about 10%. In cases in which arthrodesis of 3 vertebrae had been performed the average height of the over and underlying disks was 4.75 mm compared with an average of 5.53 mm and 5.90 mm above and below the fusion of 2 vertebrae (13 patients). This indicates a greater functional demand with greater wear in the former case. We found that the disk degeneration was not as great as could have been expected considering the long follow-up period.

The average dimension of antero-posterior osteophytes was 2.44 mm (range 0 to 9 mm) and the mean anteroinferior osteophytes measured 2.22 mm (range 0 to 7 mm). Postero-superior and postero-inferior osteophytes averaged 1.57 mm (range 0 to 4) and 1.61 mm (range 0 to 4 mm) respectively. The average size of the uncus was 4 mm superiorly (more precisely 4.41 mm right superior and 4.52 mm left superior). Inferior uncus were not considered (T1 has no uncus). The diameter of the canal averaged 16.43 mm (range 9–22 mm), and it was calculated from X-rays and CT scans.

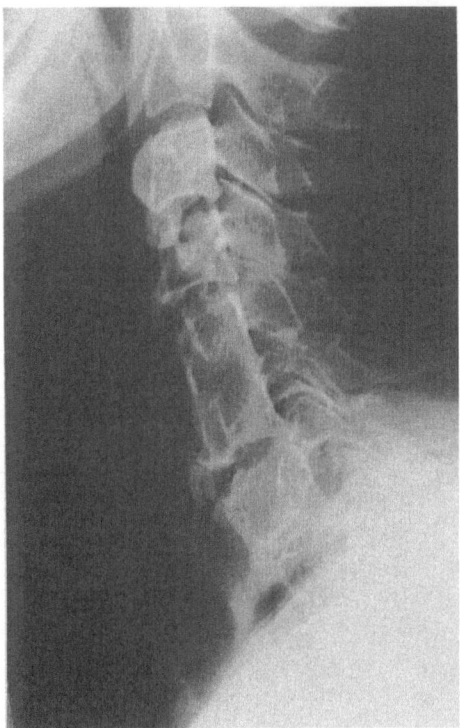

Fig. 1. C.W., woman, 42 y at surgery; present age 51 (follow-up 9 y). Fusion of C5–C6 (radiculopathy due to hard disk protrusion): the space below shows a large calcification, and posterior osteophytes

The frequent finding of prevertebral calcifications was unexpected. They were found at the level of the overlying and/or underlying disk space in 26 cases (70.27%) (Fig. 1).

From the statistical point of view, the computer generated correlation matrix contains all the variables considered. The relationship between any two of the variables can be found at the intersection of the desired horizontal and vertical axes and is expressed numerically (Pearson's r, 2 tailed test).

Significant correlations were found between disk thickness and age (inverse correlation), anterosuperior and posterosuperior osteophytes and age, (direct correlation). Obviously there was also a significant inverse correlation between age and the diameter of the vertebral canal in agreement with the prior data. An inverse correlation was found between the overlying disk height and the posterosuperior osteophytes and a direct correlation was found between the former and the canal diameter while it was inversely correlated with Nurick's post-operative score. Positive correlations were found between the various values related to the uncus and to the osteophytes.

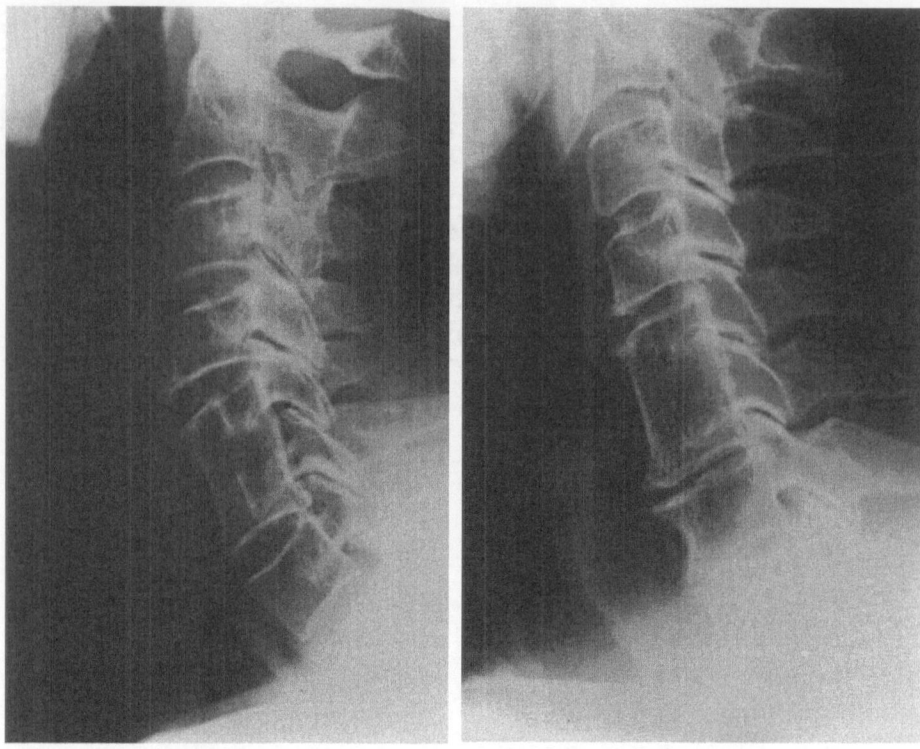

Fig. 2   Fig. 3

Fig. 2. R.C., man, 59 y at surgery; present age 75 (follow-up 16 y). Fusion of one level (C5–C6): disk spaces above and below are well preserved, despite the long period which has elapsed

Fig. 3. M.A., man, 59 y at surgery; present age 75 (follow-up 16 y). Fusion of one level (C5–C6): the disk below is reduced in height, despite the presence of osteophytes, the patient is still doing well

Discussion

The fusion of 1, 2, or 3 levels of the cervical spine with the Cloward technique causes a functional overload of the overlying and underlying disks which is directly correlated with the number of spaces fused. The overload and subsequent degeneration however are less than would have been expected (Figs. 2 and 3).

The prevertebral calcifications in front of the underlying and overlying disks, located in the anterior longitudinal ligament, are probably due to the overloading of these disks, and not to the calcification of the prevertebral post-operative hematoma. The statistical analysis highlights the important correlation between clinical result and diameter of the vertebral canal which in turn is correlated with the dimensions of the disks and osteophytes. Finally, the clinical and radiographic results reported here confirm the validity of the anterior approach with fusion of the vertebral bodies for myeloradicular decompression and stabilization of the cervical spine.

References

1. Gore DR, Gardner GM, Sepic SB, Murray MP (1986) Roentgenographic findings following anterior cervical fusion. Skeletal Radiol 15:556–559
2. Cloward RB (1958) The anterior approach for removal of ruptured cervical disks. J Neurosurg 15:602–614
3. Boni M, Denaro V (1982) Traitement chirurgical des cervicoarthroses. Valutation à distance (2–13 ans) des 100 premiers cas opérés par voie antérieure. Rev Clin Ortop 68(4):269–280

3.8. Anterior Discectomy Without Fusion for Treatment of Cervical Degenerative Disc Disease

Twelve Years Experience Based on 450 Consecutive Cases

H. Bertalanffy and H. R. Eggert, Freiburg i. Br.,
Federal Republic of Germany

Introduction

Several operative procedures for treatment of degenerative disc disease are currently available. A review of the pertinent literature reveals that apart from a few differences, the operative results are equivalent.

At the Neurosurgical Department of the University of Freiburg, discectomy without interbody fusion has been the preferred surgical method since 1976. The main advantages which led the authors to become advocates of this procedure are its technical simplicity and the lack of morbidity related to any kind of grafts.

The purpose of this paper is to demonstrate that simple anterior discectomy in our opinion constitutes an effective alternative in the surgical management of the diseased cervical disc.

Patients and Results

Four hundred and fifty patients suffering from cervical degenerative disc disease were referred to our institution between January 1976 and December 1987. Discectomy without interbody graft at one or more cervical segments was carried out in each case. Of the patients, 72% were men and 28% were women. Ages ranged from 25 to 87 years, the mean age was 50 years.

Sixty-one percent of the patients presented with the clinical picture of radiculopathy, 16% with pure myelopathy, and 23% had a combined myeloradiculopathy. In 48% the symptoms were caused by hard discs, in 40% by soft discs, and in 12% by a combination of the two types of lesions.

In 293 patients (65%) discectomy was performed at a single cervical level, in 139 (31%) at two, in 16 (3.5%) at three and in two patients (0.5%) at four levels. In total, 627 cervical discs were removed in 450 patients.

One hundred and sixty-four patients who had been surgically treated between 1976 and 1983 were followed-up clinically 1 to 8 years postoperatively, the mean follow-up time was 3.3 years. Long-term results in these patients are ranked in accordance with the criteria of Roosen and Grote [23], and were previously published in more detail [1].

For comparison of the operative outcome in this series with other results reported in the literature, the mean value of published results (according to similar criteria) was determined for 2,813 patients suffering from cervical radiculopathy and for 990 patients suffering from cervical myelopathy, presented in different publications, including several with larger series [2–12, 14–17, 20, 21, 24, 26, 28–30]. Anterior as well as posterior procedures were considered. Our own results concur with the results from the literature (Table 1).

Three hundred and thirteen patients, including 150 individuals operated on in the period 1984 and 1987, were followed-up by questionnaires, the mean follow-up time being 2 years.

According to the patients' self estimation, an excellent result (complaints relieved or markedly improved) was noted in 48% and a satisfactory result (complaints partly improved) in 31%. About one fifth (21%) of the patients questioned were not satisfied with the operative outcome (complaints unchanged or worse).

Seventy-two percent of the patients who had worked before undergoing surgery returned to their previous activity within 4 months.

One hundred and forty patients were followed-up radiologically 6 months to 9 years postoperatively, the mean follow-up time was 3.3 years. A complete fusion was noted in 75%, the fusion was incomplete in 10%, and no fusion was observed in 15% of the cases.

Fusion begins in the ventral part of the vertebral bodies (Fig. 1). Segmental mobility was measured in the levels adjacent to the segment of discectomy

Table 1. *Comparison of Long-term Results in Our 164 Own Patients with Results from the Literature*

Long-term results	Radiculopathy		Myelopathy	
	our patients	mean literature	our patients	mean literature
Excellent & good	82%	78%	55%	56%
Fair	13%	15%	25%	24%
Poor	5%	7%	20%	20%
Total (n)	109	2813	55	990

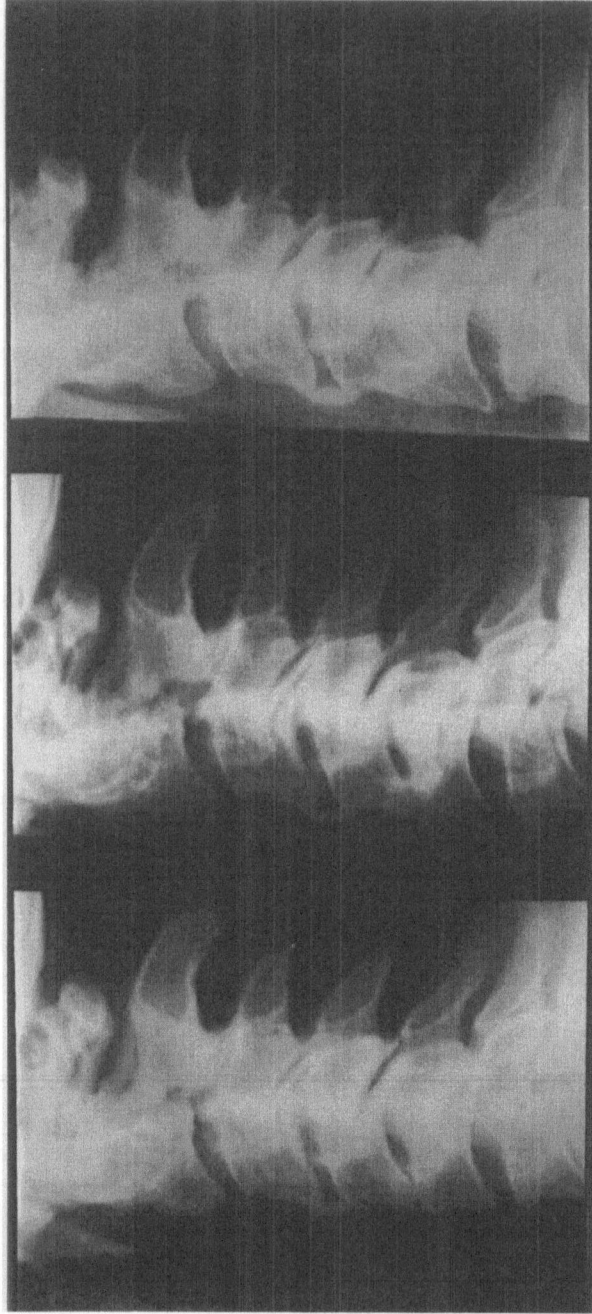

Fig. 1. Plain radiograph of a 58 year old patient at 2 days, 8 months and 3 years after simple discectomy at level C4/5

in flexion and extension. Mobility was reduced by 4° on the average in both adjacent levels immediately following the procedure. It reached the preoperative value – namely 9° on the average – at follow up in the level above, and increased by 2° on the average in the level below the segment of discectomy.

A mean kyphotic angulation of 4.8° occurred in the segment of discectomy, regardless of whether the lesion was a soft or hard disc.

In terms of the clinical long-term results, a certain correlation between degree of angulation and outcome could be observed, but this was without statistical significance.

Complications occurred in 46 out of 450 patients. Severe complications such as medullary contusion, root lesion, epidural hematoma, epidural abscess, and severe instability were observed in a total of 3% of the cases; slight complications such as Horner's syndrome, transient recurrent nerve palsy, wound infection, and local subcutaneous hematoma in 7.2%. The mortality rate was zero. Seventeen percent of the surgically treated patients complained of neck pain immediately following the procedure, which dissappeared in most cases within 1 week.

Forty patients (8.9%) were reoperated on between 2 days and 5 years after discectomy (mean 14 months). Fourteen patients had recurrent complaints due to soft or hard discs at new levels, mainly at an adjacent level below the segment of discectomy. Ten patients were operated on at the same level as in the first procedure. Surgery revealed in these cases an incomplete decompression of the neural structures.

Four patients had wound infections, as well as an instability of the cervical spine; 3 patients had a local subcutaneous hematoma, 2 an epidural hematoma and 1 individual a medullary contusion. In one patient the wrong level was operated on in the first operation and one had a meningioma of the foramen magnum, which initially had not been recognized.

Discussion

The aim of anterior discectomy is to decompress the neural components and to prevent root compression when the interspace narrows postoperatively [5, 13, 15, 18, 19, 22, 27]. To attain this goal, removal of the intervertebral disc and prolapsed disc material should always be followed by anterior bilateral foraminotomy and removal of dorsal spurs. Seeger gives a detailed description of the operative technique the way it is practiced at our institution [25].

Incomplete removal of dorsal osteophytes was the reason for progressive myelopathy in a 58 years old man, who had been operated on at level C4/5 (Fig. 1). Three years after discectomy, CT scan revealed almost complete bony fusion in the segment of discectomy, but also a persisting medial os-

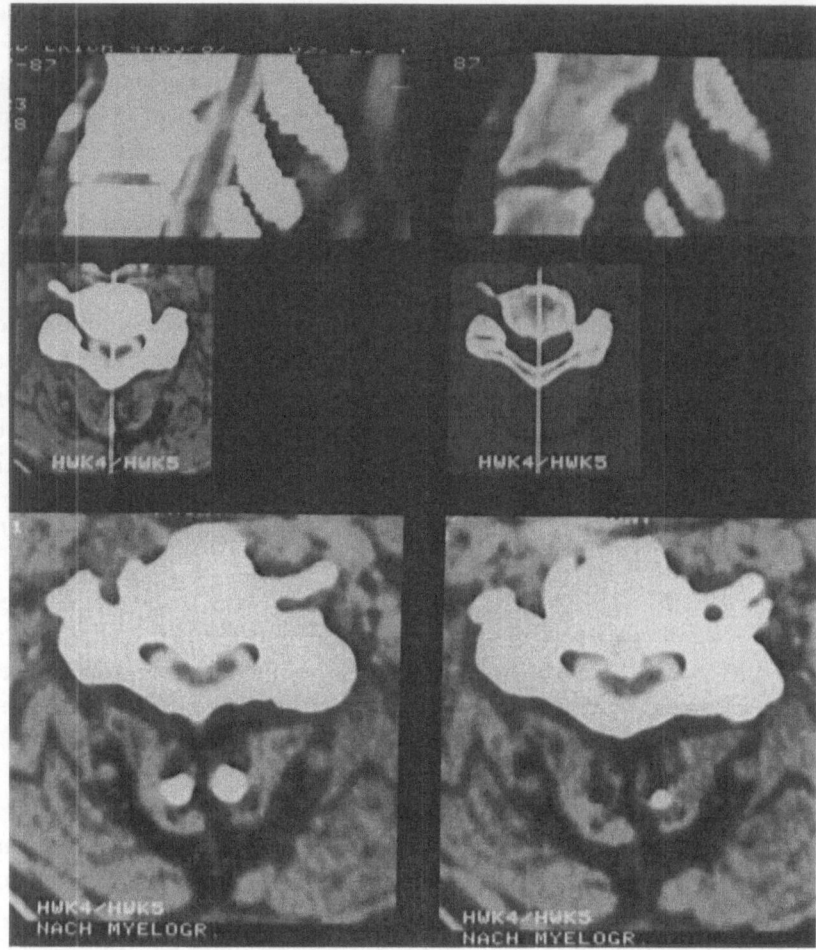

Fig. 2. Myelo-CT of the same patient as in Fig. 1, 3 years after discectomy at level
C4/5

teophyte, which caused an important cord compression (Fig. 2). This is one
of at least eight cases of this series in which no resorption of dorsal osteophytes was noted postoperatively, despite sufficient bony fusion and im-
mobility of the cervical segment.

Long-term results after discectomy were influenced by several factors.
Younger patients with radicular symptoms due to soft protrusions have the
best prognosis [1]. On the other hand, the present results demonstrate that
even older patients, with medullary complaints and multisegmental hard disc
lesions may benefit from simple discectomy. More satisfying long-term results could possibly have been achieved in some cases of this series by using
different surgical methods such as fusion techniques or posterior procedures.

However, no reliable criteria are available to determine which method is the best in each individual case. Establishing such criteria should be the subject of a randomized prospective study.

Several disadvantages are attributed to anterior discectomy, for example, postoperative kyphosis, neck pain, insufficient stability of the cervical spine, and incomplete fusion of the vertebral bodies. Our experience has shown, however, that none of these disadvantages seem serious enough to justify abandoning the method. In this series of 450 patients, instability occurred in only four cases (0.9%), requiring secondary stabilization (halo vest or spondylodesis). Postoperative neck pain of longer duration was rarely observed. Incomplete fusion and angular kyposis proved to be compatible with good and even excellent clinical outcome.

An increase in segmental mobility at the level below the segment of discectomy might be one of the reasons why most reoperations have been performed at the lower adjacent level.

The advantages of simple discectomy have already been mentioned.

Conclusions

Interbody grafts are not essential for the result in the surgical management of diseased cervical discs. Simple anterior discectomy can be applied in the different types of cervical degenerative disc disease. The chief factor responsible for poor results is incomplete decompression of neural structures.

References

1. Bertalanffy H, Eggert H-R (1988) Clinical long-term results of anterior discectomy without fusion for treatment of cervical radiculopathy and myelopathy. A follow-up of 164 cases. Acta Neurochir (Wien) 90:127–135
2. Cloward RB (1962) New method of diagnosis and treatment of cervical disc disease. Clin Neurosurg 8:93–132
3. Crandall PH, Batzdorf U (1966) Cervical spondylotic myelopathy. J Neurosurg 25:57–66
4. Cuatico W (1981) Anterior cervical discectomy without interbody fusion. An analysis of 81 cases. Acta Neurochir (Wien) 57:269–274
5. Dunsker SB (1976) Anterior cervical discectomy with and without fusion. Clin Neurosurg 24:516–521
6. Epstein JA, Carras R, Lavine LS, Epstein BS (1969) The importance of removing osteophytes as part of the surgical treatment of myeloradiculopathy in cervical spondylosis. J Neurosurg 30:219–226
7. Fager CA (1973) Results of adequate posterior decompression in the relief of spondylotic cervical myelopathy. J Neurosurg 38:684–692

8. Gregorius FK, Estrin T, Crandall PH (1976) Cervical spondylotic radiculopathy and myelopathy. A long-term follow-up study. Arch Neurol 33:618–625

9. Gros C, Privat JM, Safdari H (1984) Exérèse discale sans greffe dans le traitement des cervico-brachialgies. Acta Orthop Belg 50(1):33–38

10. Guidetti B, Fortuna A (1969) Long-term results of surgical treatment of myelopathy due to cervical spondylosis. J Neurosurg 30:714–721

11. Hankinson HL, Wilson CB (1975) Use of the operating microscope in anterior cervical discectomy without fusion. J Neurosurg 43:452–456

12. Henderson CM, Hennessy RG, Shuey HM, Shackelford EG (1983) Posterior-lateral foraminotomy as an exclusive operative technique for cervical radiculopathy: A review of 846 consecutively operated cases. Neurosurg 13:504–512

13. Husag L, Probst Ch (1984) Microsurgical anterior approach to cervical discs. Review of 60 consecutive cases of discectomy without fusion. Acta Neurochir (Wien) 73:229–242

14. Jomin M, Lesoin F, Lozes G, Thomas III CE, Rousseaux M, Clarisse J (1986) Herniated cervical discs. Analysis of a series of 230 cases. Acta Neurochir (Wien) 79:107–113

15. Lunsford LD, Bissonette DJ, Jannetta PJ, Sheptak PE, Zorub DS (1980) Anterior surgery for cervical disc disease. Part 1: treatment of lateral cervical disc herniation in 253 cases. J Neurosurg 53:1–11

16. Lunsford LD, Bissonette DJ, Zorub DS (1980) Anterior surgery for cervical disc disease. Part 2: Treatment of cervical spondylotic myelopathy in 32 cases. J Neurosurg 53:12–19

17. Mayfield FH (1966) Cervical spondylosis: a comparison of the anterior and posterior approaches. Clin Neurosurg 13:181–188

18. Martins AN (1976) Anterior cervical discectomy with and without interbody bone graft. J Neurosurg 44:290–295

19. Murphy MG, Gado M (1972) Anterior cervical discectomy without interbody bone graft. J Neurosurg 37:71–74

20. O'Laoire SA, Thomas DGT (1983) Spinal cord compression due to prolapse of cervical intervertebral disc (herniation of nucleus pulposus). J Neurosurg 59:847–853

21. Robertson JT, Johnson SD (1980) Anterior cervical discectomy without fusion: long-term results. Clin Neurosurg 27:440–449

22. Robertson JT (1978) Anterior operations for herniated cervical disc and for myelopathy. Clin Neurosurg 25:245–250

23. Roosen K, Grote W (1980) Late results of operative treatment of cervical myelopathy. In: Grote W, Brock M, Clar HE, Klinger M, Nau HE (eds) Advances in neurosurgery, vol 8. Springer, Berlin Heidelberg New York, pp 69–77

24. Scoville WB, Dohrmann GJ, Corkill G (1976) Late results of cervical disc surgery. J Neurosurg 45:203–210

25. Seeger W (1982) Microsurgery of the spinal cord and surrounding structures. Springer, Wien New York

26. Smith GW, Robinson RA (1958) The treatment of certain cervical-spine disorders by anterior removal of the intervertebral disc and interbody fusion. J Bone Joint Surg 40-A:607–624

27. Tribolet N de, Zander E (1981) Anterior discectomy without fusion for the treatment of ruptured cervical discs. J Neurosurg Sci 25:217–220
28. White AA, Southwick WO, DePonte RJ (1973) Relief of pain by anterior cervical spine fusion for spondylosis. J Bone Joint Surg 55-A:525–534
29. Williams JL, Marshall BA, Harkess JW (1968) Late results of cervical discectomy and interbody fusion: some factors influencing the results. J Bone Joint Surg 50-A:277–286
30. Wilson DH, Campbell DD (1977) Anterior cervical discectomy without bone graft. J Neurosurg 47:551–555

3.9. Osteoid Osteoma Affecting Articular Process at the Cervical Spine: Infrequent Localization and Difficult Diagnosis

C. Villas, R. Lopez, A. Arrien, and J. Zubieta, Pamplona, Spain

Summary

We present three cases of osteoid osteoma affecting the cervical spine, located in the articular process, an infrequent localization and thus a difficult diagnosis.

We found scintigraphy to be of invaluable assistance in revealing the presence of this small nodular lesion of the spine. And we found the CAT scan study useful for its precise localization of the tumor. Both modalities were used as a basis for deciding upon a viable surgical approach. Without such techniques, correct diagnosis may be made too late.

In our experience, surgical resection of the osteoid osteoma brings about immediate relief of the symptoms.

Introduction

Osteoid osteoma (O.O.) is located in the spine in approximately 10% of all cases [6, 8, 12, 15, 16, 19].

The most frequent spinal location involves the lumbar and cervical regions, with the posterior vertebral arch most commonly affected [1, 3, 9, 11–13].

Pain and muscle contractures are the most characteristic symptoms, though they are not always present. In some cases paravertebral contractures can induce scoliosis [14].

Radiologically, the lesion is represented as a radiolucent zone, surrounded by a sclerotic zone [2, 6].

Simple radiographs sometimes fail to reveal these lesions, due to overlapping of bone images and intestinal gases [1, 6]. As these lesions tend to be overlooked, the time lapse between the appearance of symptoms and diagnosis is more than 1 year in most of the series [2, 13, 17] and patients have occasionally been referred to psychiatric treatment [2].

Three new cases of O.O. are presented here, notable for their infrequent spinal location and subsequently difficult diagnosis.

Case 1

A 23 year old white male presented with cervico-brachialgia of 1 year's evolution. Onset of pain occurred nocturnally and progressed steadily over a period of one year with partial relief gained through the use of conventional anti-inflammatory analgesics. On consultation, the patient presented with parasthesias in C7. Clinical examination revealed para-spinal contracture with no evidence of neurological symptoms.

Conventional radiographs were interpreted as normal (Fig. 1a). The scintigraphy with Tc99, showed a focus of intense activity at the left articular facet of C6–C7 (Fig. 1b). The CAT scan identified a nidus, 4 mm in diameter in the proximal anterior part of the left superior facet of C7 (Fig. 1c). Surgery was performed by a posterior approach and consisted of a medial hemiface-tectomy of C6 using a high speed air drill. The nidus was identified and resected with a small currette (Fig. 1d). The cavity was filled with bone grafts taken from the upper part of the spinal process of C6.

Pain relief was complete in the immediate postoperative period and a Philadelphia orthosis was prescribed. Twenty seven months after surgical treatment the patient remains asymptomatic.

Case 2

A 23 year old white male presenting with cervico-brachialgia of 3 years evolution had undergone surgical excision of a cervical rib 5 years previously but continued to experience pain.

Our clinical examination revealed cervical contracture.

Conventional radiographs showed an irregular zone in the articular pro-cess of C4 (Fig. 2a). The scintigraphy with Tc99, showed a focus of intense activity in the right side of C4 (Fig. 2b). The CAT scan confirmed the presence of a tumor within the right articular process of C4 (Fig. 2c).

Surgery was performed by a posterior approach; the nidus was identified and resected with a small currette (Fig. 2d).

Pain relief was complete in the immediate postoperative period. Twenty one months after surgical treatment the patient remains asymptomatic.

C. Villas et al.

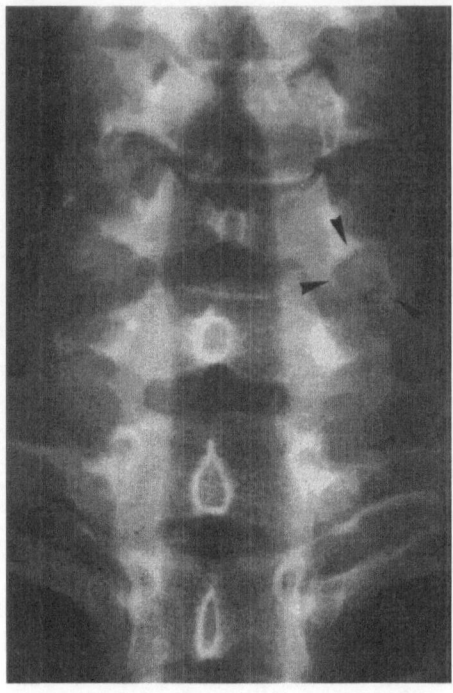

a

Fig. 1. Case 1. a) Conventional radiograph. b) Scintigraphy with Tc99. c) CAT scan.
d) Resection of the tumor

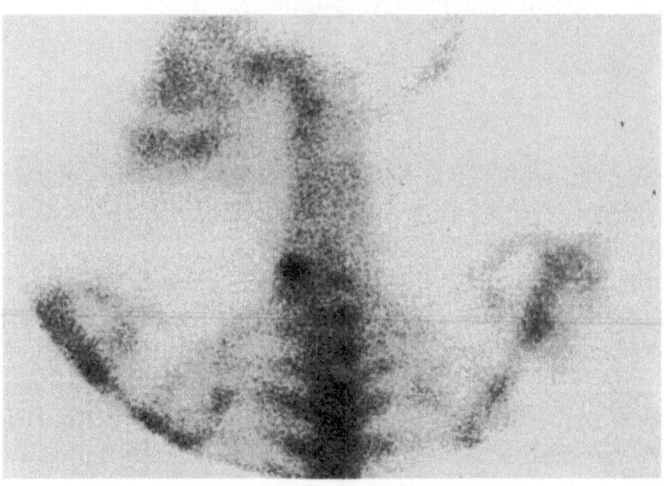

b

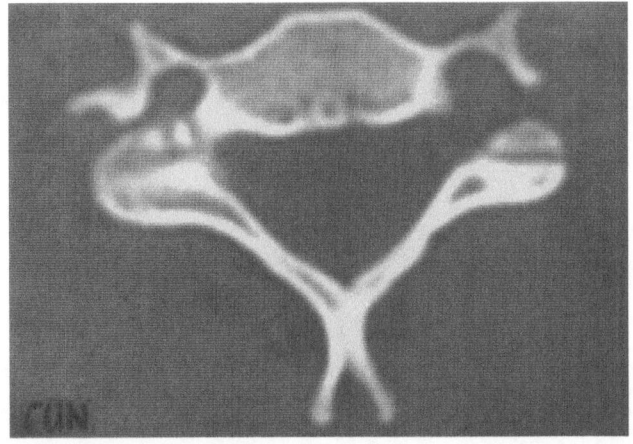

c

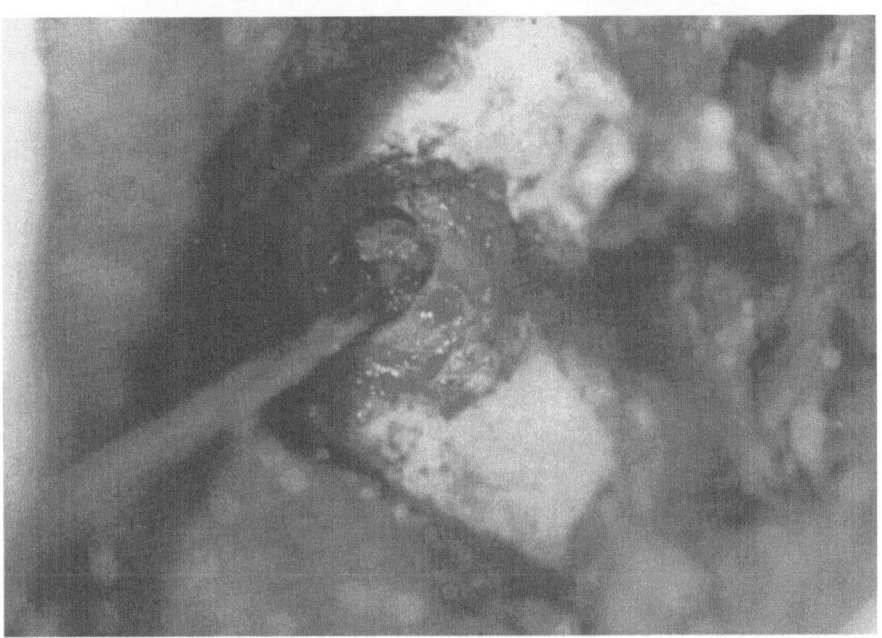

d

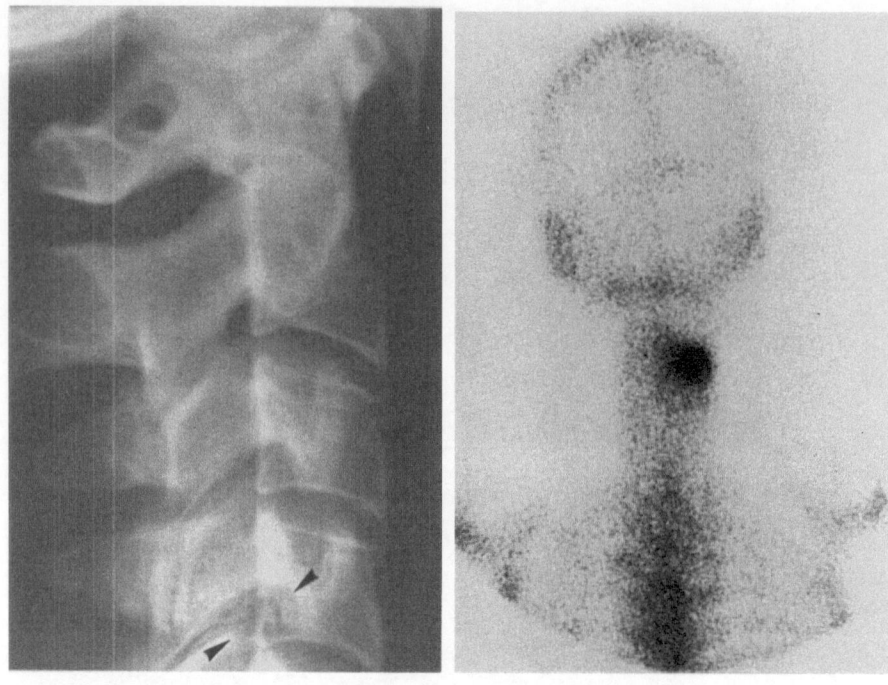

a   b

Fig. 2. Case 2. a) Conventional radiograph. b) Scintigraphy with Tc99. c) CAT scan:
preoperative. d) CAT scan: postoperative

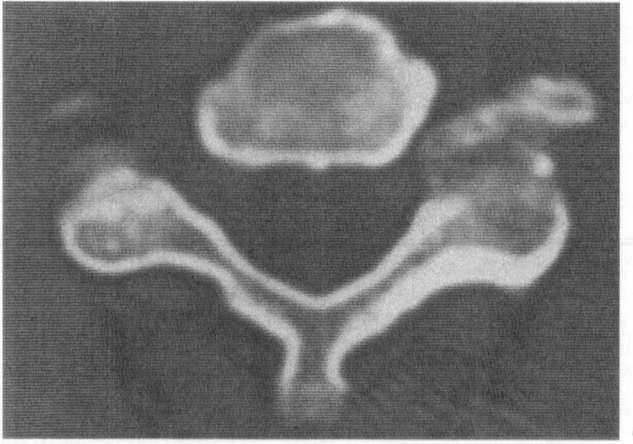

c

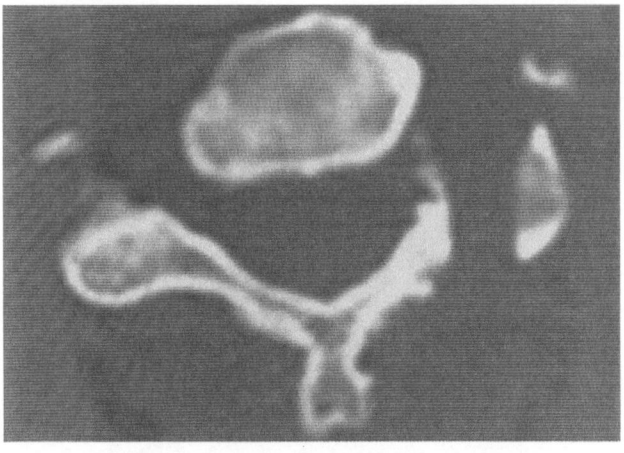

d

Case 3

A 21 year old white man presented with cervico-brachialgia of 3 years evolution. At the outset pain was predominantly nocturnal but later was to become chronic.

A myelogram was performed in a different hospital and was reported as normal but the pain persisted. Conventional radiographs showed an osteoblastic zone of approximately 1 cm in diameter located in the articular process of C6 surrounded by a sclerotic zone (nidus) (Fig. 3a). The lesion was localized with the aid of the CAT scan (Fig. 3b).

The patient rejected the proposed surgery, and was treated in another hospital.

Discussion

Conventional radiographs or simple tomographs cannot always demonstrate the presence of osteoid osteoma in the spine. In two of our verified cases presented here, conventional radiographs appeared to be normal. When the pain was partially relieved with symptomatic treatment, an incorrect diagnosis of mechanical cervical pain had been made. This delayed a correct diagnosis.

In our cases the diagnoses were made more difficult owing to the unusual location of the lesions and the difficulty in observing them with plain X-rays.

In reviewing the literature we find that only 10% of cases of O.O. affect the spine, 1.6% are located in the facet, and only 0.7% have been reported in the vertebral body [1, 8–13, 15, 17, 21].

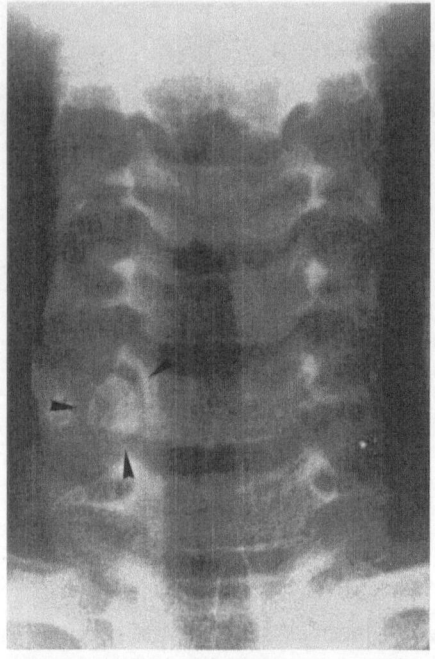

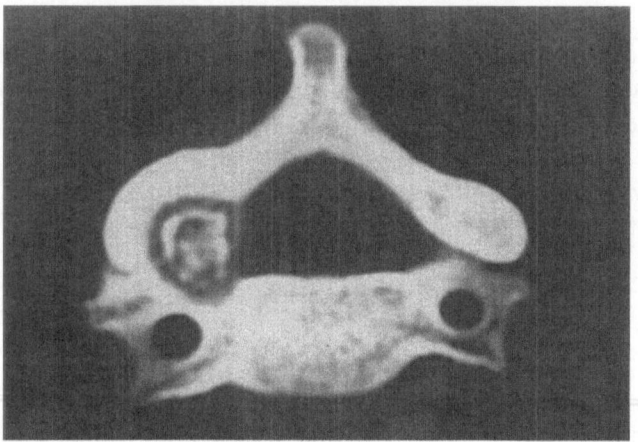

Fig. 3. Case 3. a) Conventional radiograph. b) CAT scan

We wish to emphasize the efficacy of scintigraphic studies as an aid to the early diagnosis of this painful tumor condition [9, 10, 22]. Once the lesion is precisely located, use of the CAT scan is effective.

The surgical approach can then be directed with precision so that healthy structures and spinal stability can be preserved [16, 18, 22]. Some authors prefer the use of intraoperative scintigraphy to insure total excision of the tumor [4, 5, 10, 20].

In our experience, surgical removal of the osteoid osteoma, regardless of its location, has brought about the complete relief of the symptoms [6]. Although Nelson [15] and Sim [21] considered block resection of the lesion to be necessary, our own experience leads us to conclude that marginal resection by currette is adequate. Caldicott [3] holds that osteoid osteoma can spontaneously remit on the basis of the low incidence of this lesion observed in persons over 30 years of age. When scoliosis is present, Keim [14] recommended resection so as to avoid progression of the deformity even though the lesion can remit spontaneously.

We have not been able to find any documented data concerning the follow up of these tumors which have undergone spontaneous remission.

References

1. Balasubramian E, Keim A, Majov M (1985) Osteoid osteoma of the thoracic spine with surgical decompression aided by somato sensory evoked potentials. Spine 10:396–398
2. Bas J, Escriba R, Perez L, Tamarit M, Mestre H (1983) Osteoma osteoide de localizacion vertebral. Rev Ortop Traum 27 IB:135–148
3. Caldicott W (1969) Diagnosis of spinal osteoid osteoma. Radiology 92:1192–1195
4. Colton C, Hardy J (1982) Intraoperative bone scanning. J Bone Joint Surg 64B:255
5. Colton C, Hardy J (1983) Evaluation of a sterilizable radiation probe as an aid to surgical treatment of osteoid osteoma. J Bone Joint Surg 65A:1019–1022
6. Dahling D (1978) Bone tumors. Third Ed. Ch Thomas, Springfield, Illinois, pp 86–98
7. De Santos L, Oldstein H, Murray J, Wallace S (1978) Computed tomography in the evaluation of musculoskeletal neoplasms. Radiology 128:89–94
8. De Souza L, Frost H (1974) Osteoid osteoma – osteoblastoma. Cancer 33:1075–1081
9. Ferrer Torrelles M (1960) Osteoma osteoide de la columna vertebral. Rev Clin Esp 77:10–16
10. Ghelman B, Thompson F, Arnold W (1981) Intraoperative radioactive location of an osteoid osteoma. J Bone Joint Surg 63A:826–827
11. Hershman E, Bjorkengren J, Fielding J, Allen S (1986) Osteoid osteoma in a cervical pedicle. Clin Orthop 213:116–118
12. Huvos A (1979) Bone tumors. Diagnosis, treatment and prognosis. W.B. Saunders company, Philadelphia, pp 18–32
13. Jones D (1987) Osteoid osteoma of the atlas. J Bone Joint Surg 69B:149
14. Keim H, Reina E (1975) Osteoid osteoma as a cause of scoliosis. J Bone Joint Surg 57A:159–163
15. Mac Lelland D, Wilson F (1967) Osteoid osteoma of the spine. J Bone Joint Surg 49A:111–121

16. Nelson O, Greer R (1983) Localization of a osteoid osteoma of the spine using computerized tomography. J Bone Joint Surg 65A:263–265
17. Pettine K, Klassen R (1986) Osteoid osteoma and osteoblastoma of the spine. J Bone Joint Surg 68A:354–361
18. Reis N, Zinman C, Besser M, Shifrin L, Folman Y, Torem S, Froindlich D, Zaklad H (1982) High resolution computarized tomography in clinical ortho-paedics. J Bone Joint Surg 64B:20–24
19. Schajowicz F (1982) Tumores y lesiones pseudotumorales de huesos y articula-ciones. Ed. Panamericana, Buenos Aires, pp 58–72
20. Rinsky L, Gorts M, Bleck E, Mapern A, Mirshiman P (1980) Intraoperative skeletal scintigraphy for localization of osteoid osteoma in the spine. J Bone Joint Surg 62A:143–144
21. Sim F, Dahling DC, Beabot J (1975) Osteoid osteoma: Diagnostic problems. J Bone Joint Surg 57A:154–159
22. Wedge J, Tmaang S, Macfayden D (1981) Computed tomography in localization of spinal osteoid osteoma. Spine 6:423–427

4. The Upper Cervical Spine

Cervical Spine II
© by Springer-Verlag 1989

4.1. Three Dimensional Computed Tomography of the Craniocervical Junction

C. G. ULLRICH, Charlotte, NC, U.S.A.

The radiographic evaluation of the bony anatomy of the upper cervical spine and foramen magnum region is relatively difficult. The complex bony geometry of this region makes no two-dimensional imaging technique entirely satisfactory. Multiplanar CT reconstruction (MPR) images are commonly used to aide in the interpretation of axial CT studies. The recent development of three-dimensional computer graphics images derived from routine axial CT images (3D-CT) provides a powerful new method for displaying these bony anatomic relationships. This report briefly explains the 3D-CT technique and discusses its advantages in the craniocervical junction region.

The most common technique presently used to produce 3D-CT images is the surface contour method. Simply described, the computer identifies all of the voxels which have Hounsfield number values within a range selected by the system operator. A contour (outline) of the surface anatomy is obtained by drawing a line connecting those identified voxels along the edge of the structure. Since the spatial relationship between successive axial CT images is known, a three dimensional outline of the surface anatomy is created. By using a reference light source, shading is introduced to the data, and the visual perception of three dimensions occurs. The resulting images are surprisingly life-like. 3D-CT images may be rotated to allow evaluation from virtually any perspective. Internal surfaces may be revealed by editing or "splitting" the whole spine images.

Unlike MPR images, surface contour 3D-CT images provide no density discrimination beyond identifying the voxels at the structural surface. The similar Hounsfield number values of adjacent internal soft tissue structures makes it difficult for the computer to easily identify the soft tissue surface of interest. Soft tissue surface contours can often only be produced by extensive operator editing, and therefore, are seldom used at present. Similar to MPR images, patient motion rapidly destroys the quality and value of 3D-CT images. Spatial resolution along the image's Z axis exceeding 1.5 mm to 3.0 mm is difficult to obtain in practice.

3D-CT is excellent for demonstrating the complex bony anatomy of the craniocervical junction region. The evaluation of fractures, dislocations, and subluxations is facilitated by the ability to rotate the spine image to any desired angle (Fig. 1). The "split sagittal" view is often used to demonstrate the caliber of the spinal canal, and to better delineate dislocated bone fragments and facet joints. Unstable spinal injuries can be completely evaluated from a single supine CT examination performed with the patient in traction or other external immobilization devices. The eroded demineralized bone and subluxations associated with rheumatoid arthritis are clearly seen with 3D-CT (Fig. 2). Infantile bony anatomy, including congenital segmentation

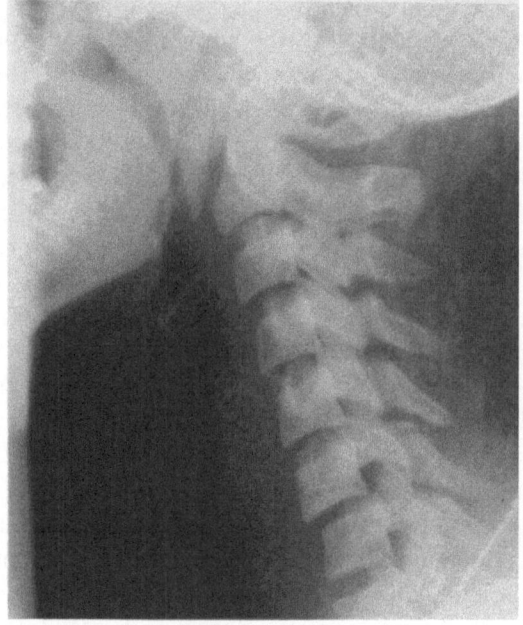

a

Fig. 1. Anterior arch of C1 fracture. A 17 year old female presented with diffuse neck pain and no neurologic deficit after an automobile accident. The lateral cervical spine radiograph (a) reveals a C6–C7 dislocation with posterior element fracture. Although alignment is normal at C1–C2, the prevertebral soft tissues are prominent. The posterior arch of C1 is not clearly seen. An axial CT image at mid-C1 (b) and a coronal multiplanar reconstruction CT image (c) show a fracture of the left anterior arch of C1. The left lateral mass of C1 appears to be slightly dislocated. The axial image shows a smooth but irregular contour to the posterior arch of C1. Anterior (d) and 60 degree rotated (e) 3D-CT images also show the anterior arch C1 fracture. The slight posterior displacement of the left lateral mass of C1 is easier to appreciate with the 3D-CT. A forward rotation ("tipped") 3D-CT image (f) displays the fracture/dislocation of the anterior arch of C1, and the incomplete posterior arch of C1. A left split sagittal 3D-CT image (g) looking inside the spinal canal shows the occipital assimilation of the posterior arch of C1 to best advantage

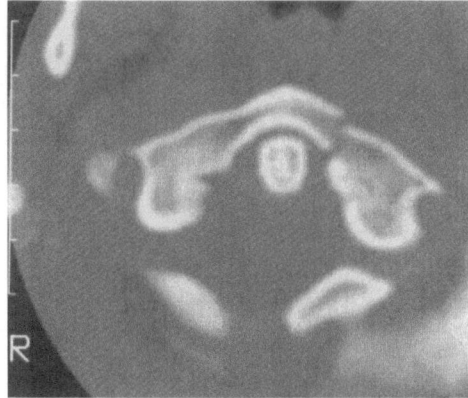

Fig. 1b

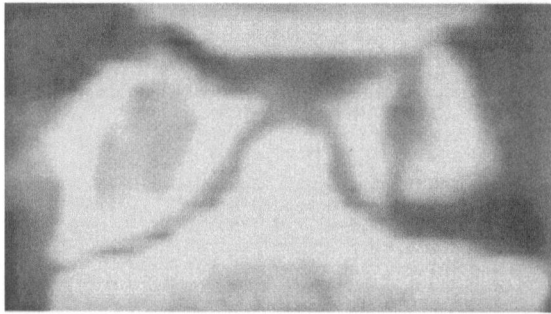

Fig. 1c

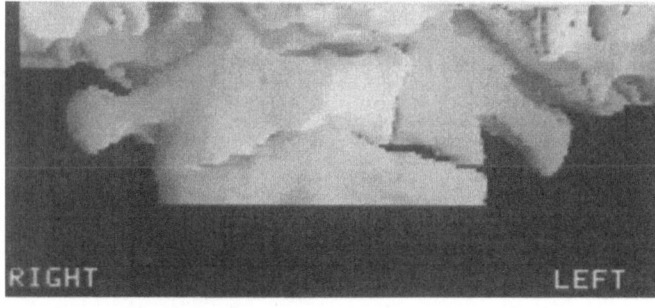

Fig. 1d

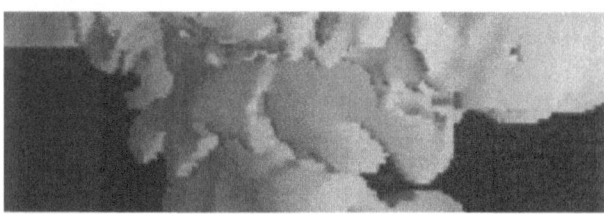

Fig. 1e

C. G. Ullrich

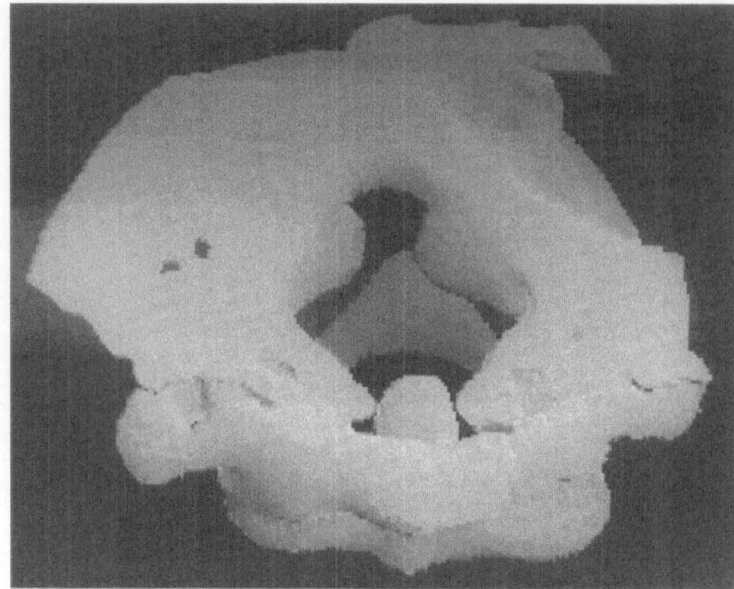

Fig. 1 f

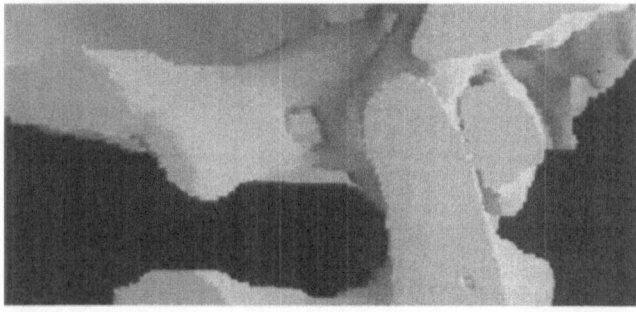

Fig. 1 g

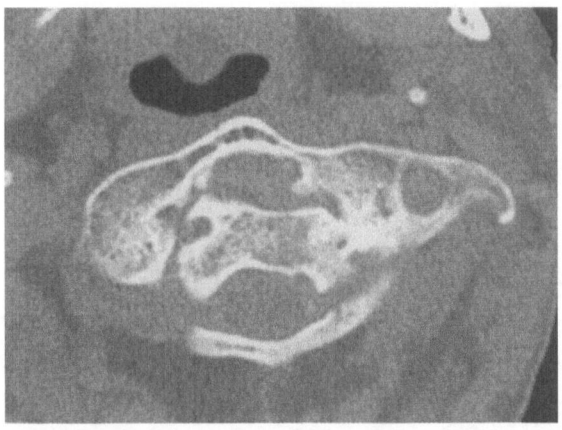

a

Fig. 2. Rheumatoid arthritis with C1–C2 subluxation. Axial CT images made at the mid-C2 vertebral body (a) and base of the odontoid process (b) show a profound forward subluxation of C1 on C2. The central spinal canal is stenotic, the base of the odontoid is eroded, and the normal atlanto-axial relationship is not identified. Sagittal (c) and coronal (d) multiplanar reconstruction images show the C1–C2 subluxation, but the anterior 3D-CT image (e) is easier to evaluate. The right lateral mass of C1 is clearly lower in position than the left lateral mass of C1. The entire C1 segment has shifted to the right relative to C2. A split coronal 3D-CT image (f), looking toward the back of the C2 vertebral body, edits away the posterior arch of C1 and C2 allowing the posterior aspect of the vertebral body to be seen. The odontoid remnant is displaced to the right along with the C1 vertebral segment. A right split sagittal 3D-CT view (g) shows the spinal canal stenosis, the eroded odontoid process, and the forward slip of C1 in relation to C2. An axial 3D-CT view from below (h) nicely demonstrates the rotational abnormality of the occiput and C2 relative to the C2 vertebral body

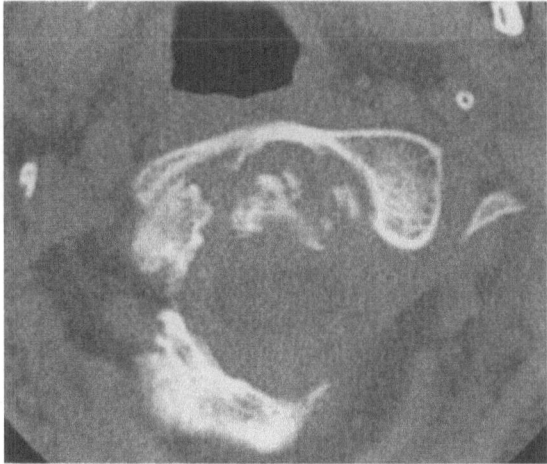

Fig. 2b

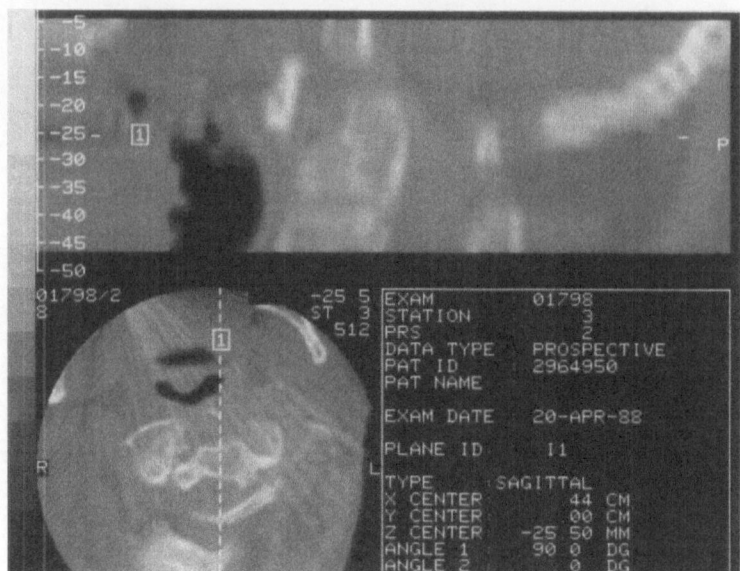

Fig. 2 c

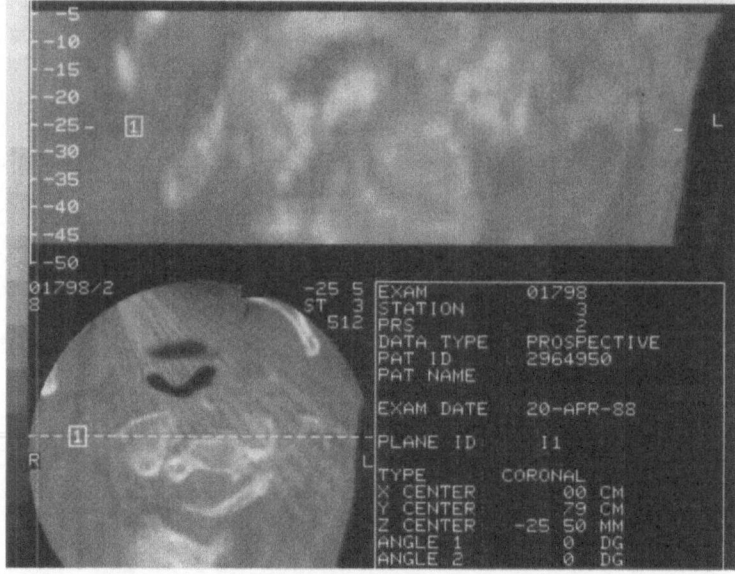

Fig. 2 d

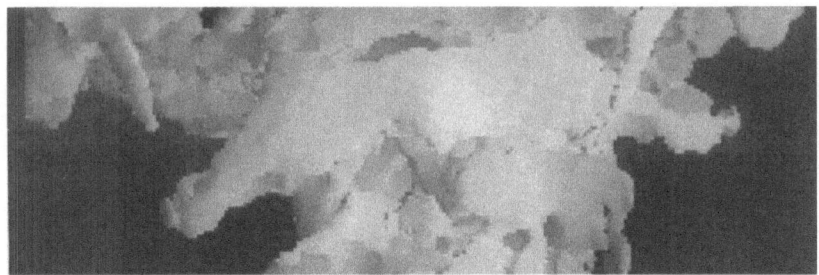

Fig. 2e

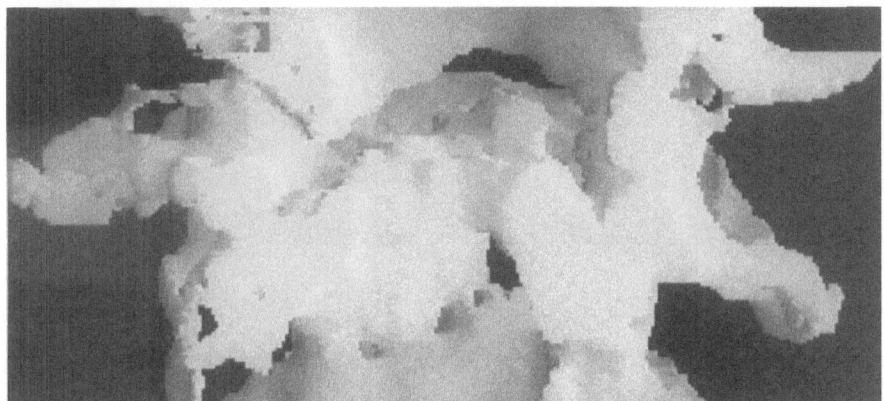

Fig. 2f

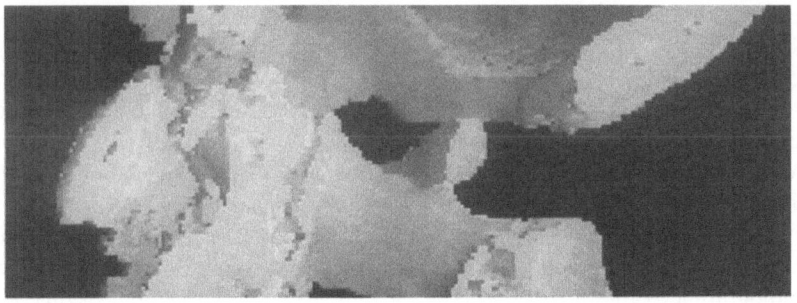

Fig. 2g

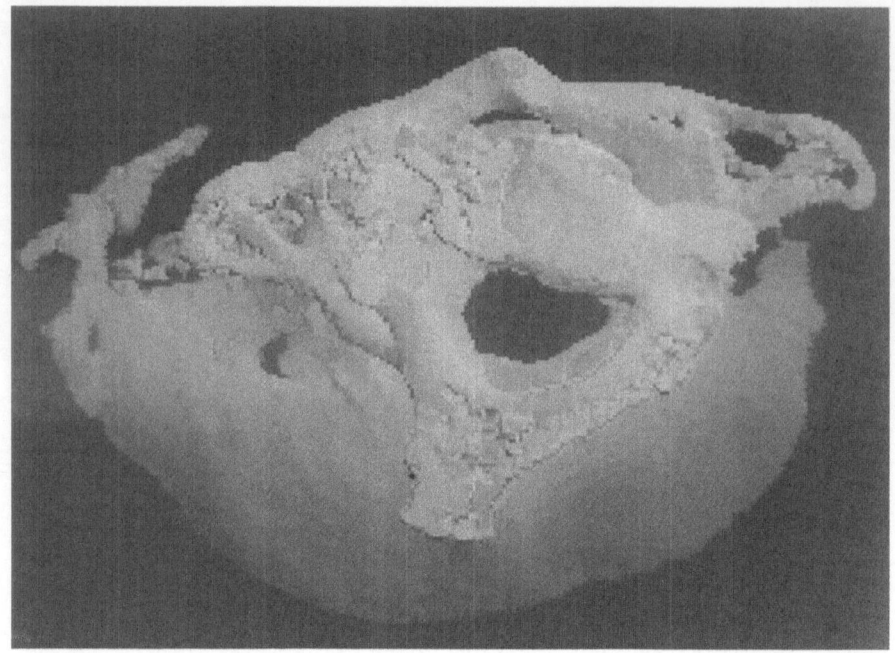

Fig. 2h

anomalies as well as trauma, may be very effectively studied with low x-ray dose CT techniques.

The medical applications of 3-D imaging are in its infancy. Even now, the potential benefits of 3D-CT images appear to be very important.

References

1. Pate D, Resnick D, Sartoris DJ, Andre M (1987) 3D-CT of the spine: practical applications. Appl Radiol May:86–94
2. Rothman SLG, Glenn WV Jr (1985) Multiplanar CT of the spine. University Park Press, Baltimore
3. Ullrich CG, Kieffer SA (1980) Computed tomographic evaluation of the lumbar spine: quantitative aspects and sagittal-coronal reconstruction. In: Post MJD (ed) Radiographic evaluation of the spine, current advances with emphasis on computed tomography. Masson Publishing, New York
4. Zinriech SJ, Rosenbaum AE, Wang H et al (1986) The critical role of 3-D CT reconstruction for defining spinal disease. Acta Radiol 369:699–702

Cervical Spine II
© by Springer-Verlag 1989

4.2. Simultaneous Rotation and Lateral Inclination of the Head: A Clinical Sign of Limitation of Rotation at the Atlanto-axial Joint

B. JEANNERET, St. Gallen, Switzerland

Observation

In a review [2] of patients with healed dorsal fusions of C1–C2 performed as described by Magerl 1987 [5], we noted a characteristic motion of their head during rotation. The rotation of the head was markedly reduced by 30 to 60 degrees and was always combined with a simultaneous ipsilateral inclination of the head of 15 to 25 degrees (Fig. 1). Head rotation was more reduced and showed less simultaneous lateral inclination in patients with degenerative changes at the lower cervical spine than in young patients with normal lower cervical spines.

Explanation of the Phenomenon

In a healthy patient, head rotation takes place at the atlanto-axial joint as well as in the lower cervical spine. Due to its anatomy, the atlanto-axial joint allows a horizontal rotation of the head during the first 40–45 degrees of rotation (Fig. 2) [3, 6]. This first step of rotation is no longer possible if the atlanto-axial joint is fused. Rotation of the head therefore is markedly reduced and takes place exclusively in the lower cervical spine. Motion segments of the lower cervical spine however, do not allow a horizontal rotation because of the orientation of their uncovertebral joints in the sagittal plane [1, 4]. As shown in Fig. 3, rotation in the lower cervical spine is always combined with an ipsilateral inclination of the upper vertebrae above and consequently of the head.

In young patients, the residual head rotation was greater than expected (up to 60 degrees). This is attributed to compensatory hypermobility of the healthy lower cervical spine motion segments after C1–C2 fusion.

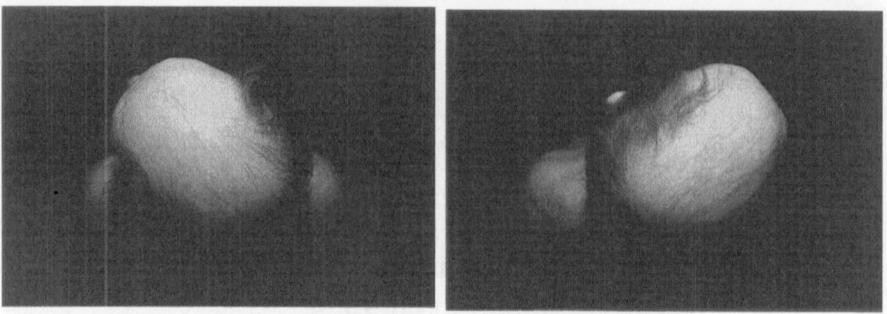

a

Fig. 1. Patients with fused atlanto-axial joints demonstrate a marked restriction of
head rotation with residual rotation of 30 to 60 degrees (a). Rotation is always
associated with a simultaneous ipsilateral inclination of the head which is visible from
the front (b), but which is more obvious when the head is faced forward in maximum
of rotation (c). The lateral inclination of the head increases simultaneously with head
rotation (d)

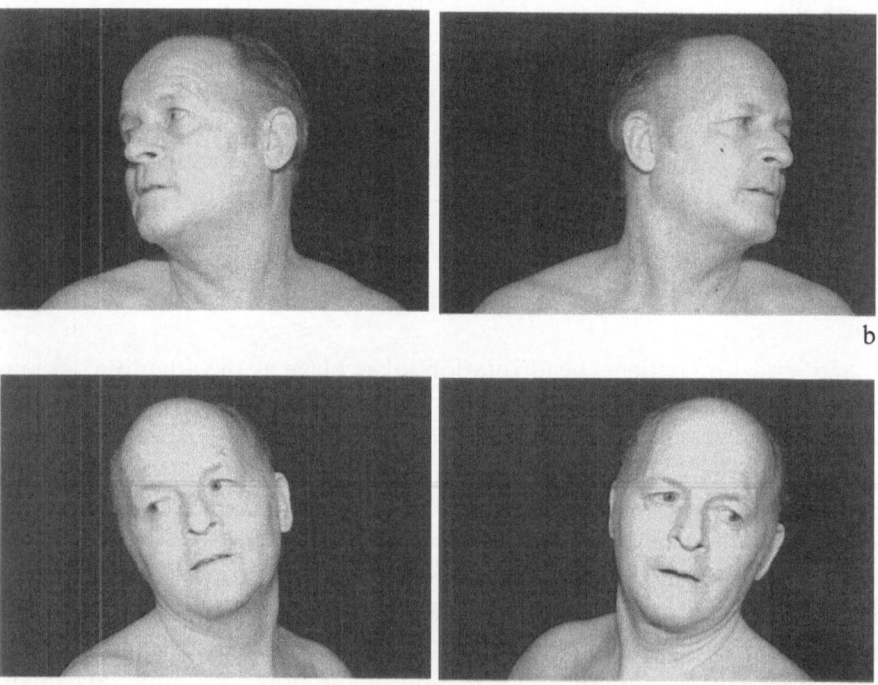

b

c

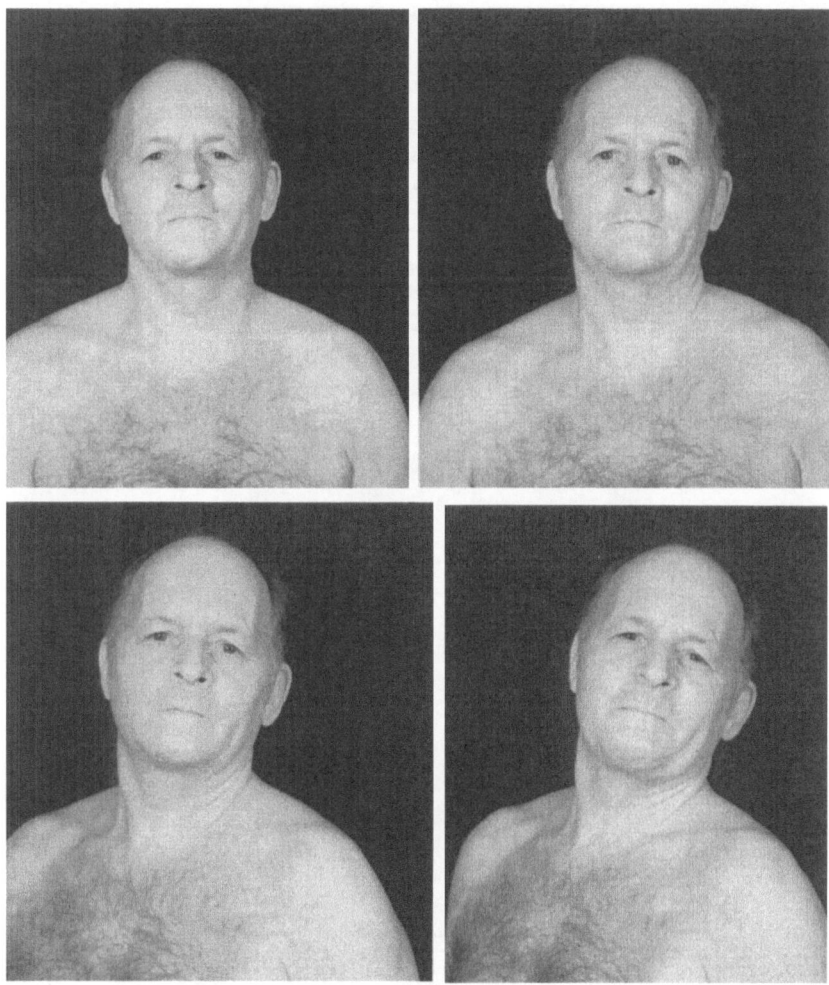

d

Clinical Application

This characteristic pattern of head motion can be used as a diagnostic sign of a blocked atlanto-axial joint [2]. The presence or absence of lateral inclination of the head during rotation is a useful aid in localizing the origin of pain and loss of movement of the head.

The patient is requested to rotate his head. If he demonstrates marked restriction of head rotation combined with a simultaneous lateral inclination of at least 15 degrees (Fig. 1), the origin of motion restriction is located at the atlanto-axial joint. If the patient shows the same amount of limitation of head rotation but without simultaneous lateral inclination (the head stays

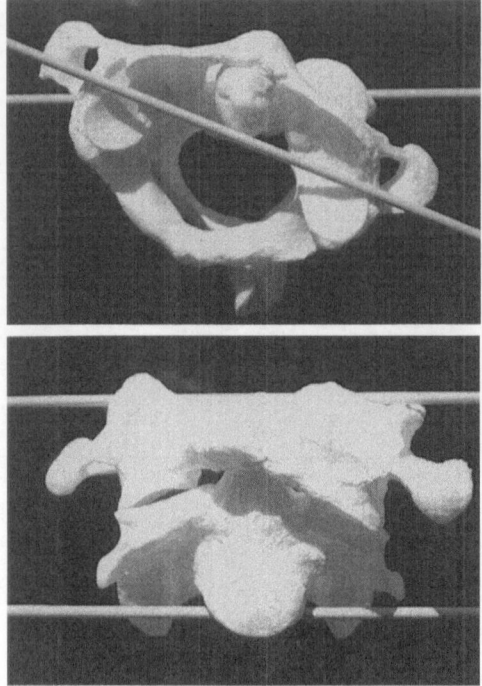

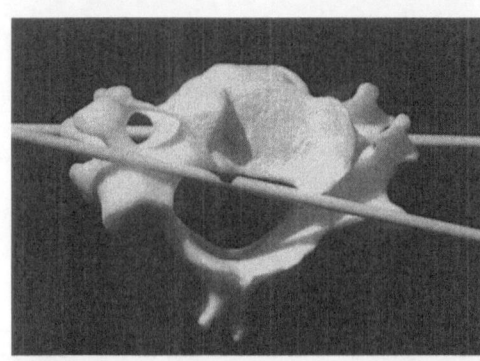

Fig. 2

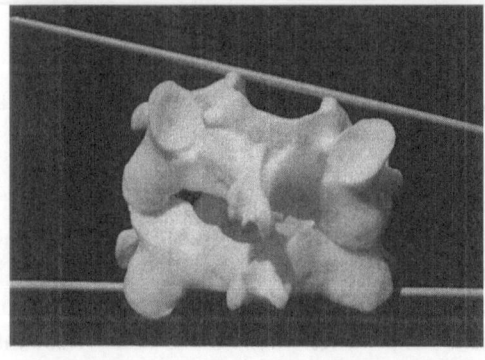

Fig. 3

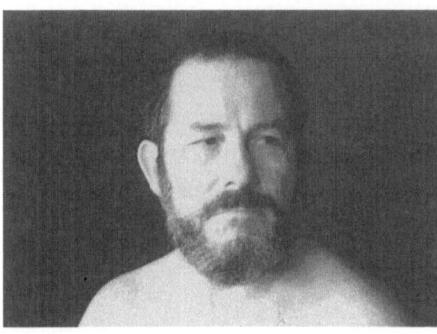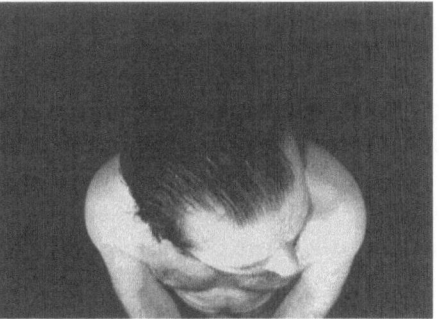

Fig. 4. This patient shows a marked and painful restricted rotation of his head, the head however remains vertical during rotation. Therefore, the source of limitation is not located in the upper, but in the lower cervical spine. This patient had degenerative changes C5–C7 which where responsible for his pain. The limitation disappeared after an anterior fusion of C5–C7 was performed

vertical during its rotation), the restricted motion is due to pain arising in the lower cervical spine from C2 to T1 (Fig. 4).

There is, however, an exception to this rule. If the whole lower cervical spine is fused in hyperlordosis or kyphosis, the plane of C1–C2 rotation is no longer horizontal, but sagittal. This rare condition may, therefore, result in a slight lateral inclination of the head during rotation. It can easily be diagnosed by plain radiography.

Fig. 2. The atlanto-axial joint allows a horizontal rotation of the head during the first 40–45 degrees of rotation

Fig. 3. Due to the orientation of the zygapophyseal joints in the sagittal plane, rotation in the lower cervical spine always is combined with a simultaneous lateral inclination of the upper vertebrae. To produce a rotation to the right, the left articular process of the upper vertebra has to move anteriorly, the right one has to move posteriorly. Since the zygapophyseal joints are orientated in the sagittal plane from anteriorly-cranially to posteriorly-caudally, the left articular process can only move anteriorly if it also moves cranially, and the right one can only move posteriorly, if it also moves caudally. This produces a simultaneous ipsilateral inclination of the superior vertebra and consequently of the head

Conclusion

As long as the whole lower cervical spine is not fused in hyperlordosis or kyphosis, a marked restriction of head rotation associated with a simultaneous lateral inclination of the head is due to a blocked atlanto-axial joint. If restricted rotation is not associated with ipsilateral inclination of the head, which means that the head remains vertical during its rotation, the source of limitation is located in the lower cervical spine.

References

1. Fielding JW (1964) Normal and selected abnormal motion of the cervical spine from the second cervical vertebra to the seventh cervical vertebra based on cineradiography. J Bone Joint Surg 46-A:1779–1781
2. Jeanneret B (1987) Simultane Rotation and Seitwärtsneigung des Kopfes. Ein klinisches Zeichen der Rotationseinschränkung im Bewegungssegment C1/2. Z Orthop 125:10–13
3. Kapandji IA (1979) Physiologie articulaire, Fascicule III, Tronc et Rachis. Maloine S.A., Paris
4. Lysell E (1969) Motion in the cervical spine. An experimental study on autopsy specimens. Acta Orthop Scand [Suppl] No 123:1–61
5. Magerl F, Seemann P-S (1987) Stable posterior fusion of the atlas and axis by transarticular screw fixation. In: Kehr P, Weidner A (eds) Cervical spine I, Strasbourg 1985. Springer, Wien New York
6. White AA, Panjabi MM (1978) Clinical biomechanics of the spine. J. B. Lippincott Company, Philadelphia Toronto

4.3. Management of the Odontoid Fractures of the Elderly

K. Liebig and D. Hohmann, Erlangen-Nürnberg, Federal Republic
of Germany

Conclusions

Comparing the different results of conservative and operative treatment of odontoid fracture in the literature with our own experiences, we prefer the double screw-technique of Böhler/Magerl.

There seems to be more odontoid fractures than traditionally reported. In our own cases during the last 7 years operation was required in 135 patients with injuries of the cervical spine. Among these were 19% suffering from odontoid fractures.

In the last two years we have treated more and more elderly people. They represented approximately 8% of all cervical spine injuries requiring operations and about half (42%) of the odontoid fracture cases which were operated on.

The prognosis of bone healing of this fracture by conservative treatment is poor. The rate of pseudarthrosis is between 6% and 60%, the average is 40%, and the chance of consolidation after the age of 40 is worse.

Conservative treatment in the classical Minerva-plaster cast or the Halo-vest fixation by Jahna and Schweigel requires immobilization between 3 and 11 months before an adequate fusion of the fracture takes place.

The long fixation times within a halo as well as other reasons made conservative treatment inappropriate for the elderly. The older age group's intolerance to prolonged immobilization and the physical restrictions of external stabilization lead us to broaden the operative indications in this age group. We used several operative techniques.

Clinical Data

From 1980 till 1987, 27 patients with an injured odontoid (except one) were operatively treated in our hospital (Table 2). Fifteen patients were between 5 and 49 years old and 11 were between 56 and 84 years old. The

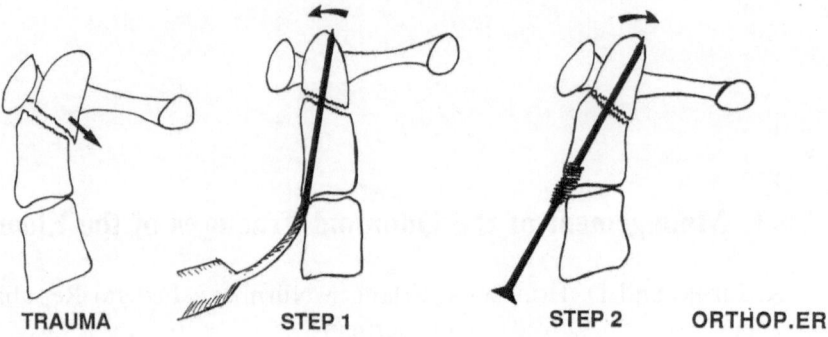

Fig. 1. Operative technique in a hyperextension-fracture

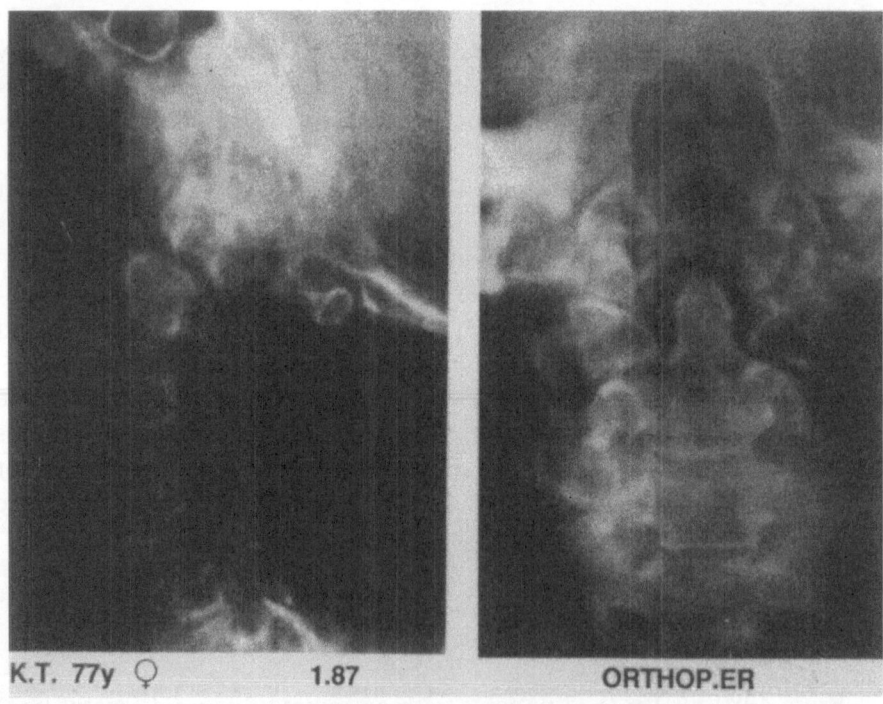

Fig. 2a. Radiographs of the cervical spine, one week after accident. Odontoid fracture of Anderson Type 2

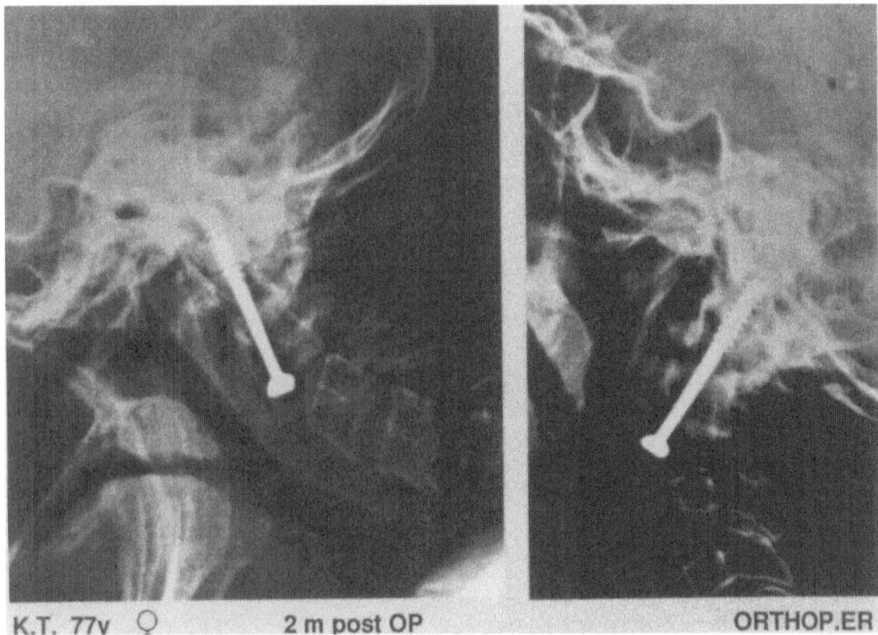

K.T. 77v ♀   2 m post OP   ORTHOP.ER

Fig. 2b. Radiographs of the cervical spine, two months post op with the Böhler/ Magerl double screws technique

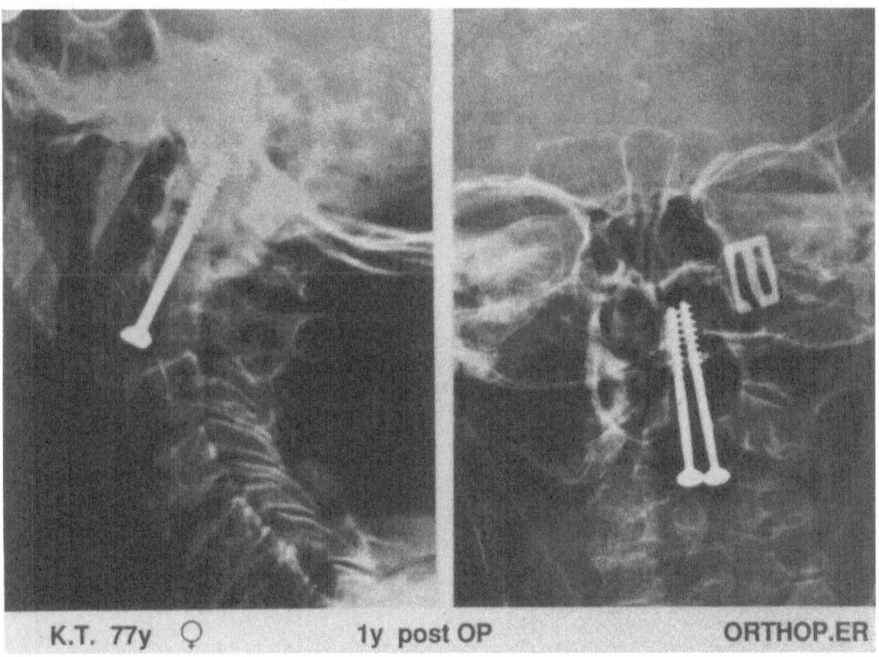

K.T. 77y ♀   1y post OP   ORTHOP.ER

Fig. 2c. One year post op and complete fracture healing

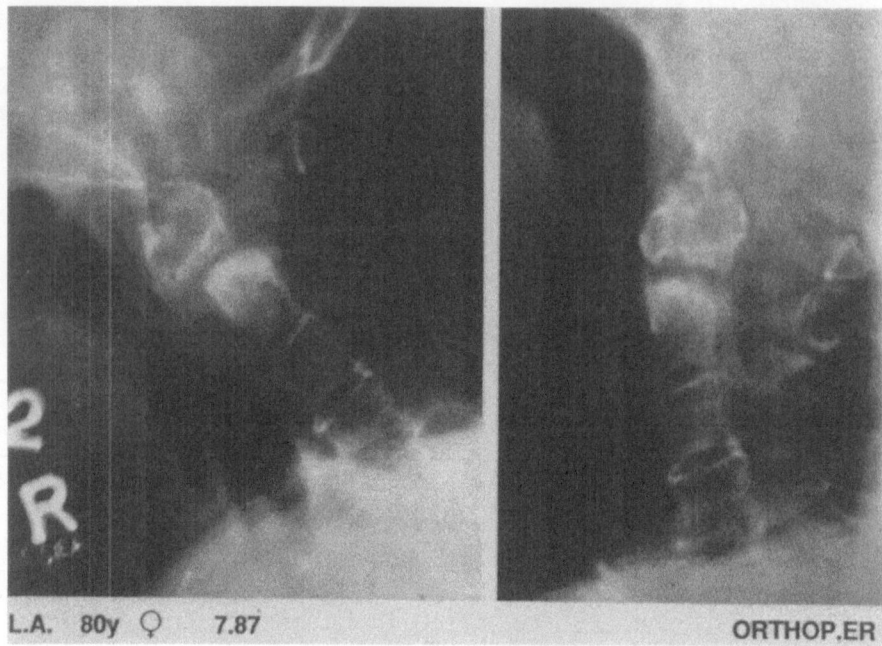

Fig. 3a. Pseudarthrosis of the odontoid, three years after accident

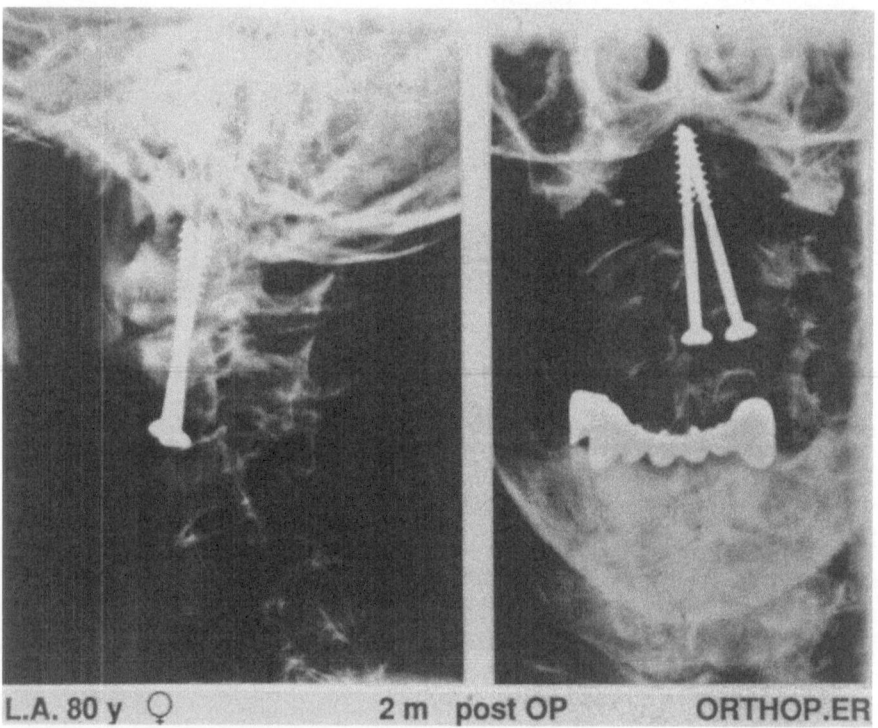

Fig. 3b. Two months post op after the double screw technique of Böhler/Magerl

younger age group had 9 fractures of type 2 by Anderson's classification, 4 had pseudarthrosis, and 2 had mobile os odontoideum.

The elderly group consisted of 7 odontoid fractures of Anderson type 2, one Anderson type 3, 2 pseudarthrosis, and one mobile os odontoideum.

In all of the young patients, the injuries were caused by traffic accidents, while in the group of the older patients we found only two having this as the cause. The remainder of the older population (9) where injured at home by falling down because of dizziness and cardiovascular troubles.

Patients with ages between of 60–80 years had special problems with regard to the operative techniques and the therapeutic results. These problems essentially were related to their age.

A posterior spondylodesis by Gallie/Brooks was done in 3 patients, an osteosynthesis by Streli-plate in 3 patients, and a double-screw osteosynthesis of Böhler/Magerl was performed in 7 patients.

The posterior spondylodesis that had been carried out in the beginning of our series, showed poor results especially in the elderly. It lead in two cases to pseudarthrosis. Because of osteoporotic bone grafts, adequate compression of the on-lay grafts required in the Gallie method, was often not possible.

There are also additional problems associated with the dissection of the musculotendinous attachments. In advanced age a progressive stiffness of the atlanto-occipital joints exists and the posterior arch of the atlas is usually fixed to the occiput.

To achieve adequate healing we were obligated to immobilize the patients with a long-term external fixation which the operative technique was ment to avoid. Two patients who had delayed fracture healing had been treated by anterior plate osteosynthesis using Streli's method.

However, the stability lasted only a short time. Despite our use of large spongiosa-screws they did not have enough hold and advanced out of the osteoporotic vertebra within a very short time.

Our favorable experiences with the younger patients using the anterior compression-screw osteosynthesis of Böhler/Magerl encouraged us to use this instrumentation in the elderly.

Since 1985 8 elderly patients have underwent operative treatment with this technique. Complications have not occurred except in one patient who died 7 days after the operation from associated complications.

Operative Technique

The approach is similar to the Cloward procedure. A tranverse half collar incision at the level of C4/5 is made. For identification of the second vertebra and introduction of the screws an X-ray image intensifier is essential. The K-wire should perforate the cortex of the top of the dens. X-ray verifies the correct position of the K-wire. The screws have a good hold in the cortex of the dens so they can be tightly pulled and thus compress the fragments.

Reduction of hyperextension fractures is only possible with flexion of the cervical spine (Fig. 1). Since drilling the screw in this position is not possible, we first drill a 2 mm K-wire through a curved canular to the top of the dens in order to temporarily stabilize the fracture. Now lordosis is possible without dislocation so that screw osteosynthesis can be completed.

Under all circumstances drilling the anterior surface of C-2 must be prevented because the screw tends to move up on the osteoporotic bone during the drilling.

Case Reports

Case 1. K.T. (Fig. 2a, b, c). A 77 year old female patient. This patient sustained an accident at home resulting in an odontoid fracture of Anderson Type 2. Operative treatment with the double screw technique of Böhler/ Magerl accomplished complete reduction of the fracture. One year postoperatively the patient has a stable screw osteosynthesis and fracture healing.

Case 2. L.A. (Fig. 3a, b). An eighty year old female patient with an accident at home three years ago (1984). The first radiographs of the cervical spine show signs of no fracture. The patient developed chronic headache and neck pain. No treatment was given until radiographs of the cervical spine in 1987 showed a pseudarthrosis of the odontoid with severe instability. Double screw technique of Böhler/Magerl resulted in rigid stability.

Results

One patient with a preoperative tetraplegia showed no recovery of the neurological deficit. We have not had any complication with the fusion. The remainer of the patients were able to leave their bed within several days. For exernal fixation they wore only a Philadelphia collar. Postoperatively the screws produced a firm compression of the fracture and sufficient primary stability.

We did not observe loosening of the screws. Bone resorption in the drill hole was seen only once, but thus occurred without any loss of stability. Two patients complained of head pain for an extended period.

The extent of fracture healing is difficult to determine from the radiographic check, because the x-ray shadow of the screws obscures the area of the fracture. Böhler maintains that fracture healing occurs in 12 weeks. Plain radiographs in extension and flexion after 3 months didn't show any instability.

Cervical Spine II
© by Springer-Verlag 1989

4.4. Transoral Surgery:
A Useful Approach to the Upper Cervical Spine

C. A. LOGROSCINO, Roma, Italy

Transoral surgery is applicable to a limited number of cases involving disorders in the upper cervical spine (C1–C2). Indeed, there were few possibilities of using this approach whose first application dates back to the pre-Christian Era and the days of Hippocrates.

Somewhat more recently it was used to evacuate retropharyngeal abscesses but these were no more than limited surgical procedures which exploited the possibility of easy exposure of the pharynx. Various reports on this approach appeared from time to time but these were actually no more than isolated events.

The first detailed account of the systematic use of the transoral approach and case presentation was given by Fang and Ong [3] of the Hong Kong School in 1962. Like most pioneering efforts a considerable number of complications were encountered and had to be resolved during the preliminary work. Yet, it must be recognized that these surgeons initiated prospects on a procedure which until that time had been considered beset with uncertainties. Transoral surgery came to be accepted as the natural anterior approach to the upper cervical spine.

The reasons for the serious complications reported in the first historic operations are not difficult to identify. Infection occurred partly as a consequence of the particular site involved (oral cavity) and partly because of the inadequacy of preoperative preparations and postoperative care. Complications involving haemorrhages (vertebral artery) were attributable to the fact that this technique still required improvement and development while respiratory failure was probably the result of insufficient assistance and diagnostic inexpertise in the delicate postoperative period.

It could well be that Fang and Ong's experience was the consequence of the enthusiasm aroused in Hong Kong by the results achieved by Hodgson and Stock [8] which made possible the anterior approach to the thoracolumbar spine for the treatment of Pott's disease.

Indications

The operation is indicated for lesions of the upper cervical spine (C1–C2); however, lesions in the clivus area can also be treated. Under normal conditions the second cervical vertebra is in the center of the field so surgery is more easily accomplished. Exposure of the higher levels (C1-clivus) is facilitated by division of the soft palate.

Resection of the hard palate allows anterior fusion and internal fixation of the occipito-cervical region ("extended transoral approach") [5].

The transoral approach thus provides more direct and central access to the upper cervical spine, also it permits satisfactory exposure in the antero-lateral sense. It must be stressed, however, that there are natural obstacles which prevent exposure in the proximal and the distal directions. On the lower side the obstacles are the tongue and the mandible. Small, fine, precise movements are needed because of these very evident space restrictions.

The presence of congenital malformations at the cranio-vertrebral junction may markedly affect the choice of surgical approach. If there is assimilation of the atlas the axis will be located higher than normally thus creating problems during the operation.

This possibility may also arise in the case of rheumatoid arthritis with the upward dislocation of the dens. This occurs as the result of changes caused by inflammation of joints.

The approach is indicated considering the site of the lesion for the treatment of various pathological situations involving acute or chronic instability (traumas, tumors, infections and malformations).

The clinical feature in other cases may be spinal cord compression, which may be acute or in gradual evolution. When the condition is acute, diagnostic investigations and the operation must be performed urgently. The level of the lesion is so proximal that it affects centres essential for life. The most serious disturbances are those affecting the respiratory system. The chronic case possibility is observed typically in congenital malformations which may degenerate slowly for years and then rapidly deteriorate.

It is important to make an exact diagnosis of the type of lesion (etiology) by means of careful diagnostic investigations (tomography, myelography, C.A.T., etc.). It is absolutely essential to ascertain the mechanism responsible for the clinical syndrome (pathogenesis). The neurological signs can be caused basically by direct compression (expansive processes) or by segmental instability.

It should be stressed that in chronic C1–C2 instability, vertebro-basilar insufficiency syndromes may be observed. The Strasbourg School (Jung and Kehr) must take credit for having drawn attention to this possibility in their very detailed report covering a vast number of cases in the orthopaedic and the traumatologic fields.

Contraindications

It is often stated that the transoral approach is anatomically invasive but we cannot subscribe to this idea. In point of fact, the transoral approach is very direct and involves no particular risks or functional sacrifices of note. The dissection made along the midline of the posterior pharyngeal wall is carried down to bone. The main limit with this approach is the restricted nature of the space available. The surgeon has very little freedom of movement for all he must do; however, this is a factor that can be overcome by experience and by adopting adequate technical equipment (microscope). There remains another limit that is insurmountable, namely, the impossibility of checking on lesions distal to C2 under normal conditions.

A contraindication that must be mentioned is the risk of infection due to the site involved, but it is felt that this is an aspect that can be kept adequately under control by appropriate preventive measures.

One of the disadvantages of the transoral approach is the need for prior tracheostomy which is not needed in the case of the extraoral approach. However if there are no risks of respiratory complications, a regular transoral intubation can be used [12].

Preopertive Preparation

A distinction must be made between urgent and planned operations. Where the former are concerned, it is impossible to lay down any hard and fast rules since each evaluation and every decision must be made case by case. If the operation can be planned, two stages are involved, namely, diagnostic investigations, to identify the etiological and pathogenetic factors, followed by the specific preparations for the operation now considered necessary. The initial task is basically to establish whether a compressive syndrome is present or whether the lesions are secondary to segmental instability.

If breathing is disturbed, the patient must be given a careful functional respiratory test. The anaesthetist must assess the patient's condition prior to the operation and take an active, responsible role in the decision whether to operate or not.

In the case of malformation syndromes, there may also be congenital anomalies of the temporomandibular joints. This circumstance must be duly noted because it may be a contraindication for transoral surgery. Preoperative otolaryngological examination is needed to exclude the presence of "foci" of infection in the pharynx. Antibiotic oral spray treatment is also one of the essential preoperative requirements.

External braces may have to be employed in some cases before the operation and these can be left in place for some time afterwards. The halo-cast or halo-vest are the ones most frequently used.

The presence of instability indicates that the head cannot be moved owing to the excessive risk of incomplete neurological involvement. When movement is possible, hyperextension without rotation of the head facilitates surgical exposure. It is advisable that rotation should be strictly neutral; the head must be secured firmly to the operating table, and great attention must be paid to protecting the patient's eyes. The anaesthetist's team and equipment must be located towards the patient's feet to give the surgeons as much space as possible near the head and to enable bulky equipment such as the microscope to be used, if necessary.

Tracheostomy, when indicated, is a separate problem; this can be temporary (the wound's being closed after the operation) or it can be maintained for a period of time. It is our opinion that the best solution is to maintain the tracheostomy for a few days and then to rapidly withdraw the endotracheal tube, since in this way an adequate margin of safety is maintained.

The surgical drapes must be careful prepared, as they must be fixed firmly around the mouth. A self-retained retractor is applied, taking great care to move the tongue which tends to limit the useful space and reducing the view of the deeper parts to some extent. Since the retractor is fixed, considerable edema of the tongue is sometimes observed at the end of the operation and the tongue cannot be contained within the oral cavity for some time. The region near the endotracheal tube is packed with surgical sponges to prevent undesired penetration of diseased or haematitic materials. Disinfection of the oral cavity and adjacent cavities must be performed, as far as possible, using products that do not irritate the mucosae.

The problem to be tackled at this point is that of illumination which can be resolved by using an operating microscope or a fiber-optic lighting system. The microscope offers the advantage of providing a picture of the field simultaneously to the surgeon and his assistant; however, it can be inconvenient when long instruments have to be used.

Surgical Procedure

This is a case of endocavital surgery performed in depth. The surgeon's room for manoeuvering is constantly limited by the restricted nature of the surgical field; movements must be small and precise. If congenital anomalies are present, a careful diagnosis has to be made so as not to run into serious difficulties during the operation. In the case of assimilation of the atlas, the axis is located at a higher level, while C3 comes into the field of transoral exposure; however, just the opposite occurs in some cases, namely, distal transposition because of the presence of deformity (kyphosis).

Dissection is performed precisely on the midline. The first decision to be made is whether or not to section the soft palate. It is usually sufficient to retract it by anchoring with a suture. When it is necessary to arrive at the proximal levels (dens of the axis, C1 or cranio-vertebral junction) the soft palate hinders visual control of the surgical field and division on the midline is necessary. More rarely, resection of the hard palate may be needed and there are no difficulties in reaching the spine. The layers to be sectioned are of little anatomic significance and blood loss is negligible. The levels involved are the pharyngeal wall, the pharynx constrictor muscle, the buccopharyngeal fascia, the anterior longitudinal ligament and the periosteum.

If the decompression is needed, identification of the dura mater may be obtained by referring to the anulus in C2–C3, after complete removal of the disc.

Two circumstances may cause problems during the course of the operation when the normal anatomic references are altered, namely, fixed rotatory deformity and aplasia of the dens. In the former case it may be difficult to find the midline required for division, while in the latter there is high risk of damage to the spinal cord as a result of inept movement of the instruments.

The vertebral artery also requires great consideration since it runs very close to the site of the operation and damage at this level is difficult to rectify. Damage to it occurs generally as a result of excessive instrumental pressure when attempting reduction of acute or chronic traumatic dislocations. The air drill can be another cause of damage especially when rotatory movements of the cutter is not halted immediately.

Internal fixation calls for separate discussion. If plates and screws are used, the site for the screws must be carefully prepared. Usually only one screw can be fixed to the dens, while one or two screws can be fixed in the body of the axis. Insertion of the screw in the dens is facilitated by partial resection of the distal half of the anterior tubercle of the atlas [11]. The dens can be perforated manually or by air drill before fixing the screw. It is commonly believed that the dens, separated from the body owing to congenital or acquired causes, is such a mobile fragment that it creates problems during perforation for internal fixation; however the capsulo-ligamentous connections are such as to guarantee quite adequate stability for the screw. It is important, to ensure that the screw does not slide laterally to the dens, the size of which is not much different from that of a phalanx. This could have fatal consequences.

Apart from the complications during the operation, sight must not be lost of those due to infection. Such risks exist because of the somewhat contaminated nature of the oral cavity. Because of the extreme thinness of the covering layers it is possible that owing to necrosis or septic complications either a bone graft or an internal fixation may project into the oral cavity. This kind of exposure may give rise to the expulsion of the extraneous matter or extension of the infection to deeper layers with even more serious consequences.

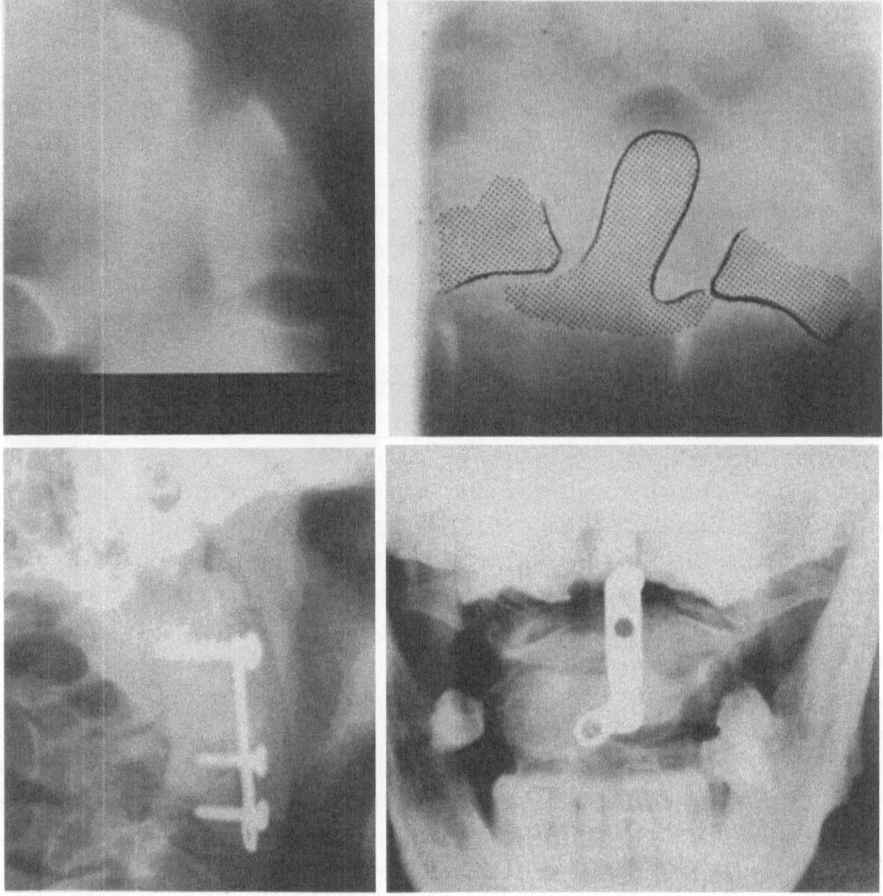

Fig. 1. Fracture of the dens associated with locked facet rotatory dislocation. Open reduction and internal fixation performed using the transoral approach

The reconstruction stage is quick and simple. A double layer is utilized, avoiding the use of material that may be reabsorbed, to prevent the risk of loosening of the wound.

Postoperative Care

The presence of an endotracheal tube provides a guarantee against complications resulting from obstructions during the postoperative stage. It is advisable to keep the tracheostomy patent while edema of the tissues or perhaps haematoma persists. If C1–C2 instability is present the patient is fitted with a halo-cast or halo-vest system which provides the necessary

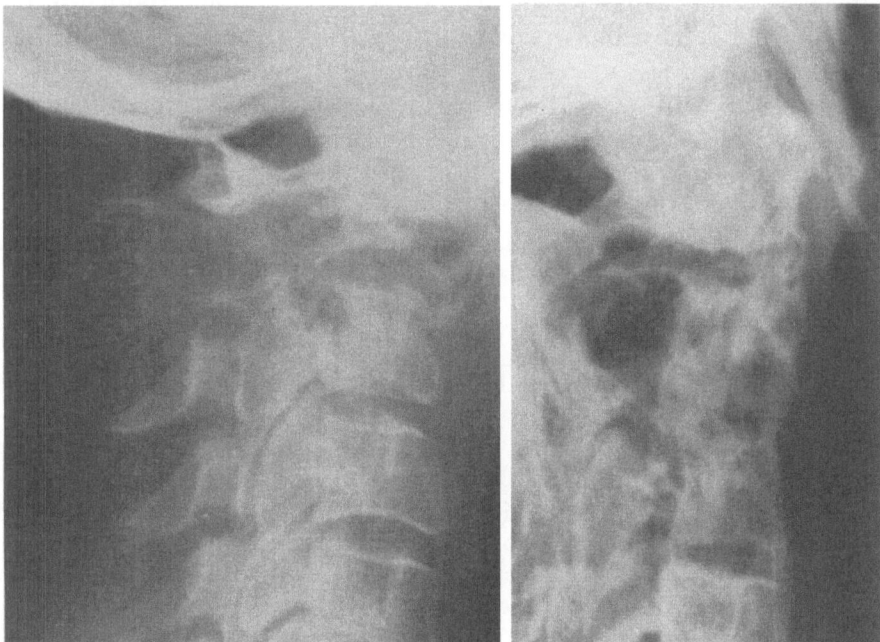

Fig. 2. Erosion of C2 by Echinococcus. Urgent decompression by transoral approach. Eight years follow up

external stabilization. Two months is generally sufficient, followed by a period of immobilization (about four weeks) in a Minerva cast.

Rehabilitation therapy is especially important and must start as soon as possible aimed at the respiratory function and recovery of use of the limbs when there is paralysis. Recovery of the respiratory function is important particularly in the case of congenital malformations which frequently result in a crisis due to insufficiency and can sometimes be fatal in this postoperative stage. In such cases, in addition to the urgent measures needed to recover from the acute episode, longterm treatment is also needed to ensure improvement in the clinical picture. Physiotherapy can provide a valuable complement to pharmacological treatment.

Conclusion

Though the transoral approach was tried from time to time in the distant past, it has not been widely adopted to date. Various reasons for this include 1) the need for tracheostomy, 2) the risks related to the anatomy of the surgical area, 3) the fact that few orthopaedic surgeons or neurosurgeons are familiar with this unusual approach, 4) the complications reported in the literature and 5) those that are feared partly as the result of over evaluation of the real risks.

There is also the success achieved by the extraoral approach which is certainly better tolerated by the patient which has markedly reduced the indications for transoral surgery.

The numerous advantages of this approach must not be ignored especially since it permits wider more direct exposure of the upper cervical spine. Its use is particularly appreciated in emergency surgery.

References

1. Alonso WA, Black P, Connor GH, Vematsu S (1971) Transoral-transpalatal approach for resection of clival chordoma. Laryngoscope 81:1626–1631
2. Andreade JR (De), McNab I (1969) Anterior occipito-cervical fusion using an extrapharyngeal approach. J Bone Joint Surg 51A:1621–1626
3. Fang HSY, Ong B (1962) Direct anterior approach to the upper cervical spine. J Bone Joint Surg 44A:1588–1604
4. Hall JE, Denis F, Murray J (1977) Exposure to the upper cervical spine for spinal decompression by a mandible and tongue splitting approach. J Bone Joint Surg 59A:121–123
5. Harms J, Schmelzle R, Stoltze D (1987) Osteosynthesen im occipito-cervicalen Übergang vom transoralen Zugang aus. In: XVII World Congress abstract book. Demeter Verlag, Munich
6. Hodgson AR, Stock FE (1956) A preliminary communication on the radical treatment of Pott's disease and Pott's paraplegia. Br J Surg 44:266–275
7. Jung A, Kehr P, Oonishi M (1968) Syndrome cervicale traumatique traité par liberation de l'artère vertebrale et uncusectomie. Mem Acad Chir 94:529–538
8. Laine E, Delandsheer JM, Jomin M (1977) Indication et possibilité de la vie transbucale-pharynge. Neurochirurgie 23:4–17
9. Logroscino CA, Nizegorodcew T, Caporale M (1980) Decompressione midollare per via transorale. In: Progr in Pat Vetebr, Aulo Gaggi Ed, Bologna, p 119
10. Louis R (1982) Chirurgie du rachis. Anatomie chirurgicale et voies d'abord. Springer, Berlin Heidelberg New York Tokyo
11. Louis R (1983) Chirurgie atloïdo-axoïdenne par voie transorale. Rev Chir Orthop 69:381–391
12. Takashi Sakou, Yoshiyuki Morizono, Norio Morimoto (1984) Transoral atlanto-axial anterior decompression and fusion. Clin Orthop 187:134–138
13. Verbiest H (1968) A lateral approach to the cervical spine: technique and indications. J Neurosurg 28:191–200
14. Whitesides TE jr, Kelly RP (1966) Lateral approach to the upper cervical spine for anterior fusion. South Med J 59:879–883

Cervical Spine II
© by Springer-Verlag 1989

4.5. Lateral Retropharyngeal Approach to the Upper Cervical Spine: Long-term Follow-up

D. M. NGUYEN, T. E. WHITESIDES, and F. C. THOMPSON, Atlanta, GA, U.S.A.

Introduction

Whitesides [6] first reported a lateral retropharyngeal approach to the upper cervical spine in 1966. The classic Robinson and Smith approach [5], medial to the carotid sheath, allows anterior exposure to C3 only. The approach can be extended proximally to allow access to the occipitocervical region. However, the surgical exposure is very limited, and injury to the laryngeal nerve may result [3]. Transoral and transpharyngeal approaches are also possible but are fraught with high morbidity and mortality [1, 4, 5]. This paper reports long-term follow-up of the Whitesides approach to the upper cervical spine.

Materials and Methods

Fourty-six cases at the Emory Clinic in Atlanta, GA, were reviewed retrospectively. The lateral retropharyngeal approach was used for anterior arthrodesis for a variety of conditions beginning in 1963. These included instability, rheumatologic disease, tumor, infection, gunshot wound, and congenital deformity. All medical records and roentgenograms were available for review.

The surgical technique is a deeper extension of Henry's approach to the vertebral artery [2]. It involves dissection lateral and posterior to the carotid sheath to reach the appropriate level (see Fig. 1). This approach has been useful for simultaneous exposure of the right and left lateral C1,2 articulations, removal of the anterior spine, fusion from C1–T1, and occasional exposure to the basiocciput area.

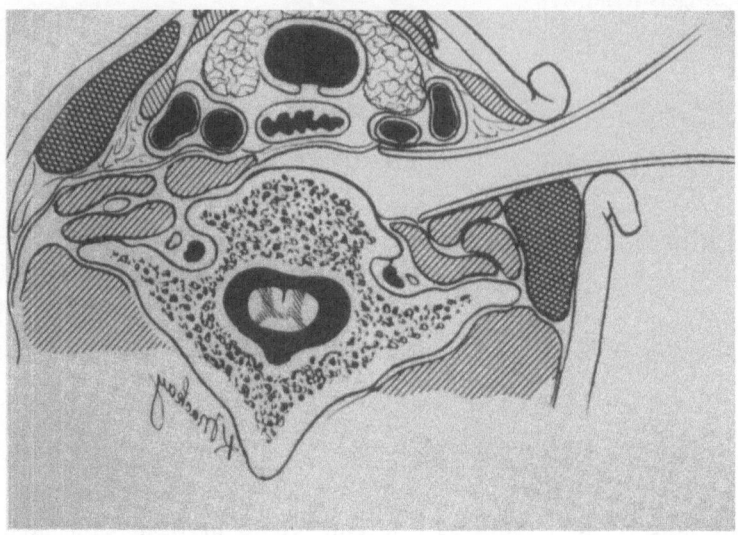

Fig. 1. The dissecting interval is lateral and posterior to the carotid sheath. Tracheostomy may be performed

Results

Fourty cases were unilateral and six were bilateral. The average age was 35.6 years old (range 5–86 y.o.). The average length of follow-up was 3.8 years (range 3 months to 20 years). Complications were minimal in the 46 cases. The infection rate was 3.0% and the total complication rate was 9.0%. Complications included one nonunion, one wound infection and two deaths. The nonunion occurred in a patient with rheumatoid arthritis. The wound infection occurred in a patient who had undergone a transoral biopsy of a giant cell tumor. The wound grew *Klebsiella* and eventually healed after debridement. The fusion was solid. One death occurred in an elderly man with myeloma of C3 who died of massive epistaxis during the first postoperative day. The second death occurred in a middle-aged woman with rheumatoid arthritis who had had an unsuccessful posterior C1, 2 fusion. The fusion mass had resorbed causing migration of the body of C2 into the foramen magnum, quadriparesis, and compression of the midbrain ganglion. The patient then underwent anterior arthrodesis and she died five days postoperatively.

Conclusion

This long-term follow-up study shows that the Whitesides route, lateral and posterior to the carotid sheath, is simple, safe, and carries minimal complications. It has a higher rate of fusion and less complications than reported for the transoral and transpharyngeal approaches.

References

1. Fang HSY, Ong GB (1962) Direct anterior approach to the upper cervical spine. J Bone Joint Surg 44A:1588–1604
2. Henry AK (1982) The vertebral artery. In: Henry AK (ed) Extensile exposure, 2nd edn. Churchill-Livingstone, Edinburgh London New York, pp 58–73
3. Johnson RM, Southwick WO (1982) Anterior cervical approaches. In: Rothman RH, Simeone FA (eds) The spine, 2nd edn. WB Saunders Company, Philadelphia, pp 106
4. McAffee PC, Bohlman HH, Riley LH, Robinson RA, Southwick WO, Nachlas NE (1987) The anterior retropharyngeal approach to the upper part of the cervical spine. J Bone Joint Surg 69A:1371–1383
5. Southwick WO, Robinson RA (1957) Surgical approaches to the vertebral bodies in the cervical and lumbar regions. J Bone Joint Surg 39A:631–644
6. Whitesides TE, Kelley RP (1966) Lateral approach to the upper cervical spine for anterior fusion. South Med J 59:849–853

4.6. A New Device for Occipito-cervical Fixation

F. Faccioli, P. Buffatti, G. Pinna, and G. Dalle Ore, Verona, Italy

Introduction

Atlanto-axial instability and dislocation, due to cranio-cervical malformations, trauma, inflammatory or neoplastic diseases, are best treated by occipito-cervical fusion. The arch of the atlas, in fact, is often unsuitable for fixation and needs to be removed to decompress the spinal cord. Several techniques have been proposed for occipitocervical fusion. Among them, the onlay construct [4], occipito-axial wiring, with or without the use of acrylic resins or bone graft [2, 3, 7, 8], and implants of various metallic devices [1, 5, 6].

The major drawbacks encountered in fixating techniques – apart from non-union – are instrument failure and prolonged immobilization. The first may be severe if the dura mater or the cerebral or spinal nervous tissue are damaged by the rupture of the metallic device. This occurs most often with the steel wires. Nervous tissue damage may also occur during insertion of these instruments. Prolonged immobilization after surgery with tedious casts, collars or Halo vests is usually necessary to achieve stabilization. This is often not well tolerated by the patients and not desirable in the elderly.

We present a technique for occipito-cervical fixation with a new instrument which ensures a solid fusion with immediate spinal stability.

Description of the Technique

The occipito-cervical fixating device is made up of seven pieces which are assembled together during surgery. The upper one is a small rectangular plate with a threaded post. A round flat cap, into which a small cylinder with a central hole is placed, is then connected with the plate. A threaded rod is screwed into the cylinder and, finally, a hook is inserted and secured by two nuts. The plate is inserted through an occipital burr hole. Tiny pin-like projections at the four corners of the plate prevent it from slipping. This manoeuvre is made bilaterally, approximately 1.5 cm lateral to the midline

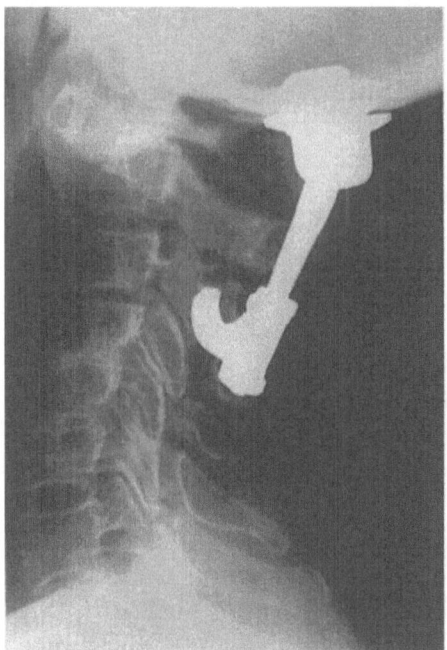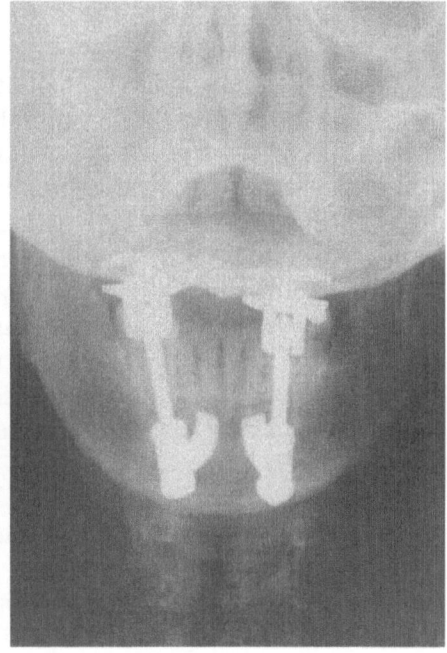

a   b

Fig. 1. a) The fixating device in place after surgery. The hooks are inserted under the laminae of C3. The posterior arch of C1 has been removed and reduction of dislocation has been obtained with enlargement of the spinal canal. b) Antero-posterior view showing the bilateral insertion of the fixating device

and lateral to the outer border of the foramen magnum. This is where the squama of the occiput is thickest. The threaded post on the plate has a variable length, according to the thickness of the bone. The round cap is then screwed and the cylinder is inserted into it. The threaded rod is screwed into the cylinder, keeping it in place. This allows enough mobility to the inferior part of the rod. The hook is then inserted on the rod and slipped under the lamina. The two nuts, which screw on in opposite directions, secure the hook which exerts a compression force. Progressive screwing results in an intra-operative reduction of the atlanto-axial dislocation. Operation is performed in the sitting position with intra-operative image intensification to check the correct position of the patient and to avoid further dislocation. The posterior arch of C1 is removed for decompression and the fixating hooks are placed bilaterally under the laminae of C2 or C3. An iliac bone graft – adequately shaped – is always placed between the occiput, the laminae and the spinous process of the vertebra involved (usually C2).

Results

The new instrument has been inserted in five patients. All presented with irreducible atlanto-axial dislocation. Four were female, one was male. Average age was 59 years (range: 48–70 yrs). In one case there was a malformation of the occipito-cervical region; in the other four cases dislocation was due to rheumatoid arthritis. All patients had varying degrees of quadriparesis associated with severe neck pain. Neither postoperative mortality nor morbidity were observed. Mobilization was encouraged on the days immediately following operation with a simple plastic collar. At follow-up (ranging from 10 months to 2 years) a remarkable disappearance of neck pain as well as motor disturbances was noted in all cases. Radiological follow-up showed a solid fusion ensured by the well placed device in all patients (Fig. 1).

Comment

Even though our experience is presently limited to a small number of cases, this new fixating device resulted in highly effective immediate and solid occipito-cervical stabilization. It avoids the risks associated with wiring procedures and allows an early mobilization of the patient, avoiding prolonged bed confinement or unpleasant external immobilization.

References

1. Cantore G, Ciappetta P, Delfini R (1984) New steel device for occipitocervical fixation. Technical note. J Neurosurg 60:1104–1106
2. De Groote M, Vercauteren M, Uyttendaele D (1981) Occipito-cervical fusion in rheumatoid arthritis. Acta Orthop Belgica 47:685–698
3. Hamblen DL (1969) Occipito-cervical fusion. Indications, technique and results. J Bone Joint Surg 49 B:33–45
4. Newman P, Sweetnam R (1969) Occipito-cervical fusion. An operative technique and its indication. J Bone Joint Surg 51 B:423–431
5. Ransford AO, Crockard HA, Pozo JL, Thomas MP, Nelson LW (1986) Craniocervical instability treated by contoured loop fixation. J Bone Joint Surg 68 B:173–177
6. Roy-Camille R, Saillant G (1972) Chirurgie du rachis cervical, osteosynthèse du rachis cervical supérieur. Nouv Presse Méd 1:2847–2849
7. Teinturier P, Levai JP, Collin JP, Terver S (1982) La luxation atloido-axoidienne au cours du rhumatisme inflammatoire chronique. Resultats de 16 arthrodeses occipito-axoidiennes. Rev Chir Orthop 68:529–538
8. Wertheim SB, Bohlman HH (1987) Occipitocervical fusion. Indications, technique and long-term results in thirteen patients. J Bone Joint Surg 69 A:833–836

4.7. Posterior Fixation of the Cervico-occipital Junction

J. Griffet, J. Lovet, M. Maestro, H. Vidal, and C. Argenson, Nice, France

The cervico-occipital junction, easily exposed by a posterior approach, can be fixed either by a metallic wiring or a short plate when only the C1–C2 level is involved, or by a cervico-occipital plate when stabilization must be extended to the skull's base.

The solidity of the fixation thus performed allows a simple post-operative immobilization by means of a soft neck brace, or rarely, by a removable plastic minerva, avoiding a disabling immobilization by means of permanent traction, a cast, or a halo-jacket [12].

Material and Method

Thirty one fixations were performed in our Department over the last nine years.

a) When only the C1–C2 level is involved, a metallic wiring uniting the posterior arch of C1 to the base of the spinous process of C2, according to Gallie's technique [7], is a simple method which has not yet caused any perioperative complications.

The embedding of an iliac bone graft between these two bone pieces provides a stable fusion, yielding a definitive fixation for rheumatoid arthritis subluxations (3 cases with a 4 years follow-up). The use of bone is preferable to methylmetacrylate in this setting [1, 2, 9].

For odontoid process fractures (type II), stabilization is ensured by 2 small plates screwed into the posterior arch of C1 and the C2–C3 [10] facet joints. These plates are removed once union is secured, in order to regain maximum rotational mobility at this level.

b) For occipito-atlanto-axial fixation, we prefer the inverted Y-shaped Fuentes plate whose upper part can be firmly fixed to the median crest of the occiput, which is the strongest part of this bone. The lower fixation, which is sometimes less reliable, requires screw-fixation into the C2–C3 facet joint, as well as the C3–C4 facet joint. Cortico-cancellous iliac bone graft is packed

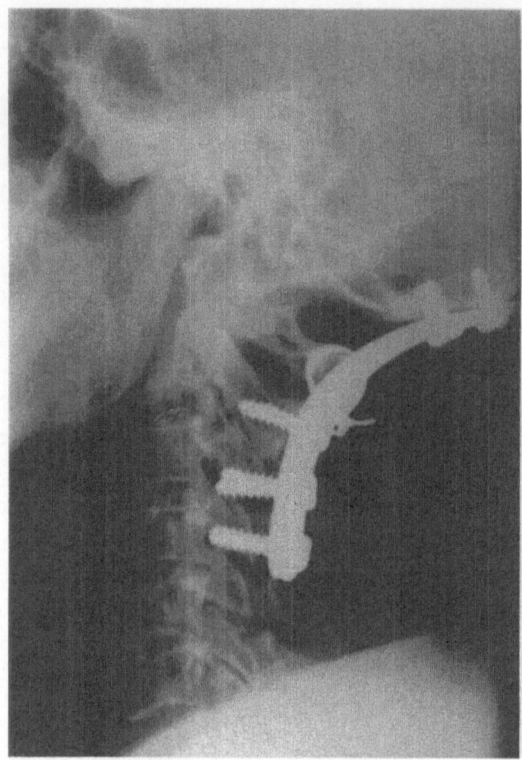

Fig. 1. Fuentes' plate in a case of metastatic bone involvement of the odontoid process. No post-operative immobilization was required

Table 1. *Postoperative Results with Respect to Pain and Mobility*

		Fracture of the dens		Rheumatoid arthritis		Severe sprain	Tumor	Congenital malformation
Fusion		C1–2	C0–2/3	C1–2	C0–2/3	C1–2	C0–2/3	C1–2
Pain	3	9	2	1	1	2	3	2
	2	2	3	2				
	1							
	0							
Mobility	3	3	1			2		2
	2	7	3	3				
	1	1	1				2	
	0				1			

Pain: 3 = no pain→0 = disabling; Mobility: 3 = normal→0 = 60% less in unbility (according to [3]): 3 = normal → 0 = 60% less in mobility on each side of the plate thus filling in the occipito-cervical angle. Cement may be used in place of bone graft in case of tumor (one chordoma and two metastatic lesions).

Results

Out of 31 cases, we have had 5 complications: one elderly patient died three weeks after surgery, one case had a superficial infection, one case with nonunion underwent again the same operative technique and subsequently united, and two cases showed incomplete displacements without neurological impairment. All the other cases fused from either temporary fixation of odontoid process fractures or from fusion for all other indications.

The mean union delay was 4 months with extremes ranging from to 3 to 12 months. We assessed our results with respect to pain and mobility. Pain was assessed using a scale ranging from 0 to 3, while mobility was assessed using Decoulx's classification [3] from 0 to 3. Results are good with respect to pain; 85% of patients are relieved and mobility is impaired only when the fixation involves the occiput.

Discussion

The discussion will deal with technique and indications.

The C1–C2 fusion *techniques* are today well established and Gallie's technique combining a metallic wiring to an iliac graft between C1 and C2 gave us very satisfactory results: The only nonunion of the series occurred in a congenital agenesis of the odontoid process. The patient underwent reoperation using the same operative technique and subsequently united.

When the occiput must be involved in the fixation, the Fuentes Y-shaped plate seems to us very suitable, and we have had neither complication nor delayed union using this technique. The fixation of the upper screws into the occipital crest was excellent.

As for indications, the temporary fixation that we had used for the odontoid fracture, using a plate fixed between C1 and C2, which required a second operation in order to remove the plate, is now replaced by direct screwing of the dens. But, a C1 posterior arch fracture combined with a fracture of the dens could remain an indication for temporary fixation of the C0–C2/C3.

A peculiar indication occured in the two cases of severe C1–C2 sprains whose diagnosis was made on the lateral X-ray view (demonstrating an abnormally increased distance between the anterior arch of C1 and the dens) and on the CT-Scan. In both cases, patients were young, and the C1–C2 fusion provided an excellent result without any loss of mobility.

Another important indication for occipito-cervical fusion is rheumatoid arthritis. Patients who undergo surgery are those with neurological signs at the outset, or those whose distance between the C1 anterior arch and the dens is greater than 8 mm, particularly if this distance increases in flexion and extension. We perform the C1 – C2 fusion, according to Gallie's technique [7], whenever there is no ascension of the dens. If ascension of the dens is seen on the lateral X-ray view (Ranawa lines [11]), we prefer a fusion involving the occiput. This last technique is also used whenever the atlanto-axial diastasis is greater than 12 mm.

Fixation by means of a metallic wiring of the C1 – C2 level or plate for the C0 – C2 levels seems to us to have greatly improved the post-operative comfort of our patients while also improving the percentage of unions.

References

1. Bryan WJ, Inglis AE, Sculco TP, Ranawat CS (1982) Methylmetacrylate stabilization for enhancement of posterior cervical arthrodesis in rheumatoid arthritis. J Bone Joint Surg 64-A, 7:1045–1050
2. Conaty JP, Mongan ES (1981) Cervical fusion in rheumatoid arthritis. J Bone Joint Surg 63-A, 8:1218–1227
3. Decoulx P (1973) Mobilité du rachis cervical. Evaluation clinique. Nouv Press Med 2, 10:557–559
4. Dunn EJ (1977) Methylmetacrylate in the stabilization and replacement of tumors of the cervical spine. Spine 2:15–24
5. Eismont EJ, Bohlman HH (1978) Posterior atlanto-occipital dislocation with fractures of the atlas and odontoid process. J Bone Joint Surg 60-A, 3:397–399
6. Fehring TK, Brooks AL (1987) Upper cervical instability in rheumatoid arthritis. Clin Orthop 221:137–148
7. Gallie WE (1939) Fractures and dislocations of the cervical spine. Am J Surg 46:495
8. Lovet J (1982) Traumatismes graves du rachis inférieur de l'adulte. Etude critique de 70 observations. Orientations thérapeutiques. Thèse de Médecine, Nice
9. Mac Afee PC, Bohlman HH, Ducker T, Eismont FJ (1986) Failure of stabilization of the spine with methylmetacrylate. J Bone Joint Surg 68-A, 8:1145–1157
10. Maestro M (1982) Nouvelle approche biomécanique et thérapeutique des fractures de l'odontoïde de l'adulte. A propos de 24 cas cliniques. Thèse de Médecine, Nice
11. Ranawat CS, O'Leary P, Pellici P, Tsairis P, Marchisello P, Dorr L (1979) Cervical spine fusion in rheumatoid arthritis. J Bone Joint Surg 61-A, 7:1003–1010
12. Wertheim SB, Bohlman HH (1987) Occipitocervical fusion. J Bone Joint Surg 69-A, 6:833–836
13. Zoma A, Sturrock RD, Fisher WD, Freeman PA, Hamblen DL (1987) Surgical stabilization of the rheumatoid cervical spine. J Bone Joint Surg 69-B, 1:8–12

5. Experimental Reports

Cervical Spine II
© by Springer-Verlag 1989

5.1. Atlanto-axial Fixation. A Biomechanical Study with CD Instrumentation

E. Dehoux, F. Deprey, Ph. Segal, and J.B. Flament, Reims, France

Introduction

C1–C2 fixation still poses many problems. We studied a series of odontoid process fractures [5] and post-traumatic C1/C2 dislocations. In our acute dens fractures series (59 cases), we used posterior wiring (with or without graft) in 30 cases. With this technique we obtained a complete reduction in 22 cases (73%) but on the follow-up X-rays we noted 12 secondary displacements of the dens (40%) and 4 pseudarthroses. We used the same operation with 10 C1/C2 dislocations, and we observed 5 postoperative slips (50%) and 2 pseudarthroses of the graft. In 1987, Perrin [4] published a short series of C1/C2 fixations of rheumatoid dislocation treated with CD instrumentation. We thought this idea was useful and before applying it, we made a biomechanical comparaison between wiring and CD instrumentation. This paper reports our results.

Materials and Methods

For this study, we took entire cervical spines of fresh or frozen cadavers. We took off all soft tissues (muscles, nerves . . .) and we kept only bones, ligaments and discs. To test the different pathologies we produced various ligament cuttings. In this way it was easy to obtain a significant instability (Roy-Camille [9]) and easy to reproduce. Instability was created by cutting the transverse, alaris and Y ligaments.

To study isolated instability beween C1 and C2, we immobilized the spine from C2 to C6 or 7 in an external fixator (Ilizarof) and we measured antero-posterior instability with a sensitive displacement gauge (1/100 mm).

To create the motion we applied increasing loads ranging from 100 grams to 2500 grams on the anterior part of the occiput. We performed measurements on 3 spines recording 5 measurements on each.

We tested several types of osteosynthesis. First, we studied a posterior wiring, like Judet's initial method of wiring, with a steel wire of 1 mm in diameter.

Second, we studied a CD instrumentation. We used pediatric material with 2 types of hooks (closed pedicular or laminar hooks) and CD rods (5 mm in diameter). We were able to make 3 kinds of construct: unilateral, bilateral and bilateral with a DTT to join the 2 rods.

Results

1. After section of the ligaments, we observed significant instability.

Untill a load of 100 g there is no displacement. Displacement appears after greater loads and it is abrupt in onset with a steep slope. Displacement reaches 7 mm with a load of 350 g (Fig. 1). We could not obtain a total dislocation, perhaps because of the persistent C1/C2 articular ligaments.

2. After posterior wiring (Fig. 2), as shown on the first curve, that with increasing load the deformation of the experimental construct reaches 2.7 mm for 2500 g. At the end of the maximum load, we discharged the load and observed that the unloaded curve didn't come back to 0 but stayed at 0.5 mm. When the system was again loaded, the deformation reached 4.9 mm and when again discharged and reloaded, the curve came back to 1.7 mm and went up to 5 mm. We didn't measure the rotational instability, but with loads of 1500 g or greater rotatory deformation appeared. This in understandable, because the wiring is very posterior and on the midline.

This kind of synthesis is deformable with deformation which increases with the repetition of the loads. This confirmed our clinical suspicion. When the deformation appears, the wiring has a tendency to wharp more and more.

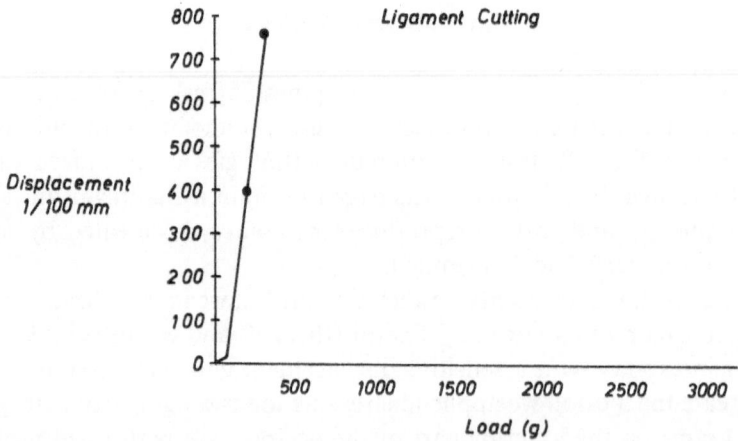

Fig. 1. Load (*g*) and displacement (1/100 mm) after ligament cutting

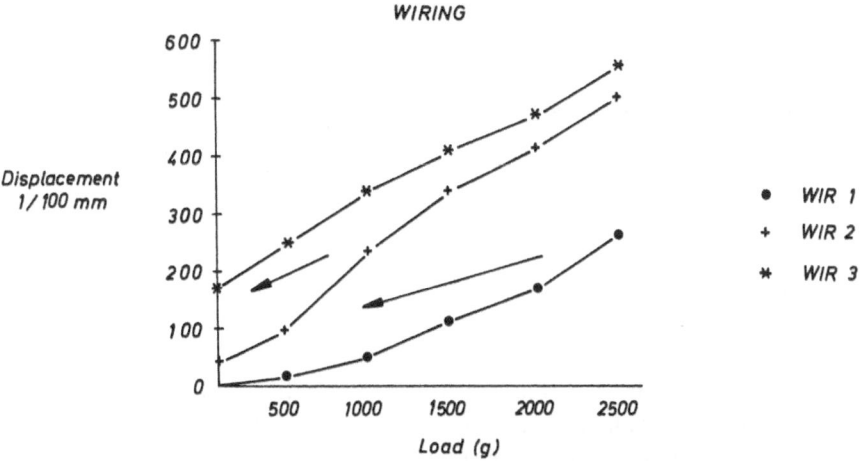

Fig. 2. Load (g) and displacement (1/100 mm) after posterior wiring

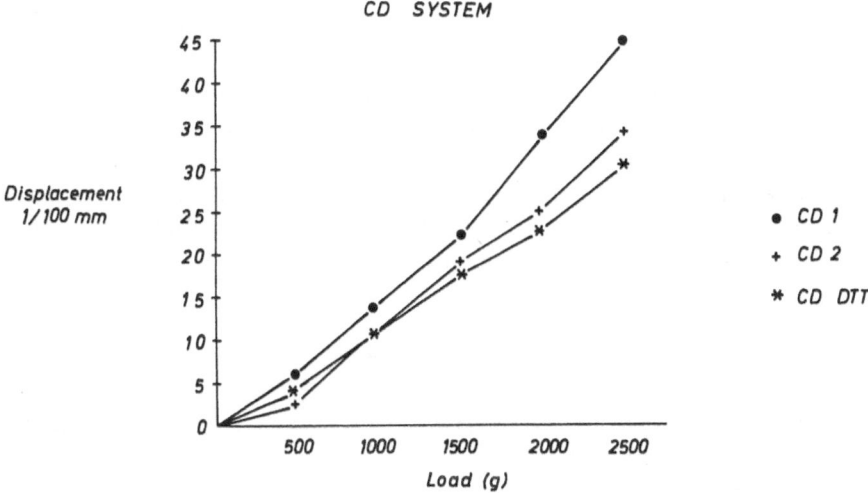

Fig. 3. Load (g) and displacement (1/100 mm) after CD-system instrumentation

3. After CD instrumentation (Fig. 3), we noted that the 3 types of con-
structs were very stiff. The curves show that 0.45 mm is reached with 1 rod,
0.35 mm with 2 and 0.3 mm with 2 rods + 1 DTT. The maximal deformation
was obtained with the unilateral construct but there is no significant difference. For each synthesis we studied a load discharge and observed in every
case that the deformation curve came back to 0. There is no cumulative
deformation as in wiring.

4. The comparison between CD and wiring is easy to describe; CD instrumentation produces much greater stability than wiring.

Discussion

Some authors do not favour the hook (Knodt or CD) because of the volume it occupies. We studied this problem during our experimentation. There was no problem of placement above the posterior arch of C1, since the cord takes up only half of the canal volume. Below the lamina of C2 the hooks stay above the ligamentum flavum and didn't invade the canal. To place the hooks above C1 it is not necessary to dissect more than 1 cm beyond the midline. The risks of injury to the vertebral artery [7] are minimal.

We compared the CD system with other stiff instrumentation like the Knodt system [2] or screw-plate of C1/C2 [7]. There are not enough publications with biomechanical evaluations to make significant conclusions. But we know that with the plate system reoperation at 6 months is required to remove the C2/C3 trans-articular screw, so to liberate this joint.

Concerning the wiring, we use the Judet wiring. Different authors have shown that other kinds of wiring can give rigid osteosynthesis but they require that the wire be placed around the lamina of C2. Other authors, as well as ourselves, believe this technique is dangerous (particularly for the risk of cord or venous injuries).

Many English-speaking surgeons use the Halo to stabilize cervical spine fractures. Some recent biomechanical tests [6] of the halo system show that the results are poor for the C1/C2 level. It seems that the halo limits only 70% of the normal motion. When there is flexion at one level, extension is created at the adjacent levels. However, the halo does create a distraction [6] but this can be injurious in cases of ligament lesions.

Conclusions

With this study, we proved the superiority of the CD system and we have went on to treat 10 patients (6 odontoid fractures, 3 C1/C2 dislocations and 1 C2 metastatic tumour). We obtained in all cases a stabilization or a consolidation of the fracture or the graft. With this stiff osteosynthesis we didn't need external support like rigid or plaster minerva and our patients were kept in only a soft collar for 6 weeks. We didn't observe post-operative complications.

References

1. Brooks AL, Jenkins EB (1978) Atlanto-axial arthrodesis by the wedge compression method. J Bone Joint Surg 60A:279–284
2. Chirosel JP (1980) Technique de stabilisation postérieure parmateriel de Knodt. 2ème symposium de pathologie rachidienne. Euromed Ed, Montpellier, pp 159–177

3. Cotrel Y, Dubousset J (1987) Congrès international CD Paris
4. Guyotat J, Perrin G, Pelissou I, Daher T, Bachour E (1987) Utilisation du matériel CD dans les instabilités C1/C2. Neurochir 32:236–238
5. Guilbot F (1987) Fractures de l'odontoide. A propos de 83 cas. Th Med Reims
6. Lind B, Sihlbom H, Nordwall A (1988) Forces and motions across the neck in patients treated with halo-vest. Spine 13(2):162–168
7. Maestro M (1982) Nouvelle approche biomécanique et thérapeutique des fractures de l'odontoide de l'adulte; A propos de 24 cas cliniques. Th Med Nice
8. O'Brien JP (1975) The halo-pelvic apparatus: A clinical, bioengineering and anatomical study. Acta Orthop Scand [Suppl] 163
9. Roy-Camille R (1986) 5èmes journées d'orthopédie de la Pitié Pathologie du rachis cervical supérieur. Masson, Paris
10. Walker PS, Lamser D, Hussey RW, Rossier AB, Dietz J (1984) Forces in halo-vest apparatus. Spine 9:773–777
11. Whitehill R, Richman JA, Glaser JA (1986) Failure of immobilization of the cervical spine with the halo-vest. J Bone Joint Surg 68A:326–332

5.2. The Relevance of Torsional Stability to Anterior and Posterior Cervical Spine Fixation Procedures – an Experimental Study

CH. ULRICH, R. KALFF, L. CLAES, O. WOERSDOERFER, and H.-J. WILKE,
Ulm/Donau, Federal Republic of Germany

Introduction

To obtain bony fusion in an unstable cervical motion segment, several anterior and posterior fixation methods are well established, and their flexional stability is compared in an experimental study in vitro [5].

Still there is no study at hand to determine the torsional stability of a human lower cervical spine motion segment under certain conditions of instability.

The purpose of the following experimental study is, therefore, to examine in vitro the primary torsional stability of anterior and posterior fixation procedures under standardized conditions of instability and to compare it with their flexional stability.

Materials and Methods

Ten fresh deep-frozen cervical spines were detached from their muscles. The motion segment C5/6 was removed, and C6 was embedded in methacrylate. We introduced the *flexion-bending load* into the unit as described before [5], but unlike the study of that time the vertical force was increased to $F_{max} = 50$ N with V = 3 mm/min. The respective tilting angle α and the lever-arm was calculated on the basis of the measured sections, b, c, Δy and F (Fig. 1). Then the average values for 10, 20, 30, 40 and 50 N were computed and printed on an x/y-recorder, to create load-displacement curves characteristic of each individual test situation.

For the *torsional testing* another ten fresh deep-frozen cervical spines were detached from their muscles, C5/6 was removed and C5 and C6 were embedded in methacrylate. Then the specimen was fixed in a special testing-machine

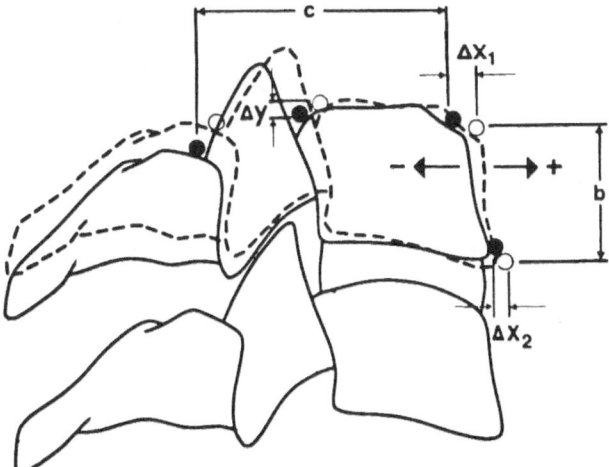

Fig. 1. Measured length used to determine the tilting angle α of the motion segment

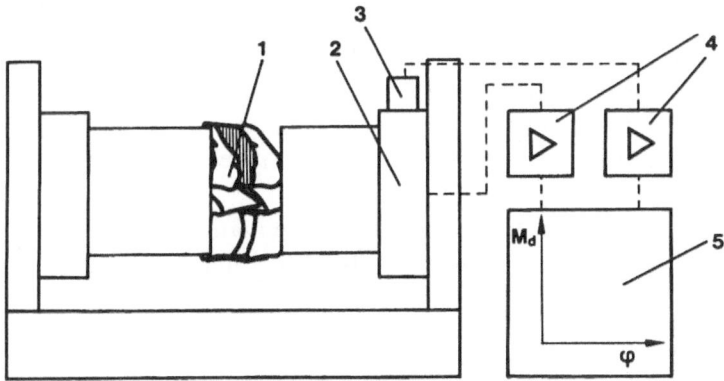

Fig. 2. Test set-up for the testing of the torsional stability. *1* Specimen, *2* mounting support, *3* RVDT (Rotatory Variable Differential Transformer), *4* amplifier, *5* x/y-recorder

[4], and a torque of 3 Nm was applied, and the torsional angle φ was directly measured by Rotary Variable Differential Transformers (RVDT's) mounted on the machine (Fig. 2). The hysteresis achieved was measured out and the individual values were computed to create the torque-deformation curves characteristic for each testing situation.

After measuring the intact spine we severed all posterior ligaments except the posterior longitudinal ligament and repeated the measuring procedure. This so called "posterior instability" was then stabilized in turn with the posterior Hook-plate, as introduced by Magerl, the posterior sublaminar wiring as introduced by Brooks, the anterior H-plate as introduced by Orozco and combined procedures (ant. H-plate/post. sublaminar wiring and ant. H-plate/post. Hook-plate).

Results

a) *Flexion* (Fig. 3)

With $M_{max} = 1.8$ Nm, which is analogous to $F = 50$ N, the tilting angle α of the intact segment was $3.66° \pm 1.85$. After posterior ligamenteous severance the tilting angle α was $3.32° \pm 1.38$. Posterior Hook-plating resulted in a narrowing of the tilting angle ($\alpha = 0.56° \pm 0.3$) just as posterior sublaminar wiring ($\alpha = 0.45° \pm 0.31$). This value dropped to $\alpha = 1.09° \pm 0.34$ with exclusive anterior H-plating; both the combined methods showed about the same stability (ant. H-plate/post. Hook-plate: $\alpha = 0.42° \pm 0.27$; ant. H-plate/post. sublaminar wiring: $\alpha = 0.45° \pm 0.26$).

b) *Torsion* (Fig. 4)

With $M_{max} = 3$ Nm the torsional angle φ of the intact segment was $3.91° \pm 1.27$. After posterior ligament severance this value dropped to $8.48° \pm 2.76$. Posterior Hook-plating resulted in a narrowing of the torsional angle to $3.42° \pm 0.66$, while posterior sublaminar wiring ($\varphi = 7.22° \pm 2.42$) and anterior H-plating ($\varphi = 5.92° \pm 2.14$) did not reach the value of the intact specimen.

Of the combined methods only the combination of ant. H-plate/post. Hook-plate exceeded the stability of H-plating alone ($\varphi = 2.08° \pm 0.26$); the

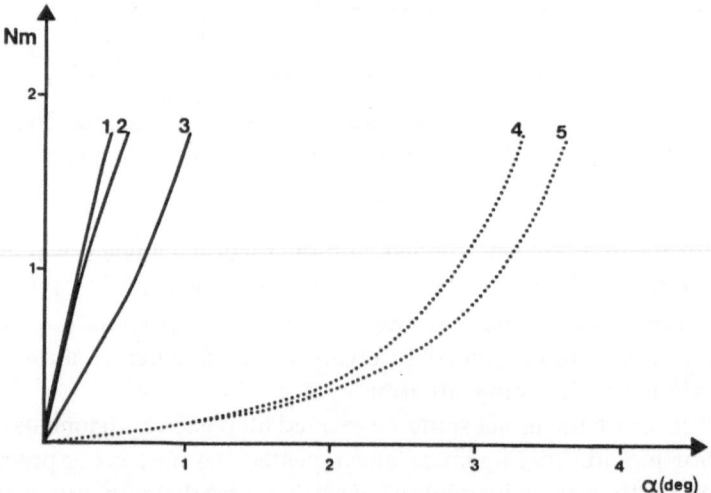

Fig. 3. Load-deformation curves for flexional stability. *1* Combined stabilization: ant. H-plate/post. Hook-plate; ant. H-plate/post. sublaminar wiring, *2* posterior Hook-plate, posterior sublaminar wiring, *3* anterior H-plate, *4* posterior instability, *5* intact segment

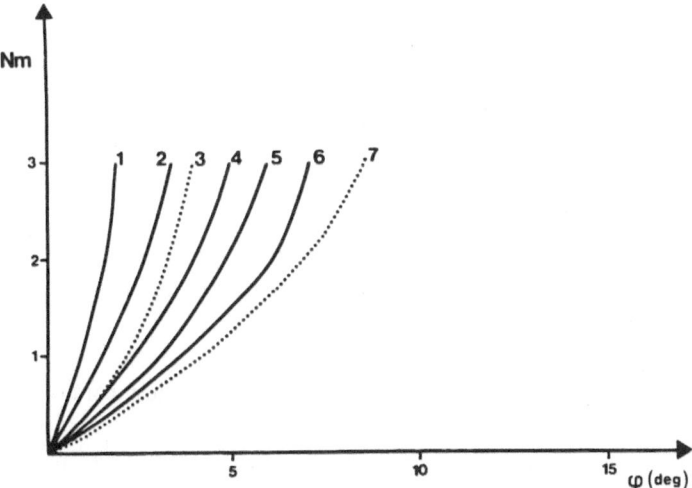

Fig. 4. Torque-deformation curves for torsional stability. *1* Combined stabilization: ant. H-plate/post. Hook-plate, *2* posterior Hook-plate, *3* intact spine, *4* combined stabilization: ant. H-plate/post. sublaminar wiring, *5* anterior H-plate, *6* posterior sublaminar wiring, *7* posterior instability

combination ant. H-plate/post. sublaminar wiring ($\varphi = 5.01° \pm 1.92$) did not improve the stability of the individual procedures decisively.

Discussion

Both the average values for torsion and flexion in an intact segment, read from the linear courses of our load-deformation-curves show about the same dimensions as the recently published measurements by CT in healthy subjects [3] for torsion or from measurements by cineradiography [6] for flexion.

Most striking is the decrease of the torsional stability after severance of the posterior ligamenteous structures, while the flexional stability is noted to raise a little under these conditions.

This phenomenon, in our opinion, is due to the pretension of the disc which is held by the Lig. flavum [2]: after severance of this structure and with the new calibration the posterior ligament is under tension by the disc itself, which results in a higher stiffness as measured.

Under *flexion*, every posterior fixation method after "posterior instability" reaches a reliable stability, all of them more stable than the intact motion segment. Even the mounting of the anterior H-plate seems to improve stability, although a fixation near or within the center of the instantaneous axis of rotation for flexion [6] is not as effective as a fixation far behind this region.

As our curves show, it is possible to improve the stability of the anterior H-plate by any posterior fixation method, but not vice versa.

Of marked interest is the *torsional* stability of the implants used. While posterior sublaminar wiring is not able to reach the torsional stability of the intact spine, only Hook-plating alone or its combination with the anterior H-plate exceeds the stability of the intact spine. It is remarkable that there is only minimal benefit for the stability if one adds an anterior H-plate to the posterior hook-plate under these conditions of instability. In addition to this we found that the torsional stability of the sublaminar wiring cannot decisively be improved by anterior H-plating, and vice versa.

In our opinion, the results highlight another aspect, which was first described by Farfan [1] for the lumbar spine, in which torsion plays an important role for the degeneration of the disc. In the presence of this, it is obvious to consider that late instability following laminectomy, which is often seen clinically [6], is a consequence of the unlimited torque to the disc. To protect the disc from the detrimental torque, a fixation with a high torsional stability seems to be imperative, as is provided by the posterior Hook-plate.

References

1. Farfan HF, Cossette JW, Robertson GH, Wells RV, Kraus H (1970) The effects of torsion on the lumbar intervertebral joints: the role of torsion in the production of disc-degeneration. J Bone Joint Surg 52A:468–482
2. Nachemson A, Evans J (1968) Some mechanical properties of the third lumbar inter-laminar ligament (Ligamentum flavum). J Biomech 1:211–219
3. Penning L, Wilmink JT (1987) Rotation of the cervical spine. A CT-study in normal subjects. Spine 12:732–738
4. Ulrich Ch, Woersdoerfer O, Claes L (1985) Experimentelle Untersuchungen zur Torsionsstabilität verschiedener dorsaler Osteosyntheseverfahren an der LWS. In: Stelzner F (ed) Chir Forum f exp u. klin Forschung. Springer, Berlin Heidelberg New York
5. Ulrich Ch, Woersdoerfer O, Claes L (1987) Comparative study of the stability of anterior and posterior cervical fixation procedures. Arch Orthop Trauma Surg 106:226–231
6. Whitehill AA, Panjabi MM (1978) Clinical biomechanics of the spine. JB Lippincott Company, Philadelphia Toronto

Cervical Spine II
© by Springer-Verlag 1989

5.3. Motion Effects on Blood Flow of the Vertebral Artery and Width of Cervical Intervertebral Foramina

U. OPPEL, G. FRITZ, H.J. STRUCKHOFF, and D. DRÜPPEL, Bochum,
Federal Republic of Germany

Summary

In six cadaver specimens flow measurements in the vertebral artery were performed in varying degrees of flexion/extension. The measurement was restricted to the pars vertebralis. Best flow was found at a position of moderate flexion (⅓ of maximum flexion).

The width of the intervertebral foramen of the cervical spine increased with flexion and decreased with extension. Taking the size at neutral position as 100%, it was 126.9% at final flexion and 77.4% at final extension.

The clinical relevance of this data was tested in a prospective randomized trial, using two cervical collars. One of them forces the cervical spine into moderate flexion. This orthosis proved to be of superior aid in conservative treatment of cervical syndromes.

Introduction

It is well known that an acute painful cervical spine often shows a non lordotic or even kyphotic posture on plain lateral X-ray. This led to our interest in the effects of flexion/extension movements of the low and mid cervical spine.

Therefore, an experimental study was performed on six cadaver specimens, selected by the following criteria.
1. no fatal accident
2. no rheumatism
3. no general bone disease
4. no metastases
5. no bony or ligamentous lesion

Experiments

After final confirmation of the above mentioned criteria by plain X-ray, the experiments were started with 10 cadaver specimens.

The first step was to dissect the atlas from the cervical spine and to prepare the vertebral artery at its entry to the costotransverse foramen of the axis. Then the proximal end of the pars vertebralis of the vertebral artery was prepared. For the nomenclature of the vertebral artery see Fig. 1 [1].

A catheter of maximum possible diameter was inserted into the proximal and distal end of this part of the vertebral artery. As a final check for the integrity of the vessel, angiograms were performed.

Four specimens had to be excluded from the study:
At angiogram two specimens showed an extensive extravasation into the paraspinal muscle for unknown reasons.
One specimen had extensive arteriosclerotic plaques. An angiogram could be performed, but there was no measurable flow during the experiment.
In one case there was only a unilateral vertebral artery, whereas the contralateral was hypoplastic.

In all six specimens examined, the pars vertebralis of the artery went from the second to the sixth cervical vertebra.

The specimens were fixed in a frame which restricted possible motion to extension/flexion excursions. To provide an orthograd perfusion the specimens were mounted upside down (Fig. 2).

Time was measured while 1000 ml of physiological saline ran through the pars vertebralis of the artery. The pressure for perfusion was a constant 150 cm water column. The range of flexion as well as extension was divided into three equal steps and three measurements were made at each stop.

In the second step of the experiment the size of the intervertebral foramen due to motion was measured. For this reason the first thoracic vertebra of the specimen was fixed at the bottom of the above mentioned frame, again restricting possible excursions to flexion/extension movements. By illuminating the intervertebral foramen from the spinal canal, a photo of the silhouette of the smallest area of the foramen was taken (Fig. 3). A motor drive camera was fixed at the frame to guarantee a constant distance between the camera and the examined intervertebral foramen. By using macroscopic equipment, the foramen had about double natural size on the film. The camera was always focused at the smallest diameter of the intervertebral canal and for each foramen focus was kept constant.

Dividing the total range of motion in equal steps, photos of the foramen D1/C7 were made at each position.

Then the first thoracic vertebra was dissected and the seventh cervical vertebra was fixed to the frame for the examination of the foramen C6/C7 in the same way. The measurements stopped at the C4/C5 level.

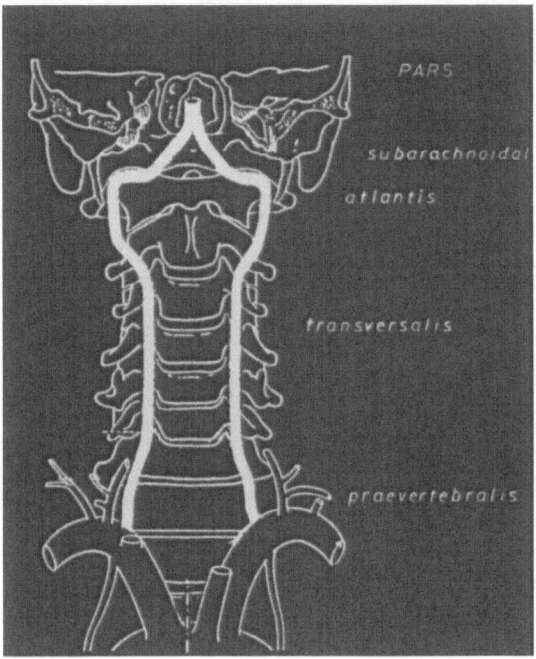

Fig. 1. Anatomy and nomenclature of the vertebral artery

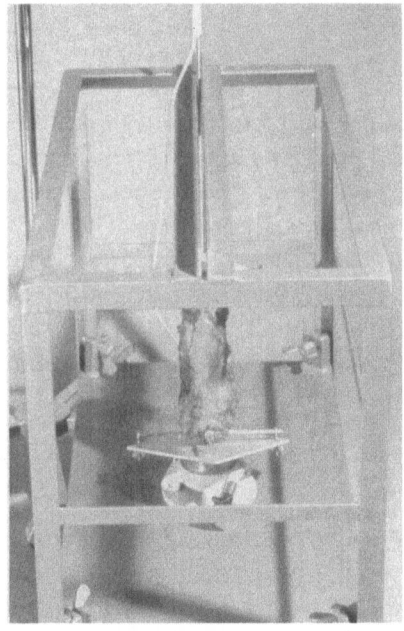

Fig. 2. Frame for the experiments, adjustable bottom, motion restricted to flexion/
extension

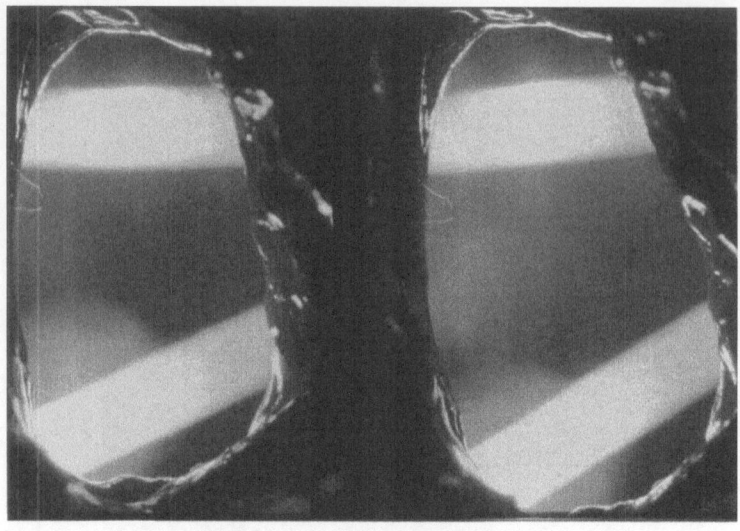

Fig. 3. Photo of an intervertebral foramen illuminated from the spinal canal: left in flexion, right in extension

Standardized enlargements gave photos which could be evaluated planimetrically.

Results

A. Vertebral Artery

The flow of the twelve vertebral arteries examined varied from 70.9 to 113.6 ml/min at neutral position (Table 1).

For further evaluation the flow at neutral position was taken as 100% and only the relative change was considered.

There was significant change in flow, due to the flexion/extension movements. The relative change of the intraarterial flow of the different specimen during motion is listed in Table 2.

As an overall result, it was found, that the maximum flow was at the first step of flexion (Fig. 4).

B. Intervertebral Foramen

For further evaluation, the size in neutral position was taken as 100% and again only the relative change was considered. First, flexion enlarged the width of the intervertebral foramen while extension reduced the size. Flexion increased the longitudinal as well as sagittal diameter of the foramen, extension vice versa.

Table 1. *Flow in the Right and Left Vertebral Artery (Pars transversalis) at Neutral Position*

Specimen	1	2	3	4	5	6
left	100.8	113.6	72.7	94.9	94.0	103.8 ml/min
right	96.0	108.1	80.2	70.9	96.6	75.1 ml/min

Table 2. *Relative Flow in the Different Arteries During Flexion/Extension, Flow at Neutral Position = 100*

Specimen		Flexion			Neutral position		Extension		
		3/3	2/3	1/3		1/3	2/3	3/3
1	left	79.3	87.4	101.8	100	93.2	86.3	82.2
	right	97.7	100.0	109.8	100	96.6	95.5	90.8
2	left	81.5	95.5	103.0	100	97.1	96.0	83.7
	right	83.4	94.3	102.6	100	97.5	93.8	84.4
3	left	95.9	110.0	111.3	100	113.1	108.1	103.0
	right	84.2	92.1	106.7	100	97.9	91.0	87.9
4	left	91.7	98.7	105.7	100	97.6	97.3	92.2
	right	94.1	102.5	115.8	100	98.3	96.6	89.8
5	left	82.7	95.9	103.0	100	102.7	97.4	93.8
	right	91.9	99.9	102.3	100	88.0	88.1	89.1
6	left	94.9	96.6	104.5	100	98.7	92.5	88.4
	right	99.1	100.4	101.5	100	100.4	99.5	99.7

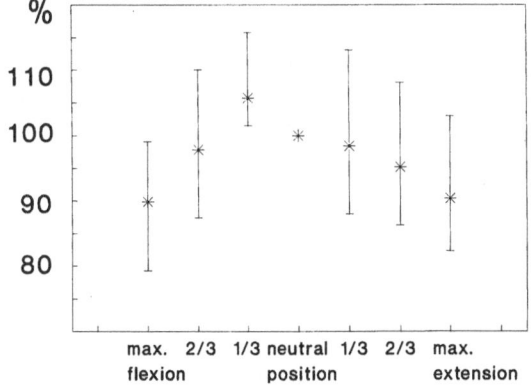

Fig. 4. Posture dependent flow in the pars vertebralis of the vertebral artery

Table 3. *Relative Size of Intervertebral Foramen at Final Flexion and Extension at the Different Levels, Size in Neutral Position 100, (n=12)*

	Maximum	Neutral position	Minimum	Different
C4/5	127.2	100	71.1	56.1
C5/6	123.5	100	80.2	53.3
C6/7	131.5	100	80.2	51.3
C7/D1	125.3	100	78.4	46.9

Second, the biggest change in width during motion was found at the C4/C5 level and constantly decreased towards C7/D1 (Table 3).

Discussion

Former studies on the posture dependent flow in vertebral arteries proved a high correlation. In all these studies the flow in the whole vertebral artery was measured and the results were explained with the diminished flow in the pars atlantis of the vessel during extension and/or adverse rotation [6]. There was no discussion as to whether or not the flow was changed in the pars vertebralis.

Primbs and Weber [5] stated that the perfusion of the pars vertebralis is unchanged during motion, but they did not explain their experiments.

The results of this study clearly demonstrate the influence of flexion/extension motion on the perfusion in the pars vertebralis of this artery. During flexion and extension these changes are not of a dimension that could affect a healthy person. But in cases of borderline perfusion these changes may contribute to vertebrobasilar insufficiency.

There was no detailed report about the size of the intervertebral foramen correlated to the posture of the cervical spine. There were a couple of radiological studies concerning the mobility of the spine for flexion and extension, but there was no report which gave an impression about the dimension of change in the volume of the intervertebral canal during motion. There was only one study with planimetric measurements of the intervertebral foramen in cases of cervical spondylosis.

Only Penning [4] gave a report about the longitudinal diameter of the intervertebral foramen during extension and flexion, as measured on lateral x-rays. He found, that the increase in longitudinal diameter between flexion and extension amounted to 20–30% over an excursion of 20 degrees. As an area is two dimensional, these results are comparable with the results of this study.

Recently Panjabi *et al.* [3] made the first study of the size of the intervertebral foramen at the lumbar spine during motion. They found that the maximum change due to segmental motion took place during flexion/extension. Flexion motion increased the foramen by 30%, while extension decreased it by 20%.

Together with the findings of this study these results show that the range of flexion/extension motion of the lumbar and cervical functional spinal units is almost the same.

Clinical Relevance

In a prospective, randomized trial, it was proved that an orthosis for the cervical spine, which forces the spine into slight flexion is of superior aid in the conservative treatment of chronic cervical syndromes, that is cases where symptoms lasted more than three months [2].

It is known that flexion of the cervical spine increases the capacity of the spinal canal for the spinal cord. In combination with our biomechanical data this might contribute to the explanation of the results of the clinical trial.

References

1. Nomina Anatomica, 4th edn (1977) Approved by the 10th Int. Congress of Anatomists, Tokyo 1975. Excerpta Medica, Amsterdam
2. Oppel U, Steffen R, Drüppel D, Panther KA (1988) Prospektive, randomisierte Studie zur Orthesenversorgung bei Cervicalsyndromen. Z Orthop (in press)
3. Panjabi MM, Takata K, Goal VK (1983) Kinematics of lumbar intervertebral foramen. Spine 8:348–357
4. Penning L (1968) Functional pathology of the cervical spine. Excerpta Medica Foundation, Amsterdam New York
5. Primbs A, Weber E (1956) Die Bedeutung des Verlaufes der Arteria vertebralis für die Pathogenese der cervicalen Syndrome. DMW 81:1800–1803
6. Toole JF, Tucker SH (1960) Influence of head position upon cerebral circulation. Studies on blood flow in cadavers. Arch Neurol 2:616–623

5.4. Morpho-anatomy and Muscle Synergies of the Cervical Spine During Head Orienting Movements in the Monkey

Ph.A. Liverneaux and F.G. Lestienne, Paris, France

Introduction

In a monoarticular movement [9] it is possible according to Wright's criteria [10], to ascribe from geometric and kinematic characteristics, a function to each one of the muscles participating in a given motor task. However, head orienting movement is usually the result of complex movements across a multijoint system controlled by more than fifteen pairs of muscles. Study of the action of these muscles requires an extensive analysis of the osteo-articular and muscle-ligament systems of the cervical cephalic segment. Such an analysis was made in cats [6, 7], monkeys [5] and humans [2]. In the same line a recent work was focused on a comparative study for several species as guinea pig, lizard, frog, chicken, rabbit, cat, monkey and human [8].

Under natural conditions a voluntary movement involves complex muscle action or "muscle synergy" which controls the spatial-temporal organization of the activity of muscles contributing to this movement [1]. Performance of a single task such as flexion or extension of the elbow joint involves a fixed pattern of electromyographic activity between flexors and extensors. However, if the conditions of the movement change such as velocity, amplitude and inertia it has been shown that a profound change in the spatial-temporal organization of the activity between flexors and extensors results [3].

Using morpho-anatomical data [4], our aim was to study during head orienting movement in the horizontal plane the plasticity of the neck muscle synergies when the conditions of the movement vary in velocity, initial head position, and associated trunk movement.

Methods

The geometry of the cervical vertebrae, articular surfaces and the morphoanatomy of superficial and deep neck muscles were studied during surgical dissection in three anaesthetized (sodium pentobarbital) rhesus monkeys

(Macaca mulatta). An X-ray generator was used on live animals to define articular amplitudes of the seven cervical joints.

Three pairs of deep muscles (RCPm rectus capitis posterior minor, RCPM rectus capitis posterior major, OCI obliquus capitis inferior) and four pairs of superficial muscles (SS semi-spinalis capitis, SC splenius capitis, TR trapezius, CO cleido-occipitalis) were implanted with bipolar electrodes. Free head movements were recorded by using a dedicated digital hardware system (Kinesigraph) via real-time video signal processing.

Results and Discussion

Anatomically and functionally the cervical spine consists of two distinct structures: a) the upper cervical spine characterized by the complex ligamentous, muscular and articular atlanto-axial structure. This complex system involves three degrees of freedom (pitch, yaw and roll) controlled by four pairs of small deep muscles (Fig. 1) b) the lower cervical spine is mainly

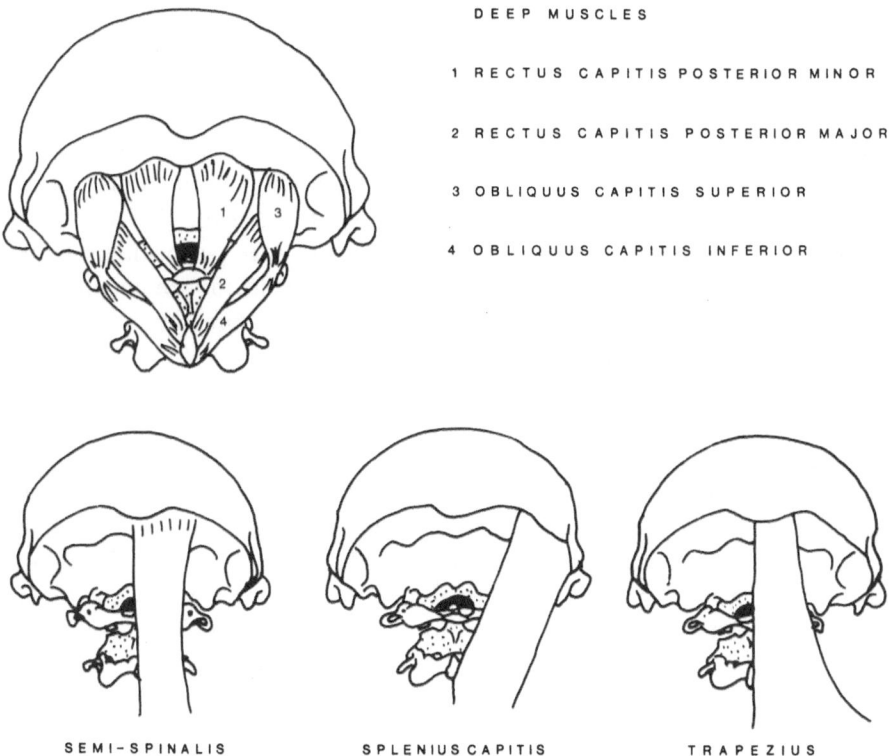

DEEP MUSCLES

1 RECTUS CAPITIS POSTERIOR MINOR

2 RECTUS CAPITIS POSTERIOR MAJOR

3 OBLIQUUS CAPITIS SUPERIOR

4 OBLIQUUS CAPITIS INFERIOR

SEMI-SPINALIS   SPLENIUS CAPITIS   TRAPEZIUS

Fig. 1. Monkey neck muscles. Suboccipital muscles (deep) and three pairs of superficial muscles

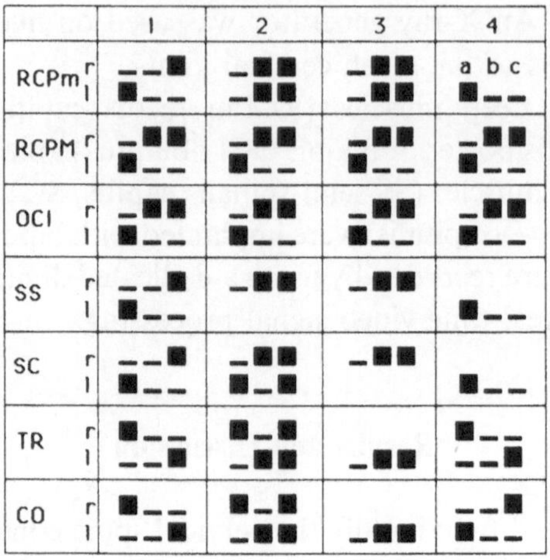

	1	2	3	4
RCPm (r / l)				a b c
RCPM (r / l)				
OCI (r / l)				
SS (r / l)				
SC (r / l)				
TR (r / l)				
CO (r / l)				

Fig. 2. Cartography of neck muscle synergies. See explanation and abbreviations in the text

responsible for two types of movements (pitch, and yaw associated with roll movements). The lower cervical spine is under the control of the superficial neck muscles. These superficial neck muscles also play an important role in the control of the mobility of the shoulder girdle and the thoracic spine.

The main characteristics of the neck muscle synergies during horizontal head orienting movements are represented in a cartography in Fig. 2.

The sequences of activity of the muscles were studied on the basis of three time intervals: before the onset of the movement (a), during the rise (b) and fall (c) of the acceleration phase. Head movements were performed for four different conditions in the horizontal plane: slow head movement initiated from the midline (1), fast head movement initiated from the midline (2), associated head-trunk movement (3), and slow head movement initiated from the contralateral side (4). Lines correspond to no electrical activity or to tonic activity and squares represent phasic activity.

Figure 2 demonstrates the existence of a well-determined chronology of the activity of the superficial and deep neck muscles. Generally speaking, the timing of activity of the three pairs of deep and four pairs of superficial muscles are well-defined and reproducible when the characteristics of the head orienting performance (velocity, direction and amplitude of the movement) and mechanical constraints (trunk fixed or free, initial head position) are identical.

However it is also clear that the chronology of the activity between the different deep muscles and between deep and superficial muscles depends upon the initial position of the head, the velocity of the movement and the accompanying trunk movement.

Nevertheless, at the level of the deep neck muscles and more precisely at the level of the RCPM and OCI the timing of the agonist and antagonist activity is practically similar whatever the velocity, the initial head position and the existence of a combined movement between head and trunk.

From this preliminary study it is possible to ascribe two different functions of the neck muscles depending upon their anatomical characteristics. Indeed it is highly possible that superficial muscles mainly deal with head postural control, while deep muscles are involved in head orientation.

References

1. Bouisset S, Lestienne F, Maton B (1977) The stability of synergy in agonists during the execution of a simple voluntary movement. Electroencephal Clin Neurophysiol 42:543–551
2. Kapandji IA (1974) Physiology of the joints. The trunk-spinal column, vol 3. Churchill Livingstone, Edinburgh, p 251
3. Lestienne F (1979) Effects of inertial load and velocity on the braking process of voluntary limb movement. Exp Brain Res 35:407–418
4. Lestienne FG, Liverneaux PhA (1988) Muscular synergies of neck muscles during monkey's head movement. J Physiol (Lond) C27 (in press)
5. Liverneaux PhA, Pellionisz AJ, Lestienne FG (1987) Morpho-anatomy and muscular synergies of sub-occipital muscles in Macaca mulatta: study of head-trunk coordination. Proceedings of IBRO. II World Congress, 16–24 Aug 1987. Neuroscience, Absts 1970 p
6. Richmond FJR, MacGillis DRR, Scott DA (1985) Muscle fiber compartmentalization in cat splenius muscles. J Neurophysiol 53:868–885
7. Roucoux A, Vidal PP, Veraart C, Crommelink M, Berthoz A (1982) The relation of neck muscles activity to horizontal eye position in the alert cat: head fixed. In: Roucoux A, Crommelink M (eds) Physiological and pathological aspects of eye movements, 1 vol. The Hague, pp 371–378
8. Vidal PP, Graf W, Berthoz A (1986) The orientation of the cervical vertebral column in unrestrained awake animals. I. Resting position. Exp Brain Res 61:549–559
9. Wilkie DR (1950) The relation between force and velocity in human muscle. J Physiol (Lond) 110:249–280
10. Wright S (1952) Applied physiology, 9th edn. Oxford University Press, London, 1190 pp
11. Zangemeister WH, Stark L (1981) Active head rotation and eye head coordination: In: Cohen B (ed) Vestibular and oculomotor physiology. Ann NY Acad Sci 374:540–559

Cervical Spine II
© by Springer-Verlag 1989

5.5. Is Chemonucleolysis in the Cervical Spine more Dangerous than in the Lumbar Spine? (Experimental Study)

P. WEHLING, Düsseldorf, Federal Republic of Germany, M.A. PAK, Düsseldorf, Federal Republic of Germany, E.N. HANLEY, Pittsburgh, PA, U.S.A., and K.P. SCHULITZ, Düsseldorf, Federal Republic of Germany

Summary

Electrically evoked compound action potentials were used to quantify the neurophysiological abnormalities caused by application of collagenase and chymopapain in rats. A branch of the sciatic nerve was stimulated with voltage impulses of constant amplitude and duration at the right external malleolus. The responses were recorded at different levels of the spine.

We used 0.1 ml of a solution of 1 ml = 1000 units collagenase (Sigma chem. comp.) and 5000 i.u. chymopapain (Woelm-pharma) for the evaluation of the neurophysiological effects. A total amount of 0.1 ml was injected into the rats spinal canal intrathrecally. The control rats were subjected to exactly the same stimulus and recording procedures but the test solution was a corresponding volume of isotonic saline.

Two hours after application there was no change in amplitude or latency of the evoked compound action potentials in the collagenase group compared to the control, although 3 of the animals developed paresis. These findings are in contrast to the increase of latency in spinal cord evoked potentials after 20 minutes in rats treated with chymopapain.

Our study indicates that collagenase acts specifically upon central nerve tissue whereas chymopapain causes nonspecific damage of central and peripheral nerve structures. We conclude that chemonucleolysis in the cervical spine by these 2 enzymes is of higher risk because here central nerve structures are close to the site of injection. This is in contrast to the lumbar spine.

Further investigation should focus on long-term follow up and on the role of the motorneuron and the ventral roots in the development of neurological complications after intrathecal injections of collagenase and chymopapain.

Introduction

Collagenase and chymopapain are enzymes used for the treatment of herniated disc disease [1]. They are also in discussion for use in cervical herniations.

These enzymes are injected into the disc, hence there might be a potential risk to nerve tissue caused by leakage of the enzyme into the spinal canal [8]. Histological findings after collagenase and chymopapain injections depend on the concentration of enzyme and on the location of injection.

Zook *et al.* found in chymopapain treated monkeys demyelination, infiltration and vascular damage in lumbar nerve roots, whereas collagenase treated animals did not show neuropathological changes compared to the control group [9]. Rydevik *et al.* showed that the neurophysiological properties of the tibial nerve in rabbits was not changed after collagenase contact [5].

Olmaker *et al.* however could demonstrate that intrathecally applied collagenase caused subarachnoid hemorrhage and paraplegia in rabbits [4].

Wehling *et al.* showed that intrathecally applied chymopapain causes acute nerve conduction slowing of lumbar nerve roots in rats [6, 7].

This study was carried out to quantify possible abnormalities caused by injection of collagenase into the spinal canal. We were interested in a comparison of collagenase and chymopapain effects on nerve tissue.

Method

A total of 19 male wistar rats (n=6 collagenase group; n=6 chymopapain group; n=7 control group) were used for the evaluation of the effects of collagenase and chymopapain on the electrophysiological recordings. Rats were anaesthesized by intraperitoneal injection of 40 mg/kg pentobarbital. In previous experiments it was verified that this type of anaesthesia did not affect the conduction properties of central and peripheral nerve tissue in the recording-stimulus area [2].

Body surface temperature was maintained at 30° C. Electrophysiological measurements were performed by a Tracor Northern-Digital-Signal Analyzer TN-1500 (Preamp Grass P511H) or by a Picker EMG 2002/1. Data were computed with a Nova3-Data General. The stimuli electrodes were concentric EEG needles (Grass) placed at the right external malleolus. We used double threshold strength. The stimuli were voltage pulses (0.1 ms-long) applied at a frequency of 91 Hz or 3 Hz. The lumbar signals were picked up by a needle which was inserted cranial to the spinal process L1 in the midline. The reference electrode for the pseudo-unipolar recordings was inserted 2 cm to the left of the L1 recording electrode. A ground electrode needle was inserted to the m. gluteus maximus on the right side. 64 xL1 responses were recorded and averaged every 20 minutes (Filters LF: 30 Hz, HF: 10 kHz). It should be mentioned that contrary to man the lumbar spine in rats is completely filled with central nervous tissue.

The observation period lasted 2 hours.

We used the clinically established ratio of 5:1 (chymo.:collagenase).

Collagenase (100 units/Sigma co.) and chymopapain (500 i.u./Woelm pharm.) dissolved in 0.1 ml isotonic saline were injected into the lumbar spinal canal between the spinal process L4 and L5 from dorsal. The intrathecal injection was carried out under visual control with the aid of an operative microscope.

The injection lasted 1 minute. The control animals were treated identically.

Results

Figure 1 shows the relative change in latency in 2 groups of animals as a function of time after application of collagenase $(n = 6)$ and chymopapain $(n = 6)$. The prolongation due to chymopapain is very clear, being about 15% relative to the mean latency before application (t-test; $p < 0.001$). In the

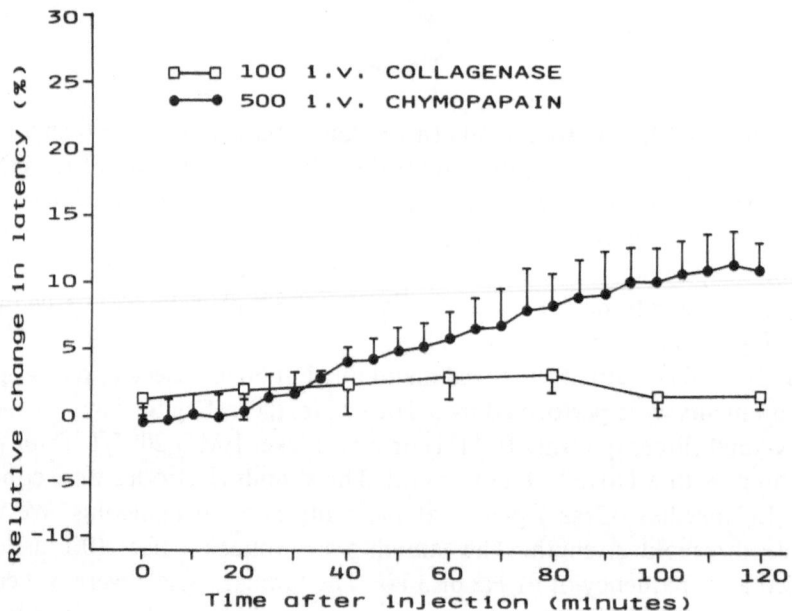

Fig. 1. Relative change in latency of the spinal cord evoked potential after intrathecal injection of collagenase and chymopapain

collagenase group no significant change compared to the control could be seen. Three of the collagenase rats and 3 of the chymopapain rats developed a paraparesis after 24 hours.

Discussion

Several authors [3, 6, 7] using the same methods demonstrated that changes in the L1-response are associated with nerve root pathology. Heninger *et al.* demonstrated in a similar model, that paraplegia in peripheral allergic neuritis is associated with an increase in latency of the L1 response [3]. This is similar to our findings with chymopapain. The conduction slowing in the chymopapain group can be explained on the basis of a membrane damaging effect [6, 7]. On the other hand no change could be observed in the collagenase group although clinical impairment occurred.

Our study indicates that collagenase acts specifically upon central nerve tissue whereas chymopapain causes unspecific damage of central and peripheral nerve structures. We conclude that chemonucleolysis in the cervical spine by these 2 enzymes is of higher risk because here central nerve structures are close to the site of injection. This is in contrast to the lumbar spine.

Further investigation should focus on long-term follow up and on the role of the motorneuron and the ventral roots in the development of neurological complications after intrathecal injections of collagenase and chymopapain.

Acknowledgements

The authors wish to thank Dr. Bennett and Dr. Lunsford, Department of Neurosurgery, Dr. Evans and Mrs. Georgescu, Ferguson Laboratory for Orthopaedic Research, University of Pittsburgh, for their help.

References

1. Brown MD (1983) Intradiscal therapy: Chymopapain or collagenase. Year Book Medical Publishers, Chicago
2. Claus D, Weitbrecht W, Neundörfer B (1985) Pentobarbital: The influence on somatosensory conduction in the rat. In: Schramm J, Jones SJ (eds) Spinal cord monitoring. Springer, Berlin Heidelberg New York, pp 90–94
3. Heininger K, Stoll G, Linington C, Toyka VK, Wekerle H (1986) Conduction failure and nerve conduction slowing in experimental allergic neuritis induced by P2-specific T-cell lines. Ann Neurol 19:44–49
4. Olmarker K, Reydevik B, Dahlin LB, Danielsen N, Nordborg C (1987) Effects of epidural and intrathecal application of collagenase in the lumbar spine. Spine 12:477–482

5. Rydevik B, Brown MD, Ehira T, Nordborg C (1985) Effects of collagenase on nerve tissue. Spine 10:562–566
6. Wehling P, Pak MA, Schulitz KP (1987) Tierexperimentelle Untersuchungen zur Diagnostik und Therapie chymopopaininduzierter spinaler Komplikationen. Z Orthop 125:427–429
7. Wehling P, Pak MA, Cleveland S, Schulitz KP The influence on spinal cord evoked potentials of chymopopain applied to the rat lumbar spinal canal. Spine, accepted for publication
8. Wiltse LL, Widell EH, Hansen AY (1975) Chymopapain chemonucleolysis in lumbar disc disease. YAMA 231:474–479
9. Zook BC, Kobrine AI (1986) Effects of collagenase and chymopapain on spinal nerves and intervertebral discs of cynomolgus monkeys. J Neurosurg 64:474–483

––––––––––

New by Springer-Verlag

F. Postacchini

Lumbar Spinal Stenosis

With a Contribution by Wolfgang Rauschning
on the Anatomy and Pathomorphology
Foreword: L. Perugia   Drawings: A. Mancini
Translation from the Italian edition

1989. With 176 partly coloured figures. 240 pages.
Cloth DM 150,-, öS 1050,-. ISBN 3-211-82111-2

I nterest in lumbar spinal stenosis has increased considerably in the last years on
account not only of the diagnostic and therapeutic problems involved, but also due to
the increasing frequency with which stenoses of the spinal canal or the nerve

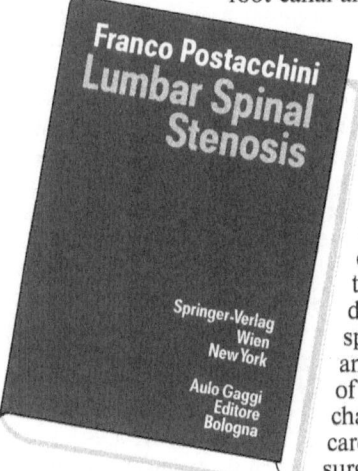

root canal are observed. In this volume the various aspects of
lumbar stenosis are analyzed, ranging from the
classification to the results of conservative and
surgical treatment. Four chapters, in particular,
deserve attention: the anatomy of the spinal
canal, the pathomorphology, diagnosis, and
treatment. The anatomy is described in detail,
particularly as far as concerns the distinction
between the various portions of the vertebral
canal and the relationship between the walls of the
canal and the spinal nervous structures. Cryomicro-
tomic pictures enhance the extremely analytical
description of the pathomorphology of the stenosic
spinal canal. The chapter on investigations provides
an exhaustive analysis of the possibilities and limits
of the old and new methods of imaging. In the
chapter dealing with treatment, the importance of
careful planning and correct technical performance of
surgery is stressed in order to decompress the nervous
structures without creating secondary pathological con-
ditions. This volume, in view of the wide variety of information it contains, is of considerable interest not only to specialists, but to anyone confronted with spinal pathology.

Jointly published by Springer-Verlag Wien New York and Aulo Gaggi Editore, Bologna
Sole distribution rights: Springer-Verlag Wien New York

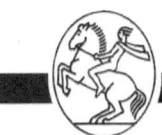

Springer-Verlag Wien New York

Moelkerbastei 5, P.O. Box 367, A-1011 Wien
Heidelberger Platz 3, D-1000 Berlin 33
175 Fifth Avenue, New York, NY 10010, USA
37-3, Hongo 3-chome, Bunkyo-ku, Tokyo 113, Japan

New by Springer-Verlag

L. Merlini, C. Granata, V. Dubowitz (Eds.)

Current Concepts in Childhood Spinal Muscular Atrophy

1989. 122 figures (240 single illustrations). 227 pages.
Cloth DM 150,-, öS 1050,-. ISBN 3-211-82131-7

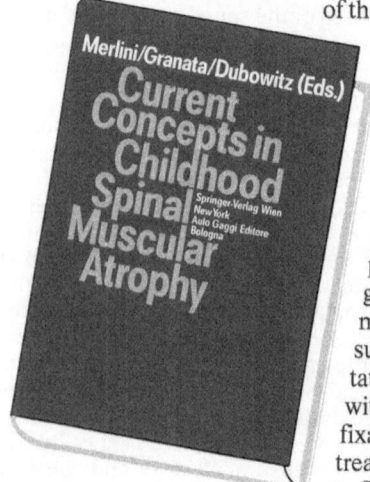

Spinal Muscular Atrophy is a childhood neuromuscular disorder with associated severe handicap and disability. Following the successful research in Muscular Dystrophy, the momentum has now swung to the Spinal Atrophies with a growing interest to basic research and new therapeutic approaches. The purpose of the book is to review and give completely up-to-date information on the various aspects of Spinal Muscular Atrophy: basic science, genetics, natural history, rehabilitation and orthopaedic surgical treatment, and psychological approach to family and patient. The different topics are dealt with by well recognized international experts. The currently emerging issues treated in depth include nerve-muscle interaction in the pathogenesis of the disorder, new strategies for gene location, new rehabilitative proposals in the management of the severe and intermediate form, surgical treatment for scoliosis. Respiratory rehabilitation in the severe form, promotion of ambulation with orthoses in the intermediate one, early surgical fixation of the spine are some of the new promising treatments presented. The multidisciplinary approach to SMA, covering every field of interest, is new. The readers can expect to find a complete information on clinical aspects, progress of research in basic science and genetics as well as on a number of the most innovative and advanced treatments in the managements of SMA.

Jointly published by Springer-Verlag Wien New York and Aulo Gaggi Editore, Bologna

Sole distribution rights: Springer-Verlag Wien New York

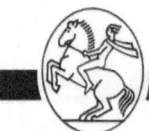

Springer-Verlag Wien New York

Moelkerbastei 5, P.O. Box 367, A-1011 Wien
Heidelberger Platz 3, D-1000 Berlin 33
175 Fifth Avenue, New York, NY 10010, USA
37-3, Hongo 3-chome, Bunkyo-ku, Tokyo 113, Japan

 # New by Springer-Verlag

Progress in Spinal Pathology

Official Publication of the Italian Scoliosis Research Group

Volume 4

E. Ascani, L. Gui, G. L. Lorenzi, R. Savini,
F. Travaglini (Italian Editors); R. B. Winter (English Editor)

Osteosynthesis in Spinal Surgery

Clinical and Biomechanical Aspects

1989. 140 figures (378 single illustrations). Approx. 185 pages.
Cloth DM 78,-, öS 550,-. ISBN 3-211-82150-3

This book series is the official publication of the G.I.S. (Gruppo Italiano Scoliosi = Italian Scoliosis Research Group), an association between highly specialized ortho-paedic surgeons which was founded about ten years ago with the aim of enhancing knowledge and research in the field of vertebral diseases, in basic science, diagnosis and therapy. Gathering the most remarkable papers presented at the annual meeting of G.I.S. the series represents the best of current practice and research in the field of Spinal Pathology throughout the whole of Italy.

From the Contents: L. Aulisa et al., Biomechanical considerations on vertebral osteo-synthesis – A. G. Frassi et al., The Harrington method: a review of 600 cases – R. Savini et al., The Luque system – C. Milano et al., The Harrington-Luque method for the treat-ment of idiopathic scoliosis – P. Bartolozzi et al., Breakage of the Harrington distractor associated with segmental stabilization: a study of possible causes – L. Catani et al., Posterior instrumentation for dorsolumbar spinal stabilization as an alternative to Harrington instrumentation – C. A. Logroscino et al., Anterior osteosynthesis – A. Solini et al., Correlations between the mechanical features of Harrington rods in steel and in titanium: possible clinical implications.

Jointly published by Springer-Verlag Wien New York and Aulo Gaggi Editore, Bologna

Sole distribution rights: Springer-Verlag Wien New York

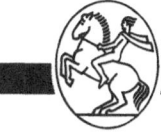

Springer-Verlag Wien New York
Moelkerbastei 5, P.O. Box 367, A-1011 Wien
Heidelberger Platz 3, D-1000 Berlin 33
175 Fifth Avenue, New York, NY 10010, USA
37-3, Hongo 3-chome, Bunkyo-ku, Tokyo 113, Japan